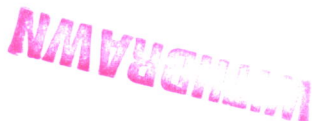

OXFORD CLASSICAL MONOGRAPHS

*Published under the supervision of a Committee of the
Faculty of Classics in the University of Oxford*

The aim of the Oxford Classical Monographs series (which replaces the Oxford Classical and Philosophical Monographs) is to publish books based on the best theses on Greek and Latin literature, ancient history, and ancient philosophy examined by the Faculty Board of Classics.

Experiencing Pain in Imperial Greek Culture

DANIEL KING

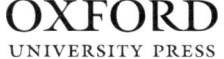

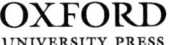

OXFORD
UNIVERSITY PRESS

Great Clarendon Street, Oxford, OX2 6DP,
United Kingdom

Oxford University Press is a department of the University of Oxford.
It furthers the University's objective of excellence in research, scholarship,
and education by publishing worldwide. Oxford is a registered trade mark of
Oxford University Press in the UK and in certain other countries

© Daniel King 2018

The moral rights of the author have been asserted

First Edition published in 2018

Impression: 1

All rights reserved. No part of this publication may be reproduced, stored in
a retrieval system, or transmitted, in any form or by any means, without the
prior permission in writing of Oxford University Press, or as expressly permitted
by law, by licence or under terms agreed with the appropriate reprographics
rights organization. Enquiries concerning reproduction outside the scope of the
above should be sent to the Rights Department, Oxford University Press, at the
address above

You must not circulate this work in any other form
and you must impose this same condition on any acquirer

Published in the United States of America by Oxford University Press
198 Madison Avenue, New York, NY 10016, United States of America

British Library Cataloguing in Publication Data

Data available

Library of Congress Control Number: 2017936882

ISBN 978-0-19-881051-3

Printed and bound by
CPI Group (UK) Ltd, Croydon, CR0 4YY

Acknowledgements

This book has had a long (and painful!) genesis. I have been guided through this process by numerous colleagues who have been generous with their time, effort, and patience; I have also been a beneficiary of the generosity of a number of institutions. I started reading about pain in the classical world during my DPhil at Merton College, Oxford. During that time, I was fortunate enough to receive the support of colleagues at Merton College, especially Rhiannon Ash and Simon Jones, and the Classics Faculty. Stephen Harrison, Tobias Reinhardt, and Jaś Elsner all read and commented on different sections of that work. Ewen Bowie and Simon Goldhill, who examined my DPhil, offered valuable advice and criticism. The manuscript was also read by an anonymous reader for the OCM series. Much of what exists now is a result of their suggestions. I would also like to thank Tim Whitmarsh. Tim read everything that I wrote as a graduate student—he provided insightful criticism on different sections of the work, timely encouragement, and help in many other ways (including curry, beer, and analysis of Michael Vaughan's batting technique). The DPhil would not have come to fruition without his efforts.

The project was substantially rewritten during my time as a lecturer at Exeter University. I would like to thank my colleagues within the Department of Classics and Ancient History, who were supportive from the outset and waited patiently for the new book to congeal into its current form. Many contributed to the research and writing through small (seemingly innocuous) comments or incisive feedback during departmental seminars; others provided a kind word or a patient ear, which was more than helpful! Exeter was also generous in arranging funding for a research assistant, Marcelina Gilka, to assist with the editing and proofreading of large sections of the manuscript; Marcelina's efforts are much appreciated. I would particularly like to thank Chris Gill and John Wilkins. Chris read and commented on a number of chapters and provided guidance and support to an inexperienced and young colleague. John also read the entire manuscript and was extremely generous with his comments and suggestions for improvement.

During the final stages of production, there were several other individuals who made substantial contributions. Jaś Elsner read and commented on further sections of the final manuscript. I would also like to thank Chris Pelling. Chris tirelessly read the manuscript twice in the lead-up to publication. The book could not have been finished without his time and patience. Charlotte Loveridge and Georgina Leighton at OUP and Donald Watt were a tremendous help in guiding a first-time author through the publication process. They too saved us from many errors and infelicitous sentences.

My gratitude also must be extended to my father, who fostered my interest in the classical world, my mother, and my sister. All have, in numerous different ways, assisted with this project and much more beyond. Finally, I would like to thank my immediate family: Claire and *les petits lutins* (Marcus and Sebastian), who have all been a remarkable source of support, love, exhilaration, and everything in between. Thank you.

Daniel King

Exeter, 2017

Contents

Abbreviations, Transliterations, and Editions	ix
Introduction	1

PART 1. DIAGNOSING AND TREATING PAIN

1. Diagnosing and Treating the Pained Body	33
2. Aretaios of Kappodokia	43
3. Galen	67
4. Diagnosis and Pain	103

PART 2. REPRESENTING PAIN

5. Refiguring Pain Symptoms	107
6. Sore Feet and Tragedy in Plutarch and Lucian	115
7. Sacred Pain in Ailios Aristeides	129
8. Pain and Language Recalibrated	157

PART 3. VIEWING TRAUMA, SEEING PAIN

9. *Ekphrasis*, Trauma, and Viewing Pain	161
10. Philostratos' Prurient Gaze	175
11. Viewing and Emotional Conflict in Akhilleus Tatios	193
12. Viewing Trauma in Plutarch	217
13. What's in a View?	233
Conclusion	237
Bibliography	243
General Index	279
Index Locorum	283

Abbreviations, Transliterations, and Editions

This work attempts to speak to a number of different audiences both inside and outside the discipline of Classics. To this end, I have translated all the quoted Greek. These translations are my own, except where noted in the footnotes. Greek terms and names have generally been transliterated as directly as possible in a Hellenized form. There are a few notable exceptions, such as Plutarch, Galen, and Lucian. It was felt in these circumstances that direct transliteration would have meant rendering some names in exceptionally unfamiliar and rather clunky form. In the text of the book, I have tried to render the titles of ancient works in familiar English form; in the footnotes and references, I follow the abbreviations listed in LSJ (with a few notable exceptions). I have also, on first occurrence, referred to modern authors by first and second name (except in one instance): I hope that this is not taken as an assertion of familiarity where it is not justified and that it does not give offence.

All Greek has been quoted from the most recent edition of the Oxford Classical Text or from the Teubner, if no OCT exists. There are, however, a number of notable exceptions to this rule. Galen, Aretaios, and Rufus of Ephesos have been quoted, where possible, from the editions of the *Corpus Medicorum Graecorum* (*CMG*) series; Soranos from the Budé; Hippokrates from the Littré. The abbreviations for Galenic works follow the standard forms that are found in Hankinson, J. (ed.) (2008), *Cambridge Companion to Galen* (Cambridge: Cambridge University Press). Where possible, I have used the Kühn volume and chapter format for references, followed by 'K' (e.g. Gal. *Loc. Aff.* viii.88-9K). Where this has not been possible because there is no Kühn edition, I have followed the conventions of the *CMG* series. Ailios Aristeides has been quoted from Keil's edition—the 'K' following these references refers to his numeration of the orations; the 'K' applied to references to Philostratos' texts refers to the Teubner edition of Kayser. The work of Akhilleus Tatios has also been quoted from the Budé.

References for non-standard editions:

Burguière, P., Gourevitch, D., and Malinas, Y. (eds. and trans.) (1988-2000), *Soranos d' Éphèse Maladies des femmes*, 4 vols. (Paris: Les Belles Lettres).

Garnaud, J.-P. (ed. and trans.) (1991), *Achille Tatius d'Alexandrie, Le Roman de Leucippé et Clitophon* (Paris: Les Belles Lettres).

Keil, H. (ed.) (1898), *Aelii Aristidis Smyrnaei quae supersunt omnia*, 2 vols. (Berlin: Weidmann).

x Abbreviations, Transliterations, and Editions

Kühn, C. (ed. and trans.) (1821-33), *Claudii Galeni opera omnia*, 22 vols. (Leipzig: Teubner).
Littré, E. (ed. and trans.) (1839–61), *Œuvres complètes d'Hippocrate*, 10 vols. (Paris: J. B. Baillière).

The following abbreviations are also used:

ANRW	(1972–), *Aufstieg und Niedergang der römischen Welt* (Berlin: de Gruyter).
AP	*Anthologia Palatina*.
Brescia	Brescia, C. (ed.) (1955), *Frammenti medicinali di Archigene*. (Naples: Libreria Scientifica Editrice).
Calabrò	Larizza Calabrò, G. (ed.) (1961), 'Frammenti inediti di Archigene', *Bollettino del comitato per la preparazione dell'edizione nazionale dei classici greci e latini* 9: 67-72.
Daremberg	Daremberg, C. and Ruelle, C. (eds. and trans.) (1879), *Œuvres de Rufus d'Éphèse* (Paris: J. B. Baillière).
Deichgräber	Deichgräber, K. (ed.) (1965), *Die griechische Empirikerschule, Sammlung der Fragmente und Darstellung der Lehre* (Berlin: Weidmann).
DK	Diels, H. and Kranz, W. (eds.) (1951–2), *Die Fragmente der Vorsokratiker*, 4 vols. (6th edn; Berlin: Weidmann).
Euporista	Wellman, M. (ed.) (1907-14), *Euporista*, in M. Wellman (ed.), *Pedanii Dioscuridis Anazarbei de materia medica libri quinque*, vol. 3 (Berlin: Weidmann).
Garafalo	Garafalo, I. (ed.) (1988), *Erasistrati fragmenta* (Pisa: Giardini).
Gärtner	Gärtner, H. (ed. and trans.) (1962), *Rufi Ephesii quaestiones medicinales* (CMG, Suppl. IV; Berlin: Akademie Verlag).
Gedanken	Winckelmann, J. (1756), *Gedanken über die Nachahmung der griechischen Werke in der Malerey und Bildhauer-kunst* (2nd edn; Dresden and Leipzig: Walther).
Ideler	Ideler, J. L. (ed.) (1841), *Physici et medici graeci minores*, 2 vols. (Berlin: Reimer).
IG	(1913-40), *Inscriptiones Graecae*, (2nd edn; Berlin: Reimer).
IK	(1972-), *Inschriften griechischer Städte aus Kleinasien*, vols. 12–16: *Die Inschriften von Ephesos* (Bonn: Habelt).
Iskander	Iskander, A. (ed. and trans.) (1988), *Galeni de optimo medico cognoscendo libelli versio Arabica* (CMG, Suppl. Or. IV; Berlin: Akademie Verlag).
L	Blümner, H. (ed.) (1880), *Lessing's Laokoon* (Berlin: Weidmann).

LIMC	Ackermann, H. and Gisler, J. *et al.* (eds.) (1981–99), *Lexicon iconographicum mythologiae classicae* (Zurich: Artemis).
LS	Long, A. and Sedley, D. (eds. and trans.) (1987), *The Hellenistic Philosophers*, 2 vols. (Cambridge: Cambridge University Press).
LSJ	Liddell, H., Scott, R., and Jones, H. (1996), *A Greek–English Lexicon* (9th edn, with revised supplement; Oxford: Oxford University Press).
Mannebach	Mannebach, E. (ed.) (1961), *Aristippi et cyrenaicorum fragmenta* (Leiden: Brill).
Nauck	Nauck, A. (ed.) (1889), *Tragicorum graecorum fragmenta*, (2nd edn; Leipzig: Teubner).
Pfaff	Wenkebach, E. and Pfaff, F. (eds. and trans.) (1956), *Galeni in Hippocratis epidemiarum librum VI commentaria I–VI* (CMG, V 10, 2, 2; Berlin: Akademie Verlag).
Simon	Simon, M. (ed. and trans.) (1906), *Sieben Bücher Anatomie des Galen* (Leipzig: J. C. Hinrichs'sche Buchhandlung).
SVF	von Arnim, H. (ed.) (1903-5), *Stoicorum veterum fragmenta* (Leipzig: Teubner).
Tecusan	Tecusan, M. (ed. and trans.) (2004), *The Fragments of the Methodists: Methodism outside Soranus*, vol. 1: *Text and Translation* (Leiden: Brill).
Usener	Usener, H. (ed.) (1887), *Epicurea* (Leipzig: Teubner).
van der Eijk	van der Eijk, P. (ed. and trans.) (2000-1), *Diocles of Carystus: A Collection of the Fragments with Translation and Commentary*, 2 vols. (Leiden: Brill).
von Staden	von Staden, H. (ed. and trans.) (1989), *Herophilus: The Art of Medicine in Early Alexandria* (Cambridge: Cambridge University Press).

Introduction

> He [Sophokles] did not portray Laocoön as more stoical than Philoctetes or Hercules. Stoicism is not dramatic, and our sympathy is in direct proportion to the suffering of the object of our interest. If we see him bearing his misery with nobility of soul [Elend mit großer Seele ertragen], he will, to be sure, excite our admiration [Bewunderung]; but admiration is only a cold sentiment [kalter Affekt] whose barren wonderment excludes every warmer passion [wärmere Leidenschaft] but every other clear conception [deutliche Vorstellung] as well.
>
> Lessing, *Laokoon*, 154[1]

Classical representations of pain resonate in modern culture. When Gotthold Lessing speaks of Sophokles' lost tragedy *Laokoon*, he challenges not only modern readings of ancient representations of pain, but also their place in modern Western thinking. Lessing's words are energized by their polemical relationship with the work of his predecessor Johann Winckelmann. In his *Reflections on the Imitation of Greek Works in Painting and Sculpture*, Winckelmann had argued that the Laokoon statue was a paradigm of the Greek representation of suffering: 'the pain of his body and the greatness of soul', Winckelmann wrote, 'are distributed equally over the entire structure of the image.... Laokoon suffers, but he suffers like Sophokles' Philoktetes; his pain reaches our souls, but we wish that we could bear suffering like this

---

[1] The full German title is *Laokoon oder über die Grenzen der Malerey und Poesie* (originally published in 1766). The German is from Blümner's 1880 edition of Lessing's text, abbreviated hereafter to *L*. The English is taken from McCormick's translation: Lessing (1984), 9. All future references to Lessing are taken from Blümner's edition.

great man.'[2] Winckelmann's treatment was predicated on what he saw as the way in which Greeks represented suffering: the Laokoon was defined by the contrast between the visible physical pain so apparent on the priest's body and his calm and noble soul revealed by the fact that he does not scream in agony. This tension defined Winckelmann's aesthetic appreciation of Greek art: the Laokoon demonstrated the Greek qualities of 'noble simplicity and quiet grandeur' ('edle Einfalt, und eine stille Größe').[3] For Lessing, the situation is more problematic. He points out that Greek poetry is littered with heroes and gods who express their pain through screams, groans, and weeping: to be Greek and to demonstrate nobility of soul is, for Lessing, to scream.[4] Lessing's view of Greek art is defined, unlike Winckelmann's, by the contrast between poetry and plastic art. Poetry, unlike art, is capable of expressing these vocal elements of pain. His focus on 'clear conception', at this point, is part of his argument for the need to understand both the message and medium of ancient pain representation.

Laokoon and Philoktetes—no less than the two critics Winckelmann and Lessing—have played a pivotal role in the Western intellectual consideration of pain. These two iconic ancient representations lie at the heart of classicism, Western aesthetic thinking, philosophy of language, and ethics.[5] Winckelmann and Lessing are particularly familiar to modern classicists. Nonetheless, for all their familiarity, they continue to ask challenging and confronting questions for the history of pain. Both interrogate the cultural status of classical pain.

---

[2] Winckelmann, Gedanken, 22: 'Der Schmerz des Körpers und die Größe der Seele sind durch den ganzen Bau der Figur...Laokoon leidet, aber er leidet wie des Sophokles Philoktetes: sein Elend gehet uns bis an die Seele; aber wir wünschten, wie dieser große Mann, das Elend ertragen zu können'. The full German title is *Gedanken über die Nachahmung der griechischen Werke in der Malerey und Bildhauer-kunst*. German quoted from the 2nd edition of 1756 (original 1st edition: 1755).

[3] Winckelmann, Gedanken, 21–2, where he also outlines the connection with Laokoon and his great soul. For the centrality of pain to Winckelmann's reading of the group, see Richter (1992), esp. 43–9.

[4] For the scream as a natural expression of pain and its representation in Homeric heroes: *L* 152–3. For the explicit analysis of Winckelmann's comparison with Sophokles' Philoktetes, see 151–2.

[5] For German classicism's fascination with the Laokoon, see Richter (1992). On the centrality of Winckelmann to classicism, see Harloe (2013). For philosophy of language: Ferber (2010) and Weissberg (1989). Ethics: Scarry (1985) and Sontag (2003). For the influence of Sophokles' treatment of physical pain on later Western literature, see Budelmann (2007).

Is it an object of modern admiration? A model for our own suffering? Or an object of sympathy or other 'warm passions'? Both authors probe how we should react to ancient suffering and navigate our own. The Laokoon offered, for Winckelmann, a model of how 'we' should suffer. For Lessing, the problem with admiration is that it undermines both other forms of emotional engagement with the ancient material and a clear understanding of it. Understanding the nuances of ancient pain—its place in that culture and ancient reactions to it—involves navigating the complex modern reception of it.

This twin challenge lies at the heart of this book. *Experiencing Pain* offers an investigation into Imperial Greek culture's understanding of pain. In his famous treatment of second- and third-century-CE Roman society, E. R. Dodds argued that the Imperial period was defined by 'anxiety'. Dodds' view was designed to speak to the nature and importance of the individual's inner life in the transition period between the pagan and Christian worlds.[6] His words, however, reflect a then current view of the Imperial period as one beset by physical, cultural, and moral deterioration.[7] Glen Bowersock, in his *Greek Sophists in the Roman Empire*, also claims that the period was one afflicted by a disease which Galen could do nothing about.[8] In such a scholarly climate, it is little wonder that Ailios Aristeides (alongside other ill individuals) was considered a paradigm for his culture's fascination with the failing body. These scholarly readings stress the body's decline to emphasize cultural maladies; the *sōma* becomes a metaphor for the degeneracy of the period and the decline of classical antiquity.[9] This book contributes to the debate about pain and suffering's place in Imperial society by rephrasing the connection between an interest in the pained body and cultural decline. This society was deeply interested in the nuances of physical agony and pain; this fascination reflected, however, an interest in pain's social ramifications. Physical pain was a sociocultural experience. It had its roots in the physiological nature of the body, but also incorporated broader aspects of cognitive, emotional, and social experience. How one felt about one's own perceptions, how it was communicated to others, and how others reacted to it mattered for this society. These

---

[6] Dodds (1965), 3–4.   [7] Gleason (1995), xviii.
[8] Bowersock (1969), 75.
[9] Gleason (1995), xviii: 'we are invited to physiognomize the age, drawing inferences from the visible imperfections of the body... to the rot within.'

aspects of pain experience ensured that the physiological perception was moulded by, and helped to shape, relationships between the pain-perceiver and others: physical pain provoked emotions, transformed language, and helped to create and to deny interpersonal relationships. How one navigated pain lay at the heart of this community and its imagination of itself.

The second half of Lessing's challenge is also critically important. Imperial writing on pain continually articulates its social ramifications, positioning the experience between self and 'other'. One implication of this is how modern viewers react to such images of pain. The first person plural of Winckelmann's formulation is significant because it brings home the continuing relevance of his provocation: does Winckelmann just mean to refer to his contemporary society, or does his statement resonate with more recent readers, continuing to involve wider communities which share his fascination with Greek art in his interpretation of the Laokoon? So, too, with Lessing's criticism of his predecessor. The texts and representations treated throughout this book not only ask modern readers to re-evaluate the ancient historical situation, but to examine critically their own positioning in relation to classical pain. How does classical pain affect us? How do we position it within our own society? Significantly, too, they ask us to interrogate self-reflexively how we position ourselves against the representational and art-critical tradition, especially figures such as Winckelmann and Lessing (and their readings of ancient art and pain).

Returning to the history of pain in antiquity is an urgent exercise. Pain, atrocity, and other forms of human misery continue to occur at alarming levels in our own society. Philosophical, political, and ethical thought continue to question this proliferation of violence. Two of the most famous examples of this ethical objection and resistance to suffering—Elaine Scarry's *The Body in Pain* and Susan Sontag's *Regarding the Pain of Others*—start from classical material. Scarry's monumental work—which has been especially influential in shaping modern readings of pain and language—starts from (what she sees as) the inarticulate screams of Philoktetes.[10] Susan Sontag's heartfelt call for a re-evaluation of the images and representation of suffering begins from a familiar point:

---

[10] Scarry (1985), 5–10; for further treatments of Sophokles' pain in modern literature, see Morris (1991), 249.

Introduction 5

The iconography of suffering has a long pedigree. The sufferings most often deemed worthy of representation are those understood to be the product of wrath, divine or human. (Suffering from natural causes, such as illness or childbirth, is scantily represented in the history of art; that caused by accident, virtually not at all—as if there were no such thing as suffering by inadvertence or misadventure.) The statue group of the writhing Laocoön and his sons, the innumerable versions in painting and sculpture of the Passion of the Christ, and the inexhaustible visual catalogue of the fiendish executions of the Christian martyrs—these are surely intended to move and excite, and to instruct and exemplify.[11]

Sontag's return to the Laokoon is telling: 'pedigree', in this context, figures Laokoōn's antiquity and also its privileged status within the history of Western aesthetics. As she continues, the connections with classical material continue to proliferate—she lists 'the repertoire of hard-to-look-at cruelties from Classical antiquity' and the reception of mythic accounts of torture such as Titian's depiction of Marsyas and Goltzius' representation of Kadmos' companions' destruction by the dragon.[12] More importantly, she uses these examples of ancient (and more recent) material to contrast the representation of suffering and atrocity in other contexts like war. Unlike the images of atrocities wrought during war, these iconic works do nothing to help the viewer protest or deplore suffering.[13] My point in elaborating Sontag's famous critique of representation in her *Regarding the Suffering of Others* is that navigating contemporary responses to suffering, misery, and pain requires positioning oneself against the classical tradition. For all its confrontation of Winckelmann and Lessing and the 'pedigree' of classical images, Sontag's reference to admiration and instruction chimes with their view. Rewriting contemporary responses to modern and ancient agony involves a critical repositioning of its classical representation.

1. PAIN EXPERIENCE

Over the last fifty years, scholarship on pain has expanded at a considerable rate in scientific and humanist disciplines. Despite this

---

[11] Sontag (2003), 40. [12] Sontag (2003), 41–2.
[13] For the references to more classical material and the contrast with images of war, see Sontag (2003), 41–2.

proliferation of critical work, however, pinning down the notion of pain remains as difficult as ever. For neurologists and biologists—who often claim to be moving closer to a universally applicable definition of pain perception—it is understood in primarily physicalist terms: a 'neurobiological sensory function of the brain and spinal cord.'[14] This view stresses the universality and consistency of pain across cultures and historical periods: 'all pains are created equal'.[15] Yet cultural anthropologists, historians, and philosophers continue to challenge this reductionist approach.[16] The variety and amount of scholarship on pain in different contexts and cultures calls attention to the variety of meanings, experiences, and models of understanding that define what it means to feel pain.

This study of pain is designed to contribute to the elaboration of a particular historical context in the ancient world; it also participates in discussions which explore the relationship between biological and cultural visions of pain in a modern context. Increasingly, scholars from multiple disciplines have been willing to approach pain from an ambivalent perspective in which the perception holds a middle ground between cultural metaphor, psychological and emotional experience, and biological or neurological reality.[17] As Sarah Coakley suggests:

> We know, for instance, that the expressions of personal response to pain (even when measureable 'objectively' under test conditions) are bewilderingly varied, not only between individuals but also between cultures. It seems that our particular sensitivity to pain, and the anxiety that attends it, is not simply a matter of genetics, physiology,

---

[14] Woolf (2007), 27 and, for the rejection of other approaches, 27 and 35. For similar claims for 'universal' pain, see Hardcastle (1999) and Fields (2007). For the concept of 'nociceptors' or 'pain fibres' which are, from a neurological and biological perspective, responsible for the perception of pain, see Woolf (2007), 30–1.

[15] Hardcastle (1999), 7.

[16] For examples of the increasing cultural-anthropological discourse on pain, see Morris (1991), DelVecchio Good et al. (1992), Kleinman, Das, and Lock (1997), and Glucklich (2001). The most recent and informative attempts to combine the cultural-historical and scientific approaches are Aydede (2005), Coakley and Shelemay (2007), and Bourke (2014). Bendig (2000) is also a good example of this in a nineteenth-century context. For a brief overview of the evolving discourse, see Hide, Bourke, and Mangion (2012) and the articles contained in the special issue of *Interdisciplinary Perspectives on the Long 19th Century* entitled *Perspectives on Pain*.

[17] Coakley (2007), 1: '[i]t has long been acknowledged that pain (like the brain itself) occupies a strange liminal position between biology and culture'. A similar approach to pain is adopted in Aydede (2005), ix–xvi.

and circumstance, vitally important as these are, but also one of learned 'hermeneutics': the way we interpret our pain is all important for the mode of our suffering of it.[18]

These words, quoted from the introduction to *Pain and Its Transformations*, represent one way of conceptualizing pain that continues to hold sway in modern anthropological and historical work on the subject. When she talks of the mode of suffering, Coakley speaks to a model of pain which combines the realities of the body (flagged by reference to 'genetics' and 'physiology') and the contexts of interpretation, what she designates as 'learned hermeneutics', which we inherit from our cultural context. While Coakley attempts to bring together two divergent models for approaching pain, her formulation is beset by considerable difficulties. There is, it seems to me, too much stress placed on the opposition between the 'learned hermeneutics' of interpretation and the science (facts? realities?) of genetics and physiology. Are not physiology and genetics forms of hermeneutics, learned like other metaphorical representations and understandings of the body? Her division between the two categories, for all its sympathy to a complex multilayered reading of pain, treats the body as ahistorical and interpretation as something that impacts on it; experience (her 'mode of suffering') is, on this reading, a combination of an *a priori* reality and cultural interpretation.

One of the reasons for exploring the limitations of Coakley's formulation is to stress the ways in which it simultaneously challenges the discussion of pain in antiquity and threatens to limit it. In the context of the Imperial period, pain has been predominantly viewed through two different perspectives.[19] One privileges a 'history of ideas' approach which attends closely to theoretical understandings of pain in scientific and philosophical contexts; the second adopts a more cultural-historical framework which plots pain's evolving representation and meaning. The first is, perhaps, best exemplified by Roselyne Rey's *History of Pain*, which, in the context of the Imperial

---

[18] Coakley (2007), 1–2.
[19] There are a number of studies that focus on specific areas of Classical (and Archaic) representations of pain. For ancient medicine, especially Hippocratic material: King (1988) and Horden (2008). For Homer: Holmes (2007). For other Archaic poetry: Allen (2009). For tragedy, there is a wealth of material (I note only a few): Budelmann (2006) and (2007), and Kosak (1994). For a brief survey of the issues in relation to tragedy, see Budelmann (2014), 941–3.

period, focuses on the theories of different medical figures, especially Galen, Aretaios of Kappodokia, and Celsus. Rey's discussion of Galen's diagnostic categorization epitomizes her approach:

> [w]hether circumscribed to one area or diffuse, steady or shifting, acute or chronic, the multifacets of pain could nevertheless be deciphered. The success of this classification system was undoubtedly due to a number of reasons: it rested, for its definitions, on the solid logical foundations of an Aristotelian system of classification which made it possible, through a complex combination of attributes, to account for the extreme diversity of observable phenomena and to reach sensible conclusions. It also had the ambition, or aspiration of better understanding the reality of sickness through the help of this system, and of providing medicine with a rational foundation and basic certainties which had previously been the object of considerable disagreement.[20]

The objectives of Rey's project and its implications for her reading of pain are clear. The phenomenon is, firstly, seen from the perspective of its incorporation into a rational system of thought. But there is also an underlying interest in the reality of pain. Her passage suggests that, for Galen, pain is something to 'be deciphered' only; its 'reality' or its 'extreme diversity' is simply there to be catalogued; 'the reality of sickness' suggests that diagnosis comprised the classification and, thus, the understanding of a biological phenomenon of disease and its symptoms. Rey, to be sure, points to the important ancient medical practice of cataloguing and classifying different symptoms. It is also the case, however, that what is missed in this reading is any sense of the cultural context of Galen's method or views: what the patient feels or what pain means for her, how it is negotiated by different people who are affected by it, and what it means in the context of an individual's life are not discussed. For all the nuances of her analysis, Rey's study promotes a top-down intellectual reading of Galen's (and others') treatment of pain.

What Rey's study lacks, of course, is a subtle understanding of the way in which pain might be managed in medical contexts, how it is shaped by different relationships or different visions of the body's

---

[20] Rey (1995), 36, along with 35, for further elaboration of the 'rational system'. For similar treatments of medicine as focused on cataloguing, see, in relation to Hippokratic medicine, Horden (2008), 296: medicine 'step[s] aside from the religious and ethical frameworks within which pain can acquire meaning'. For further discussions of medical 'theories of pain', see García Ballester and Moreno Rodriguez (1982) and Le Blay (2006).

biology. How do all these various factors play out within the historical context of doctor–patient relationships and diagnosis? How are the ideas and approaches of this context related to other areas of the cultural landscape? The history of ideas model might contribute to understanding what constitutes pain in a limited sense of its philosophical or scientific definition, but does little to elaborate pain's place within this culture. Some of these questions are taken up by Judith Perkins' work, *The Suffering Self*, which offers an important example of the cultural-historical perspective. Perkins' primary objective is to trace the transformations in the cultural concern with the suffering body throughout the first three centuries CE. Her wide-ranging study maps a discursive struggle over the representation and interpretation of a body liable to 'suffering and pain';[21] she traces the transition during this period from (what she sees as) a classical to a Christian model of the pained individual; in the former, the mind exercises control over the body and the experience of pain is downplayed; in the Christian context, pain is given greater and more positive treatment.[22] The 'triumph' of Christianity, she argues, needs to be understood in terms of this transition: it would be, she holds, around a type of represented subject, 'the suffering self, that Christianity as a social and political unity would form and ultimately achieve its institutional power'.[23] I will return to questions of Perkins' Christian focus a little later. In the present context, I want to concentrate on her reference to suffering. Perkins' study has the benefit of analysing the ways in which the experience of suffering is embedded in cultural discourses that extend beyond, and cut across, medicine, philosophy, and literature. In a sense, *The Suffering Self* explores the cultural interpretations ('learned hermeneutics' in Coakley's terms) which shape the nature of suffering. The concern with the representation of the self as a sufferer, however, fails to treat the question of suffering in sufficient detail. Is suffering equivalent to, or can it be effectively assimilated into, pain? Perkins' approach ultimately takes the complexities of the body's experiences of pain as given; despite its apparent placement at the centre of her study, the experience of pain is often left in abeyance.

The reason for connecting these two accounts of pain in the Imperial period with the work of Coakley is to point out how one

---

[21] Perkins (1995), 3.   [22] Perkins (1995), 3.   [23] Perkins (1995), 3.

modern view challenges scholars to bring together multiple ways of thinking about pain in any given community. It stresses the need to combine the specificity of Rey's approach with the broader cultural grasp of Perkins'. At the same time, however, Coakley's formulation highlights the possibilities presented by the ancient context. Coakley's framework and other recent approaches to pain which depend on bringing together interpretation and physiological reality do not work effectively in the ancient world. They are ineffective, in no small part, because the body's reality is debatable. Attending to the Imperial world reveals how culturally specific the modern discourse of pain is because it is dependent on a particular vision of the relationship between science, culture, and the body.

In light of this, I investigate three questions over the course of this study: (1) How are accounts or theories of pain integrated into representations of the body's reality? Put another way, I interrogate how the notion of pain and representations of the body's reality mutually inform each other. To what extent does thinking about pain in a particular way depend on interpreting or understanding the body in a particular light? How does that view of the body then influence what can and cannot be perceived by the individual? (2) How are these two mutually related phenomena allied to other aspects of pain, such as its intellectual and affective impact on the individual and those around them? I probe the ways in which the perception of pain is transformed by various emotional and cognitive responses to it, and how the pain-perceiver is positioned by others' reactions to either it or them. (3) How are these various issues incorporated into the representational world of the first three centuries CE?

This study investigates (what I will term, for convenience) 'embodied pain experience' or, more briefly, 'pain experience'. One of the reasons for thinking about pain in these terms is to stress the importance of the combination of theories about pain *qua* pain with broader aspects of experience. Physical trauma, corporeal destruction or deterioration, and changes in the states of the body were commonly assumed to cause pain. This physiological element of pain, however, only tells part of the story. What it means for the individual—how they navigate those perceptions within the context of Imperial society, or incorporate them into their understanding of their own lives—is also important in defining the experience of pain. I should stress (again) that it is not a case of superimposing onto a physiological reality a set of higher-level metaphorical and social meanings: my point is that these multiple levels are inseparable and mutually constitutive.

Such an approach to 'embodied pain experience' is underpinned by three interpretative cruxes, which will be germane to this study. In the first instance, I raise a number of questions about Imperial views of the body itself: how is pain related to a growing awareness of, and interest in, the anatomized body? Secondly, I probe the relationship between language and that body: how do ancients represent the connection between pain and language? If language and narrative offer one vehicle for socializing or communicating the physiological aspects of experience, then how does the relationship between language and the *sōma* influence pain experience? How, in short, does it define the cognitive and affective aspects of pain experience? Finally, I turn to the affective and interpersonal aspects of the experience. How does pain make one feel about one's own body or others feel about the pain-perceiver? Thinking about pain in these terms speaks to the history of emotion and its complex relationship with the individual's body and the community.

a. Imagining a/the/Every Body

The history of the body in antiquity, and the Imperial period in particular, is a substantial discourse, and it is one that continues to grow.[24] Much of this interest has been spurred on by the third volume of Michel Foucault's *History of Sexuality: The Care of the Self*, which suggests that the Imperial period should be seen as a watershed in the ancient cultural concern with, and practices of, the body.[25] Significantly, that discourse has until recently played down the way the body operates as the *locus* of sensory experience in which the body's physical perceptions and sensory activities are located within a broader cultural context. The emerging discourse of sensory studies has been driven by the desire to analyse more effectively aspects of

---

[24] Porter (1999), 1 for the way in which the fascination with the classical body has discovered itself. For an overview of the field in its early form, see Porter (1991). For more specific studies on antiquity: Gleason (1995), Wyke (1997) and (1998), Porter (1999), Gunderson (2000), Rimell (2002), König (2005), and Garrison (2012). One of the most influential texts on the emergence of the ancient body for this study is Holmes (2010), on which, see further below (text to nn. 30–1).

[25] Foucault (1986).

quotidian existence that are excised from traditional history and from the history of the body.[26] As is implicit in the discussion of 'pain experience', this study starts from the question of physical pain—i.e. the perception or *aisthēsis* of pain in the body. While this concern for the body's *aisthēsis* does not attempt to reclaim the real sensory experiences of a past culture, it does investigate some of the ways in which perception was conceptualized or represented as a physiological process. My interest in *aisthēsis* is, therefore, twofold. I want to try and broaden the understanding of the body by contributing to a discussion of sensory perception in a number of interconnecting cultural discourses. I also want to elaborate how sensory perception was integrated into frameworks of meaning and understanding: *aisthēsis* combines (and by implication, its historiography should emerge from) representational practices and ideas, physiological theory, and social and cultural *praxis*.

It is central to my argument throughout this book that embodied pain experience was underpinned by the emergence of a particular understanding of the physical *sōma* in this period, which I will call the anatomico-aesthetic model of the body. This view combined anatomically-driven understandings of the structure and nature of the *sōma*, the aesthetic appreciation of the body, and the consideration of the individual's ethical qualities. This approach to the body incorporated a range of different strands of cultural discussion and thought.

In terms of its concerns with anatomy and perception, this conception of the body was shaped, partly, by the inheritance of Classical (and older) material. The writers of the Imperial period draw explicit connections with the finer points of physiological thought in Plato, Aristotle, and their immediate successors. Galen's views about pain, for instance, are based on ideas he attributes to Plato and Hippokrates about perception and change within the human body.[27] The works of Aristotle, especially *On the Soul*, also contributed significantly to Imperial writers' understanding of the internal processes

---

[26] This has focused largely on the question of smell, but has included other elements of the human sensorium. This study has been particularly influenced by the work of Meyer (2010), Throop (2010), Butler and Purves (2014), and Bradley (2015). For the traditional silencing of the history of sensory experience in humanistic disciplines, see Butler and Purves (2014), 2.

[27] The critical passages are Gal. *PHP*. v.636–7K and *Caus. Symp.* vii.115–17K. The *Caus. Symp.* passage is drawn largely from Pl. *Ti.* 64d, although it refers to Hippokrates as well. For a similar Platonic view of pain, see *Phlb.* 32a–b.

Introduction 13

of perception and their interpretation of pain.[28] Similarly, when Imperial writers from medical and other contexts—Aretaios, Galen, and Plutarch, for instance—discuss the process of pain perception, they look to the Hellenistic philosophical schools, especially that of the Cyrenaics, and imagine themselves engaging in active debates about the nature of pain or perception with pre-Socratic natural philosophers such as Demokritos.[29] Thinking about the body's capacity for the perception of pain drew heavily, or, at least, was determined to present itself as drawing heavily, on Archaic and Classical philosophical, medical, and scientific traditions.

One area where the Imperial period's conception of the body does diverge from these pre-Hellenistic models is the intensity of their anatomical knowledge about the internal body. Under the Empire, writers connect the perception of pain with the *minutiae* of physical processes and anatomy in ways which broke with the Classical past. Brooke Holmes's study, *The Symptom and the Subject*, illuminates clearly the ways in which Archaic and Classical writers—driven by debates about the nature of the universe—locate disease inside the body.[30] For medical writers, she notes, the body has many cavities; the emergence of the symptom requires individuals 'to see' inside a body which is comprised of 'a hidden space of bones, sinews, and joints, hollows and channels'.[31] There is some evidence that thought about the human body and its internal qualities was informed by the practice of animal dissection. Aristotle and Diokles of Karystos, for example, appear to have engaged in dissecting different animals, from which they extrapolated about the internal make-up and structure of the human body.[32] While they imagined, however, the internal spaces of the body, this early engagement with the *sōma* remained both largely speculative and sporadic. In contrast, for the writers of the

---

[28] Arist. *de An.* 416b34–424b. For Galen's connection with Aristotelian theories about pain perception, see García Ballester and Moreno Rodriguez (1982).

[29] See, e.g., Plut. *Non Posse* 1087–8 for his argument with Epikouros' view of pain. For Galen's argument with the Atomists on the basis of pain: Gal. *Hipp. Elem.* i.418–9K and *PHP* v.636–7K. There is further discussion of Aretaios' and Galen's engagement with philosophy in Chapters 2 and 3 respectively.

[30] Holmes (2010), 126–47 on the symptoms of disease and their capacity to reveal the internal workings of the body; 9–29 on the way in which symptoms allowed doctors to see inside the body.

[31] Holmes (2010), 126.

[32] On Aristotle's practices: Kollesch (1997), 370. For Diokles' treatise on anatomy, see Gal. *AA.* ii.282K (= Frag. 165 van der Eijk).

Imperial period, the process of taking hold of the body in terms of the *minutiae* of its internal functions, composition, and structure was fundamental to how they conceptualized pain. This process of anatomizing the body was most strongly displayed in medical discussions by rational doctors who were driven to discover in the internal body the *aitia* of particular diseases or conditions. Imperial rational medicine (for all its sectorial differences) was characterized by the consistent use of a type of locative diagnosis in which diseases and symptoms were understood in relation to the anatomical make-up of specific parts of (or places within) the body, the function of different organs or parts of the body, and their relationship to each other. That approach to diagnosis was built upon a precise understanding (or imagination) of the internal structures of the body, and was often linked explicitly with anatomical discoveries of the Alexandrian doctors and anatomists Herophilos, Eudemos, and Erasistratos.[33] Especially important in the Imperial context was the elaboration of some aspects of the nervous system and the description of the fine detail of internal membranes, organs, and structures of the *sōma*.[34] Medical culture views the body with an anatomical specificity not seen in the pre-Hellenistic period.

This interest in the internal body and its anatomy leaked into other areas of Imperial culture. The body was submitted to a type of scientific-aesthetic gaze in which looking at—and, more importantly, inside—the body was widespread. In this context, the spectacular display of the destroyed body had particular resonance. Gladiatorial displays opened the body, revealing its insides to large audiences across the Empire. These performances were, of course, linked closely with the science and practice of anatomy. Galen's own career (as well as those of others before him) included time as a professional doctor treating the wounds and injuries of gladiators in Pergamon.[35] His account of the experience draws explicit connections between the destruction of the body and its subsequent viewing in the arena and his own anatomical displays; his practices during his time at

---

[33] For the importance of Hellenistic anatomists to Imperial doctors, see Rocca (2003), 42–7.

[34] For the importance of the Alexandrian discovery of the nervous system, see, e.g., Gal. *Loc. Aff.* viii.212K (= T. 80 von Staden), along with Rufus of Ephesos: Ruf. Eph. *Anat.* 71–5 (pp. 184–5 Daremberg = T. 81 von Staden) and *Onom.* 149–50 (p. 153 Daremberg = T. 125 von Staden).

[35] Gal. *Comp. Med. Gen.* xiii.599–601K; Gal. *Opt. Med. Cogn.* 9.4–8 (pp. 103–5 Iskander).

Pergamon drew upon his anatomical training and contributed further to it.[36] Just as the spectacularity of the destroyed body linked gladiatorial display with anatomy, the visuality of the opened body was reiterated at other points on the cultural landscape. It is arguable that public anatomical displays were held throughout the Empire.[37] Textual representations of anatomical demonstrations certainly stress the theatrical qualities of the violent activity. In Galen's two exhaustive accounts of his anatomical thought and procedures—*On the Usefulness of Parts* and *On Anatomical Procedures*—he often refers to the audiences and spectators (*theatai*) of demonstrations.[38] In the case of *On Anatomical Procedures*, especially, he provides extended, vivid accounts of the process of destroying the body of various animals as if they were human bodies; he constantly encourages his readers to imagine that they are looking inside the human *sōma*.[39] It is in this context that the interest other texts or writers show in the body should be understood: peering inside the damaged or opened body emerges as a common trope in this period. Akhilleus Tatios' account of the body and now famous concern with the relationship between external and internal aspects of the *sōma* are embedded in an anatomical fascination with the body in the culture at large.[40] In a similar

---

[36] Gleason (2009), 108–10, for the connections between the two contexts, and Debru (1995).

[37] For the medical competitions of the so-called 'Megala Asklepieia' at Ephesos in the second century CE: *IK* 1161, 1162, 1163, 1165, 1166, 1167, which list victors in various medical competitions (*agōnes*). Competitions appear to have included displays of ability and training in *suntagmata* (treatises), *problēmata* (problems? diagnoses?), *kheirourgia* (surgery), and *organa* (equipment?). Medical competitions or public displays are implied at Plut. *Adulat. Amic.* 71a, which refers to 'doctors who perform surgeries in the theatre for contracts' (οἱ χειρουργοῦντες ἐν τοῖς θεάτροις ἰατροὶ πρὸς ἐργολαβίαν). Galen also seems to suggest anatomical competitions at, e.g., Gal. *AA*. ii.642–3K, *Opt. Med. Cogn.* 9.6–7 (p. 105 Iskander), and *Praen.* xiv.625–6K (NB the reference to ἀγών here). For discussion, see Gleason (2009), 89 and 92–100.

[38] For references to *theatai*: e.g. Gal. *AA*. ii.669K, *UP*. iii.631K.

[39] On homology of animals and man: Gal. *AA*. ii.219K and 221–2K. On the careful positioning involved in the analogy of human and animal: Gleason (2009), 86–7 and 111–13. For the 'spectacle' or the 'the audience/spectators': Gal. *AA*. ii.221–2K on looking at corpses; *AA*. ii.220K on autopsy and osteology at Alexandria; and discussion of visual observation at *AA*. ii.223–4K; also *AA*. ii.225K for Galen as an observer at Satyros' demonstrations. For the anatomical display as *epideixis*, see: von Staden (1995b), 51–65.

[40] For the fascination with inner and outer elements of the body in this text, see Zeitlin (2012).

fashion, Philostratos the Elder's reading of visual culture in the *Imagines* is allied to this way of viewing the body.

Just as looking at the anatomized body was important for medicine, so too was its aesthetic appreciation. For Galen, the ideal of the healthy body was the statue of the Doryphoros by Polykleitos. According to *Art of Medicine*, the acme of a well-balanced physique was that described in the *Kanon* of Polykleitos (i.e. the Doryphoros), which manifests 'every form of symmetry' (συμμετρίας ἁπάσης, *Ars. Med.* i.343.2K); in *On Temperaments*, Galen obliquely praises the statues of the *Kanon* of Polykleitos as offering a model of the body which demonstrates symmetry and has been well made.[41] Medical health, aesthetic beauty, and moral appreciation are all combined in these comparisons. At other moments, he points out that physiological symmetry (*summetria*) between (among other things) body parts, muscles, and physical structures is vital to maintaining good health.[42] It is no accident that the quality of proportion is also fundamental to aesthetic appreciation of the artistic representation and the individual. The notion of 'good proportion' or 'symmetry' appears to have been critical to Polykleitos, and his predecessors' notions of sculptural and aesthetic beauty.[43] In addition to providing a basis for both medical and artistic readings of the beautiful body, the term also carries implications of moral and psychological 'good order'.[44] The quality *summetria* is a marked term that cuts across multiple discourses' ways of gazing at the body.

I do not want to suggest that this anatomico-aesthetic model was the only way of approaching the body in this period. There is much medical activity that is not as focused on anatomy as Galen was, such as the therapeutic work and ideas of Methodist doctors.[45] Rhetorical training

---

[41] Gal. *Temp.* i.565–6K. Both texts emphasize the *summetria* of different aspects of the body (including various organs and structure, as well as physical qualities like the wetness and dryness of the body) and praise its aesthetic and ethical qualities.

[42] Gal. *San. Tu.* vi.2K and 7K for the 'symmetry' of humours and organs; *San. Tu.* vi.13K for repeated connections with health.

[43] Hurwit (1995), 10–11 and 21 for its importance to the *Kanon*. Pliny claims that Euphranor wrote a treatise *On Symmetry*: Plin. *NH*. 35.129. Cf. his discussions of Apelles' interest in proportion at 35.79–80. For the connection between Classical medical views of the body and the work of Polykleitos, see Leftwich (1995).

[44] See Pl. *Phlb.* 64e for the link between symmetry and 'beauty' (κάλλος) and 'virtue' (ἀρετή).

[45] References to pain symptoms litter, e,g. Sor. *Gyn.* ὀδυνή: i.5.29, 5.35, iii.2.92, iv.4.28, 6.30. ἀλγεῖν: i.14.46, ii.3.5–6, 5.26, iii.2.50, 4.41, 4.99, 5.26. ἄλγημα: i.3.22, 7.34,

and practice also provided alternative ways of approaching and managing the body and its condition through corporeal training, vocal exercises, and diet.[46] What is telling, for my purposes, is the way in which this reading of the body—this anatomico-aesthetic concern—is closely allied with the history of pain perception in this culture. Much of the thinking about pain in multiple cultural discourses partakes of this way of understanding the body.

b. Pain and Language

A second aspect of my interest in the emergence of pain experience concerns the way in which it is integrated into different cognitive and emotional frameworks through the medium of language and representation. Pain's articulation or communication in language or narrative has been a central theme of modern philosophical and ethical debates about pain and suffering and their place in historical and contemporary cultures.[47] The pain–language nexus is important because of language's capacity to shape how pain is integrated into relationships between people: it allows for the recognition of others' perceptions, builds emotional relationships, and underpins the treatment of the pained individual.[48] While debates about the pain–language nexus continue to define the understanding of pain in contemporary discussions and in some ancient contexts, such as Athenian tragedy, not enough attention has been paid to similar questions in the Imperial period.

In her influential work, *The Body in Pain*, Scarry argues that pain is inherently resistant to the process of socialization, that it is unshareable. This unshareability of pain is defined by its unavailability to

17.24, 17.27, 22.8, iii.2.106, 2.157, 4.21, 4.79, 7.19, 11.19, 13.18. Cf. the treatment of gout and *podagra* in Aretaios. (*SD.* iv.12) and Caelius Aurelianus (Cael. Aur. *CA.* v.ii. 43 and 50–1 (= Frags. 94–5 Tecusan), where the focus is shifted to methods of treatment rather than explanation.

[46] Gleason (1995), 84–91, although, as Gleason points out, rhetorical *askēsis* was heavily informed by medical concepts of the healthy body.

[47] Most contemporary discussions begin with Scarry (1985). The interest in pain and language in a modern context can be taken back, however, to debates between Herder, Rousseau, and Condillac in the eighteenth century. On this debate: Weissberg (1989) and Ferber (2010).

[48] I use 'other' in the rather unsophisticated sense of those who were exposed to individuals who felt pain.

linguistic or narrative representation. Because pain is not 'for' or 'of something', it lacks referential content and therefore breaks down traditional understandings of linguistic reference.[49] Physical pain, Scarry argues further, 'does not simply resist language, but actively destroys it, bringing about an immediate reversion to a state anterior to language, to the sounds and cries a human being makes before language is learned'.[50] This inaccessibility to language raises questions about the possibility of understanding and empathizing with others' pain:

> for the person in pain, so incontestably and unnegotiably present is it that 'having pain' may come to be thought of as the most vibrant example of what it means to 'have certainty', while for the other person it is so elusive that 'hearing about pain' may exist as the primary model of what it is 'to have doubt'. Thus pain comes unsharably into our midst as at once that which cannot be denied and that which cannot be confirmed.[51]

Scarry's formulation, then, confronts the possibility of the cultural history of pain in stark terms. If pain is characterized by its resistance to knowledge and sharing, then how might we conceive both of genuine empathy and action and the cultural history of pain?

Scarry's assertions about pain's incommunicability are predicated on a particular approach to a referential theory of language in which the capacity to indicate the full nature of inner perceptions and sensations is downplayed. Scarry's suggestion that pain has the capacity to destroy language, to my mind, ignores the way different cultures offer individuals a range of resources and strategies for communicating their pain to others; and, indeed, the ways different cultures represent the pain others perceive. Pain perception maintains, I hold, a close productive relationship with narrative and language; that relationship helps shape the cultural positioning of the experience and individuals' navigation of their pain.

In order to approach the pain–language relationship in Imperial society more productively, I turn to recent anthropological work which stresses the subtle and positive relationship between narrative and physiological or cognitive experience. As Arthur Kleinman, Veena Das, and Margaret Lock explain in their work *Social Suffering*, the performative aspects of language and speech genres within

[49] Scarry (1985), 5.   [50] Scarry (1985), 4–5.   [51] Scarry (1985), 4.

Introduction 19

particular communities help 'in moulding the experience of suffering so that certain experiences of pain and grieving become expressible while others are shrouded in silence'.[52] They argue that it is possible to see that language and pain maintain a close relationship, each working to form the other:

> while experience is shaped by representations it can also push against these representations—resisting language, bending it in new directions, and distorting the received ways of expressing distress and desperation so that these distortions themselves transform the experience of suffering.[53]

Kleinman, Das, and Lock propose, then, a model which prioritizes the performative and mutually transformative relationship between language and pain.

The words of *Social Suffering* provide a starting point for the work of this study. In what follows, I turn to a number of specific ways of expressing pain from across the Imperial period. I maintain a particularly close focus on the terminology used to describe the perception. One reason for this close philological focus (whatever gestural self-positioning is implied by this) is to avoid overuse of the concept of suffering. As I suggested, the metaphor of suffering (like a number of others, such as torture) covers a range of possible experiences, many of which do not involve physical pain. The second reason for doing so is that there are, across different cultural contexts, some consistent ways of discussing pain in the Imperial period. Variations of the nouns *ponos*, *algos*, and occasionally *lupē* (and their verbal and adjectival forms) are consistently used to designate pain in different literary genres. The weighting given to the various possible meanings of some of these terms provides some access into this culture's thinking about the nature of pain: when, for instance, do the tragic implications of *ponos* receive explicit emphasis and in what contexts are such connections played down? Certain perceptions of pain are also modified by technical or common terminology such as 'numbing' (ναρκώδης), 'biting' (δακνώδης), or 'pulsing' (νυγματώδης). These terms, while especially common in medical contexts, also appear in different cultural and literary settings. Certain conditions also have specific terminology which differentiate the perceptions of pain in one condition or part of

---

[52] Kleinman, Das, and Lock (1997), xiii–iv.
[53] Kleinman, Das, and Lock (1997), xiv.

the body from another. The types of language which authors choose (and the capacity of such language to link the perception and experience of pain with certain cultural themes) are particularly telling.

The second aspect to this work's focus on language concerns the ways in which pain and broader aspects of narrative representation help to communicate the experience. If Perkins (and others) think about the representation of pain, what they do not do is give enough attention to the possibilities, difficulties, and effects of representation itself. One objective of this study is to emphasize the emergence of an intimate relationship between the body and the process of articulation. The body is presented, repeatedly, as having a profound influence on the types of speech that the pained individual is capable of: pain and other experiences of the body deny and facilitate as well as authorize and dehumanize different forms of speech. Imperial society continually investigates what types of linguistic register or speech act—the scream, clear medical terms or the structured medical description, the rhetorical allusion or quotation—effectively communicate pain and, in so doing, facilitate recognition and understanding or more affective reactions among others. Does silence communicate effectively and how might one overcome or engage with incomprehensible language or those who do not, ostensibly, appear to have the capacity for human language? These are questions to which ancient authors repeatedly return.

There are two further points to note about this interest in language and representation. In the first instance, the engagement with pain language goes beyond interest in the use of particular archaizing dialects. Scholars of the 'Second Sophistic' have been particularly alert to the ways in which elite members of Imperial society have employed the use of Attic (and other dialects) to stress their *paideia*.[54] There is no doubt that the linguistic purism associated with this period is consistently used to emphasize social and cultural supremacy among elite Greek males. It should be recognized, however, that the interest in the language of pain and the questions surrounding the capacity to communicate pain were not always bound up with the authorization of a particular dialect. Many of the issues that inhere in the Imperial debates about linguistic purism—educational status, social and cultural authority, and Greek identity—continue to play a

---

[54] Swain (1996), 27–42 on the importance of 'purism' and 43–64 with Schmitz (1997), 69–93.

role in the discussion of pain, its communication, and its interpretation. These issues are not, however, phrased in the terms which have become familiar to critics of this period.

The second issue concerns the way in which the interest in language (and representation) implicates audiences or readers. Authors repeatedly probe the capacity of language to facilitate understanding between pained individuals and their audiences within different narrative scripts (i.e. intra-diegetic readers or audiences): they dramatize the reactions of individuals to those who feel pain. They are also determined, in many instances, to shape the relationship between pain and pained individuals and external (extra-diegetic) readers. Importantly, that process implicates modern readers just as much as ancient ones. If representation shapes processes of recognition, then so too does it help to mould affective reactions to pain among such audiences: the question of where internal and external audiences of pain narratives are placed in terms of their affective responses to others' pain is a question over which this society spent considerable interrogative energy.

c. Pain, Understanding, and Feelings

Pain moulds—and is shaped by—cognitive and affective elements of experience which help not only to define what pain means for the individual, but also to construct relationships between people. The intersection between the body's perceptions and broader experience links the sensory aspects of the body with the history of emotions.

One of the most apparent ways in which pain's broader consequences might be seen concerns the cognitive reactions and understandings of the other towards those who feel pain. Scarry suggests, for instance, that pain's resistance to language means that it might be seen as the epitome of one's doubt about an other's experiences. The difficulties and possibilities of imagining or understanding others' feelings or perceptions was a subject of considerable thought in Imperial culture—it was problematized in a number of different generic contexts, epistemological traditions, and cultural settings. Diagnostic recognition offered a very specific form of philosophically informed understanding and knowledge. Galen and other rational doctors draw on a long tradition of philosophical thought about the extrapolation of information about the body and its internal conditions from the visible signs of the body and their understanding of the way the body works.[55] Recognizing or diagnosing the diseases of the body involved imagining the internal conditions of the individual based on what patients claimed to feel, the discernible symptoms of the body, and the understanding of the body's anatomy. That sense of recognition was often critically re-examined or rephrased in different cultural contexts. Ailios Aristeides, for instance, continually attempts to construct a sense of recognition concerning his painful symptoms that is explicitly defined by its extension beyond the nature of medical diagnosis. As we shall see, these approaches to recognition are set against those types of understanding which are developed in other literary contexts, such as Plutarch's *On Flesh-Eating* or Philostratos' *Imagines*. What is common to these different aspects of recognition is the continued insistence on the ability of one to imagine the perceptions and experiences of others. That imaginative act raises further important questions about how individuals in this community relate to each other on the basis of that information. Even in some diagnostic contexts, the process of recognition moves beyond a straightforwardly detached cognitive process of intellectual classification and therapeutic activity and determines how the doctor might engage with—act towards, associate with—the patient before them. Confronting some of the ways in which one imagines the pain of others brings into question some important communal values for members of this society, especially related to the applicability of justice towards other members of the community, the importance of pity, and *philanthrōpia*.

The second issue raised by the impact of pain on the broader aspects of the individual and their relationship with others concerns the affective elements of pain. The history of emotions has emerged as one of the more invigorating and productive areas of classical scholarship in the last decade.[56] Although it has, understandably, been a consistent and long-held object of interest in some philosophical and theoretical contexts, the study of the *pathē* has, in recent years, broadened to include areas of cultural activity and literary practice that have not traditionally been connected with the emotional landscape of antiquity. Two aspects of the treatment of emotions hold

---

[55] On the epistemological context of diagnosis from sign inference, see Hankinson (1995) and Holmes (2010), 121–46.
[56] The discourse on emotions has expanded considerably: I note only a few important works: Konstan and Rutter (2003), Konstan (2001), (2003b), (2006), Chaniotis (2012), Chaniotis and Ducrey (2013), and LaCourse Munteanu (2013).

particular interest. The first concerns the way in which narrative contexts help to elaborate the complex interplay of emotions in different situations. I am particularly interested in the way in which different types of narrative emphasize (or downplay) the presence of certain emotions in situations in which the individual feels pain. The second element of the discussion of emotions that I turn to in this context is Martha Nussbaum's notion of 'moral intelligence'. Throughout her *Upheavals of Thought*, Nussbaum argues for what she terms the 'cognitive-evaluative' model of emotions.[57] In this context, emotions are seen in terms broadly reminiscent of a Stoic model in which the *pathē* are types of value judgement about the world. For Nussbaum, emotions provide ways of understanding or interpreting the world; they are ways of determining what matters in the individual's life and what one thinks about others. In linking pain perception with the individual's emotions and their affective evaluation by others, writers of the Imperial period explore larger questions about social interaction, values, and ethical action. Pain's integration into the emotional life of the individual and communities cut to the quick of this society's vision of itself.

There are two ways in which I want to explore the emotional dimension of pain perception through this Nussbaumian framework. Firstly, I suggest that affective elements help shape pain experience precisely because they locate pain perception within the broader context of one's own life. The emotions of fear (*phobos*), hope (*elpis*), and despair (*athumia* or *apistia*) are remarkably common across the representation of pain. These emotions (and quasi-emotions) locate pain perception within an understanding of what matters for that individual. As we shall see, that process often has a dramatic impact on how the individual feels about, and negotiates, their body.

Secondly, the emotional aspect of pain experience helps to define the relationships that the pain-perceiver is incorporated into. As I have suggested, narrative descriptions of pain perception dramatize the responses of internal audiences and guide external reactions towards those who feel pain. These reactions are often explored in

---

[57] For the term 'cognitive-evaluative': Nussbaum (2001), 23. For a general elaboration of her view of emotions and moral intelligence, see 19–88, esp. 19–24. Nussbaum's approach represents something of a common trend in modern studies of the emotions: see Konstan (2001), 8–10.

terms of the *pathē* felt by viewers. Emotional reactions link the pained person and the other in combined engagements with pain. Plutarch famously writes in his *Sympotic Questions* that we look upon the ill and the dying 'with distress' (ἀνιαρῶς), but their artistic representation with pleasure.[58] Plutarch's words are energized by an engagement with the Aristotelian idea that one sees or encounters reality differently from its mimetic representation. We will discuss this passage and the issues it raises further, but for the present context, I want to point out the ways in which viewing or encountering another's painful experience could be seen in terms of distress and difficulty on the part of the viewer. As we shall see, in some medical contexts, the idea of feeling emotions or distress 'in common' with the patient is underscored.[59] These emotional reactions govern how non-pained individuals conceptualize themselves (or are represented) as doctors, viewers, or ethical individuals.

Other affective responses shaped this relationship. Of particular importance are reactions such as 'shock' or 'amazement' (commonly designated by cognates of *thaumazein*), as well as 'pity' (*eleos* or *oiktos*), and pleasure or desire (commonly designated by cognates of *hēdus*). Across the diverse cultural contexts of this book, we will see that these emotions are developed (or eschewed) by authors to suit different agenda. What remains consistent, however, is the interest in using emotion to figure both the other's understandings of what the pained individual is going through and also the relationships between those who feel pain and those who view them. The quasi-emotional reaction of amazement or wonder, in particular, raises questions about the intellectually confusing or overwhelming power or qualities of the object viewed. Very often, it is used to construct a type of power relationship between those who feel pain and those who do not.

Pity, too, speaks to the ways in which relationships between the pain-perceiver and other are constructed. In scholarly discussions of

---

[58] Plut. *Quaest. Conviv.* 674a: 'we view the dying and the ill in a distressing way' (ἀνθρώπους ... ἀποθνήσκοντας καὶ νοσοῦντας ἀνιαρῶς ὁρῶμεν). Plutarch reiterates the point moments later at 674b: 'And when we see a consumptive person we are disturbed, but statues and drawings of consumptives we view with pleasure' (καὶ φθισικοὺς μὲν ὁρῶντες δυσχεραίνομεν, ἀνδριάντας δὲ καὶ γραφὰς φθισικῶν ἡδέως θεώμεθα).

[59] For medical compassion and pity in Hippocratic works, see Kosak (2005) and Porter (2014), esp. 35–48, for a good introduction to the question of pity in the Imperial period.

ancient emotions, pity has received a considerable amount of attention.[60] The emotion offers an excellent starting point for thinking about the ways in which pain and difficulty impact not only on the individual themselves, but also on those who surround them. Much of the scholarly discussion of this emotion has centred on the view of pity articulated in Aristotle's *Rhetoric*, where he famously defines the emotion as a type of pain felt towards the undeserved suffering of others, which the viewer feels might happen to him or someone close to him.[61] Importantly, this view of pity links viewer and viewed in a number of ways. It involves assumptions that must be made on the part of viewer about whether or not the pitied person deserves that which has befallen them: it demands intellectual judgements about what has happened and the character of those who are exposed to certain events. At the same time, Aristotle's definition emphasizes the ways in which the pitier conceptualizes their relationship with the pitied or their susceptibility to events or experiences which are deserving of pity: according to the *Rhetoric*, pitier and pitied are connected by the shared possibilities of human vulnerability. Aristotle's model of pity is, to be certain, specific to the context of Classical Athens. As Chris Pelling has pointed out, there is a range of articulations of pity during the Imperial period, many of which do not map easily onto the Aristotelian framework.[62] Nevertheless, it offers a useful starting point for thinking about the ways in which pity connects the pained and other in Imperial society. The concept of pity, in a range of different contexts, becomes a vehicle for exploring the ways in which the pained individual is conceptualized and integrated into different relationships with those around them.

The question of the reader's pleasure, finally, also relates to the ways in which the pained and other interact. The suggestion that the representation of pain—its *mimēsis* in rhetoric, art, or

---

[60] See, e.g., Konstan (2001), Sternberg (2005b), and Blowers (2010).
[61] Arist. *Rh.* 1385b13–16: ἔστω δὴ ἔλεος λύπη τις ἐπὶ φαινομένῳ κακῷ φθαρτικῷ ἢ λυπηρῷ τοῦ ἀναξίου τυγχάνειν, ὃ κἂν αὐτὸς προσδοκήσειεν ἂν παθεῖν ἢ τῶν αὑτοῦ τινα, καὶ τοῦτο ὅταν πλησίον φαίνηται ('Let pity be a certain distress towards an apparent evil, either destructive or distressing, which happens to one who does not deserve it, which one might expect oneself or certain of one's friends to experience, and this when it appears near'). For discussion of this passage, see Konstan (2001), 128–36.
[62] Pelling (2005) and Porter (2014), 34–48, for a slightly different approach to pity in the Imperial period.

drama—could be received pleasantly by those who view or listen to such representations can be traced back at least to Aristotle's *Poetics*.[63] Aristotle's casting of the effects of *mimēsis* on the viewer were, of course, taken up by writers in the Imperial period. Plutarch's discussion in book 5 of the *Sympotic Questions* returns to the Aristotelian formulation which stresses the pleasurable viewing of mimetic representations. In Plutarch's words, while we might be distressed by viewing those who are really in pain, we view their mimetic representation with pleasure.[64] Plutarch's distinction between these different aesthetic responses to those who feel pain and those who are represented as feeling pain helps to position the pained within the aesthetic and moral spectrum of ancient society. The ways in which pleasure is formulated as a viewing response to those who might be in pain or those who are represented as feeling it speaks volumes about the ways in which pain and the pained were viewed by others in this society.

2. REIMAGINING THE IMPERIAL PERIOD

The discussion of pain experience will, I hope, help to redefine how we approach the Imperial period. Scholars have attempted to connect the Greek culture of the first three centuries CE with the emergence of Christian ethics and culture. The body has played a central role in this positioning, helping to figure the Imperial period as either the end of classical antiquity or the beginning of the Christian late antiquity; it has been seen as an important site for the construction and reification of the political and social authority of these two cultural movements. This scholarly frame has undermined the complexity with which we approach the experience of pain: Foucault and Perkins, as well as Peter Brown and Brent Shaw (among others), have all attempted to show how the interest in the body and its pain contributes to a new cultural understanding of the self and its relationship to society in Christian culture.

---

[63] Arist. *Po.* 1448b10–12.
[64] Plut. *Quaest. Conviv.* 674b: ἀνδριάντας δὲ καὶ γραφὰς φθισικῶν ἡδέως θεώμεθα ('but statues and drawings of consumptives we view with pleasure'). See n. 58 for the full quotation. For a similar point: Plut. *Quomodo Adulesc.* 18c–d.

Foucault's *Care of the Self* offers a useful starting point for analysing that critical vision. For Foucault, the medical and philosophical interest in corporeal pleasures was built on an understanding of the body as a site of social and political interest and ethical and hygienic action. Medical discourses and philosophical exhortation continually encouraged individuals to attend to the control and management of the body in an attempt to form themselves as ethical subjects; because elites were denied the opportunity for the political and public honours available under the Republic, they turned towards the management of the self through the practice of attending, intensely and constantly, to the experiences of the body.[65] Foucault's model of ethical concern with the body has been attacked from a number of different angles by (among others) Maud Gleason and Jason König.[66] Nevertheless, his suggestion that the body operated as a site of cultural concern has been broadly adopted and developed by scholars. Brown, in particular, has advanced this view by showing how codes of sexual practice were a medium for resistance to the current political authorities within the Roman Empire among different Christian and Jewish communities.[67] For both Foucault and Brown, the body was a site of cultural definition and political action throughout the Imperial period.

If the work of these two scholars has emphasized the centrality of the body to the cultural life of the Imperial period, then that model has also facilitated a particular historical mapping of that culture between the Greco-Roman world and Christian late antiquity. Foucault's ultimate aim in the *Care of the Self* was to place the ethics of Greek philosophers and writers alongside their later Christian counterparts. He writes of the codes surrounding the body:

> [b]y focusing only on these common traits, one may get the impression that the sexual ethics attributed to Christianity or even to the modern West was already in place, at least with respect to its basic principles, at the time when Greco-Roman culture reached its culmination. But this would be to disregard fundamental differences concerning the type of relation to the self and hence the forms of integration of these precepts in the subject's experience of himself.[68]

---

[65] Foucault (1986), 85–6.
[66] Gleason (1995), xxv–vi and (slightly differently) König (2005), 14. For more general criticisms of Foucault's *Care of the Self*, see Goldhill (1995), xi–xii.
[67] Brown (1988), 5–32 on the austere sexual codes of antiquity.
[68] Foucault (1986), 144 and 39.

28   *Introduction*

Foucault's placement of ancient ethics appears to emphasize the disjuncture between ancient pagan and Christian concern with the body. Yet his suggestion that the relationship is defined by similar codes but a different 'relation to the self' appears ambiguous and (as Virginia Burrus points out) goes a long way to paving the way for a reintegration of Christianity into ancient ethical concern with the body and pleasure.[69] More significantly, what interests me is the framing of Foucault's investigative task, which emphasizes the comparison of the two cultural systems. Foucault's ultimate aim was to place ancient ethics on a trajectory which led to the development of Christian (and, ultimately, modern) sexuality.

The stance that Foucault adopts at this point is matched by Brown's, who sees in the sombre codes of antiquity the origins of a Christian concern with austerity.[70] What matters here is not the specific relationship between the codes and culture of the body that Foucault and Brown (in their different ways) document. These approaches attempt to place the body within a teleological account of ancient culture in which pagan society is evaluated in terms of the bodily practices and belief system which emerged in Christian communities of late antiquity. The Christian late antique society becomes the cynosure against which the pagan world is understood.[71] The implications of this approach are twofold. Firstly, it warps our interest in the cultural practices and concerns of the Imperial period: the significance of different phenomena is evaluated in terms of their relationship with, or contribution to, the development and success of later historical or cultural forms. Secondly, it assumes a teleology to the practices of pagan culture in the first three centuries CE. Such an evolutionary model promotes and solidifies a scholarly complicity in the triumphant history of Christianity.

The teleological model impacts directly on the way scholars have approached the history of pain and suffering in this period. In his article 'Body/Power/Identity', Shaw turns to the question of Christian resistance and self-definition through the endurance of pain. For Shaw, the trials and executions of Christians use force (represented

---

[69] Burrus (2004), 2–4.   [70] Brown (1988), 21–3.
[71] The teleology of Brown's view is most explicitly stated in his *Making of Late Antiquity*: his aim is to map 'in the late second, third, and early fourth centuries the emergence of features that were far from clearly discernible at the time ... and which finally came together to form the definitively Late Antique style of religious, cultural, and social life that emerged in the late fourth and early fifth centuries'. Brown (1978), 1.

in the painful destruction of the body) to inscribe political ideology and power on the body of the condemned.[72] Shaw's central argument is that individuals used the patient endurance of torture and suffering imposed by others to resist the imposition of cultural ideology by political authorities; by mobilizing cultural codes which valorized 'endurance' (ὑπομονή), writers (and the individuals they represented) were able to reverse the political relationships (that are assumed to be?) inherent in the infliction of bodily pain and torture.[73] Once again, pagan texts are mined for the discourses which explain the success of Christian culture: according to Shaw, the process of resistance through patient endurance ensured that individual instances of political domination through torture failed and contributed to the ultimate failure of the pagan political authorities.[74] Shaw points to Akhilleus Tatios' *Leukippe and Kleitophon* and the presentation of Leukippe's resistance and confrontation of her master (and would-be rapist) Thersandros as evidence for a change in the ethical codes which figure resistance to power.[75] Shaw's use of Akhilleus Tatios' novel co-opts the novel into the construction of Christian ethics which emerge during the final stages of the Imperial period.[76] It is, of course, hard to deny that this specific text might have participated in or influenced (or been influenced by) the development of Christian culture. My concern emerges from the fact that reading the treatment of pain and suffering in Akhilleus Tatios serves to reify a complicity with the ultimate success of Christian culture and ethics; secondly, it circumscribes the complexity of the ancient text and limits potentially

---

[72] Shaw (1996), esp. 275–8. For a similar reading: Potter (1993), 52–3.
[73] Shaw (1996), 278–84; 291–300; cf. Table 1 at 310.
[74] Shaw (1996), 311:

[t]he body was indeed the site of a struggle. The spectacular trials and executions of the Christians are but an extreme instance of the use of force to elicit a certain public behaviour from subject bodies, to inscribe one sort of ideology on the body. In this case, it was rejected. Not only did such attempts fail in individual cases—the cumulative effect of individual acts of resistance compelled a final failure in the long term.

[75] For Shaw's use of Akhilleus Tatios and other classical authors, see Shaw (1996), 269–84 and 295–6. The critical scene is Ach. Tat. vi.20-2, in which Leukippe gives an impassioned speech in defiance of torture by Thersandros. For an alternative reading: Morales (2004), 199–203.

[76] A point made more poignant by the fact that this novel appears to have been co-opted by ancient writers into the construction of Christian ethics: NB the epigram attributed to either Photios or Leon: *AP.* ix.203, along with Goldhill (1995), 100–2.

instructive readings made apart from Christian sources. Can we evaluate Akhilleus Tatios' treatment of pain and suffering without focusing on the way it contributes to the emergence and dominance of Christian culture? Shaw's study intersects, especially, with Perkins' *The Suffering Self* and its focus on the emergence and success of the Christian triumph.[77] What becomes significant is that which contributes to that evolution of the Christian world view.

Shaw is not alone in stressing the close relationship between torture, the pained body, and power regimes. There is no doubt that this particular dynamic—which Christian and classical scholars (following Foucault and Brown) have been determined to see in the treatment of the body in this society—is one element of pain's complex story.[78] Importantly, however, it is only one aspect. This culture's interest in pain extended far more widely than traditional accounts acknowledge. While there are no doubt occasions on which power is linked to the creation and infliction of pain on the individual's body, it is also true that the connection is not inherent. Part of what this project aims to do is to emphasize the limitations of thinking about pain in those terms. The second major concern of this investigation reflects how pain was linked to bigger questions about how one felt about it. What mattered for this society was the social and affective questions that emerge from the confrontation with pain. How one feels pain, how one feels about it, and how others feel about those who experience it matter. The complexity of this culture's engagement with pain and its concern for those who felt pain needs to be understood apart from the (at the time, deeply uncertain) emergence of Christian ethics and the valorization of the poor.

---

[77] See, e.g., Perkins (1995), 3.
[78] See duBois (1991) for another example of the interest in torture and power in a classical setting, and also Ballengee (2009).

Part 1

Diagnosing and Treating Pain

1

Diagnosing and Treating the Pained Body

There are few Imperial discourses more centrally concerned with pain than medicine. If the period was defined by anxiety over the condition of the body, then that concern was often focalized through a medical lens.[1] Medical culture under the Empire was, as scholars have recognized, characterized by different scientific, religious, and philosophical ideas; such ideas circulated in a multifaceted, variegated landscape of practitioners, patients, and healing practices.[2] Within that landscape there were different ways of conceptualizing and explaining the pained body. Medical treatises on diagnosis, as well as treatises concerned with specific conditions and their therapy, were produced by doctors from different philosophical sects—Pneumatists, Empiricists, Methodists, and others steeped in traditions of rational medicine. They present varying interpretations of both what pain is and how doctors and patients should engage with it. Inscriptions, charms, and votive offerings deposited in Asklepieia and other healing sanctuaries around the Roman world attest to widespread belief in the religious and the magical treatment of pain and other symptoms; personal accounts of illness and the images of pained bodies (and especially specific body parts) from these sites

---

[1] Dodds (1965), 3–4 for the phrase 'age of anxiety' and Bowersock (1969), 74–5 for the disease infecting Imperial society. For discussion of this theme, see the Introduction (text to nn. 6–9). On the importance of medicine to Imperial culture, there is considerable material: see, e.g., Bowersock (1969), chapter 4, esp. 79, or Nutton (2004), 191–235 for a brief introduction to various sects and their significance under the Empire.

[2] For the variety of medical practice, see van der Eijk, Horstmanshoff, and Schrijvers (1995). For more a specific general introduction to, and discussion of, the importance of Methodism, see Nutton (2004), 186–201 with Cels. *de Med. praef.* 53–7, along with the fragments collected in Tecusan. Empiricism: see Frags. 249–308 collected in Deichgräber. Pneumatic sect: Wellmann (1895b).

give voice to the great numbers of individuals who felt pain and who sought alleviation through divine intervention.[3] I approach medical culture through two related figures—Aretaios of Kappodokia and Galen of Pergamon—who wrote (probably) in the second century CE and whose medical practices are linked in some way to rational, anatomically-informed medicine; while the view of medical culture adopted is limited to one (albeit quite broad) vein of the complex medical landscape of this period, it will offer an important view of how pain was integrated into medical discourse at large.

Medicine's interest in pain is long-standing. The Hippokratic work, *On the Art of Medicine*, suggests that pain is an important aspect of the doctor's concern with the internal conditions of the ill body and that its removal is one of the objectives of the medical art.[4] The interest in tracing symptoms of pain within the ill body might have had a long history, but it takes on a particular tenor in the Imperial period. This investigation focuses on the central role that pain plays in the nexus of ideological assumptions and clinical practices that scholars understand as diagnosis and therapy: how is pain integrated into, or understood within the context of, diagnostic and therapeutic practice? Investigating pain through this lens turns directly to the three issues I raised in the Introduction concerning physiological pain: post-Alexandrian interest in the anatomy of the body; Imperial debates about language and narrative and their relationship to the body; and, finally, the relation to the broader psychological and emotional impact and experience of pain. These elements combine to create a particularly distinctive Imperial medical interest in pain experience.

Rational diagnosis focuses on the physicality of patients' ill bodies. Diagnosing and 'reading' pain involves accounting for the intricacies of the body's anatomical structure, its capacity for sensory perception,

---

[3] For the relationship between medicine and religion, see, e.g., Israelowich (2012), chapters 2–3. Petsalis-Diomidis (2005) and (2010) for specific discussions of Ailios Aristeides. For healing-cult votives, see Edelstein (1967) and Chaniotis (1995).

[4] Cf. Hp. *de Arte.* 3, which is critically modified to refer to pain at *Fist.* 7: ἢν ... ἀπαλλάσσηται τῆς ὀδύνης, ἀρκείτω ('if ... there is a release from pain, let this be sufficient'), and in *Aff.* 2.3–4 and 4: ἢν ... ἡ ὀδύνη ἀπολείπῃ, ἀρκέει ('if ... the pain goes away, it is sufficient'). On Hippokratic medicine and pain, see Horden (2008), Byl (1992), King (1988), and Rey (1995), 17–23. Of course, the Hippokratic texts themselves were working within long-established intellectual and cultural traditions of medical interest in pain: cf. Hom. *Il.* 4.190; on the status of pain in Homer: Holmes (2007), 45–84, and for Archaic poetry generally: Allen (2009).

and combining these with the notion of pain itself. As I touched on in the Introduction, many of the ideas about pain perception articulated by Imperial writers can be traced, in their broad form, to earlier Archaic and Classical material. The vocabulary and the interpretive framework for much of Aretaios' and Galen's approach to the body is drawn from Aristotle's work on biology and natural science; these later writers draw heavily on Hippokratic writings about painful symptoms and their connection with certain organs or internal areas within the *sōma*.[5] Having said this, the Imperial medical gaze perceived the body with an anatomical intensity and precision that was not possible for pre-Alexandrian medicine.[6] The work of Alexandrian investigators—Herophilos, Erasistratos, and others— helped to elaborate the internal spaces of the body with remarkable nuance and precision. It is clear that Galen drew heavily, for instance, on Herophilos' work on the liver, and on the nervous system and its connection with the brain as well as other areas of the body.[7] According to Rufus of Ephesos, Erasistratos appears to have differentiated effectively between those nerves which are sensory and those which are responsible for motor activity.[8] This work contributed to a more precisely elaborated understanding of the body and its internal structures and, in so doing, laid the foundations for the understanding of the possibilities of pain perception and its connection with the intricate nuances of the body's structure. In exploring and delineating the details of pain's presence within the spaces of the body, the medical

---

[5] For Galen's connection with Aristotle, see Debru (2008), 265-6 for a brief introduction. Hankinson (2008d), 210-36 provides a broad overview of the influence of Hippokratic and Aristotelian thinking on Galen's philosophy of nature. The importance of both Aristotle and Hippokrates to Galen is demonstrated by the volume of commentaries he wrote on both: Flemming (2008). For Galen's references to Hippokrates in relation to specific anatomy, see, e.g., Gal. *Loc. Aff.* viii.79K.

[6] Especially important here is von Staden (1989). On Galen's debt to earlier anatomists: Rocca (2003), 42-7 and (2008). For the actions of the anatomists and their connection with the rational approach to causes and signs: Cels. *de Med. praef.* 23-6 (= T. 63a von Staden). For the revival of anatomical knowledge in the second century CE: Rocca (2003), 42-3.

[7] For the importance of Herophilos' work on the nervous system: Gal. *Loc. Aff.* viii.212K (= T. 80 von Staden) and *AA*. 9.9 (pp. 8-9 Simon = T. 82 von Staden). On the liver: Gal. *PHP*. v.543-4K (= T. 115 von Staden). On the uterus: Gal. *Ut. Diss.* ii.895-6K (= T. 114 von Staden). For further discussion of the impact of the discovery of the nerves, see von Staden (2000).

[8] Ruf. Eph. *Anat.* 71-5 (pp. 184-5 Daremberg = T. 81 von Staden) and *Onom.* 149-50 (pp. 153 Daremberg = T. 125 von Staden).

writers of the Imperial period reveal their heavy debt to the anatomical discoveries of the Alexandrian revolution.

The interest in anatomy leads to the second element that marks out medicine in the first three centuries CE: the focus on the way in which patients report or recount their perceptions of pain. Rational medicine integrates patients' language and reportage of their felt sensations of pain with anatomical theory. Language and anatomy are combined to shape how the doctor explains pain perception and its diagnostic significance; the anatomical view of the body is not contradicted or undermined by the importance of narrative; rather, they mutually inform and support each other. Consequently, the diagnostic significance of pain is elaborated through three related issues: who speaks within the clinical encounter; in what terminology patients and others describe their (or others') symptoms; and how those symptoms are explained and represented by doctors. Rational medicine—which operated in a world devoid of more modern instruments for evaluating the body and its conditions—relied heavily on the relationship between language and the body. Aretaios and Galen (among others) navigate the limits of their science by managing medical language as well as the narrative-based interactions between doctor and patient.

The concern to integrate reportage, narratives, and pain terminology with anatomical theory inflects a third aspect of Imperial medicine—the devotion to developing and managing the experience of pain. The two elements described above form an important part of the way in which doctors and patients relate to each other and, critically, how they both understand and manage the broader questions of pain's impact. Pain is presented as a phenomenon which not only changes patients' emotional and psychological states, but also shifts the dynamic of their relationships with the doctor and those around them; it influences how others view and react to them and their pain. This sense of experience—its impact on the individual and those around them—becomes a key discursive battleground: doctors stake their professional authority on precisely how that relationship develops.

Taken together, these three elements raise an important, though largely undiscussed, point. From a medical perspective, experiencing pain involves all of these aspects. As we shall see, doctors and patients combine a conception of pain as physiological phenomenon grounded in the anatomy of the body, the nuances of felt sensation and its reportage and explanation, and more holistic views about the ways in which individuals navigate pain from an affective and interpersonal perspective. They develop a view of pain which emphasizes the combination of physiology, language, and the complexities of the interactions of the doctor–patient relationship.

1. DIAGNOSIS, NARRATIVE, AND INTERPERSONAL RELATIONSHIPS

The elaboration of this view of pain has ramifications for a number of broader issues in the history of medicine. Because pain is central to the diagnostic process, shifting the scholarly understanding of pain requires developing a more supple view of this central aspect of clinical practice. In beginning from a focus on diagnosis, this chapter turns to a remarkably understudied area. In the last three decades, the question of how to approach diagnosis has become one of the major issues of contemporary cultural analysis; in relation to Imperial culture, however, there remains little work on the subject. I emphasize three points. Firstly, that medical diagnosis—for all its scientific and epistemological foundations—was broadly a process of narrative recognition and explanation. Secondly, that recognition, narration, and explanation have to be understood not only within their scientific and epistemological context, but also as practices grounded in the broader sociocultural sediment of Imperial society. They were predicated on social relationships and interactions, ideas and understandings drawn from the culture around medicine. Finally, that the intricacies of this narrative situation ensured that pain was related to a holistic view of the patient. By drawing out the narrative basis of scientific diagnosis (and the treatment of pain), I hope to bring into the limelight questions about the subjective nature of experience and perception, as well as the idea of the patient as an individual who has a relationship with those around them.

These issues have become particularly important within contemporary debates about medicine, especially in medical anthropology, in particular Arthur Kleinman's work, *Patients and Healers in the Context of Culture*. Kleinman's 1980 study inspired a range of different approaches to the study of historical medical cultures, but also initiated a sea change in the way in which scholars, doctors, and the public have understood contemporary medical practice.[9] According to Kleinman, health-care systems are characterized by, among other things, 'the management of particular illness episodes through communicative operations, such as labelling and explaining'.[10] Such operations fit illness into a culture's semantic system by elucidating an individual's physical symptoms, providing aetiologies, narrating the course of illnesses through time, explaining their severity, and labelling their particular form.[11] Clinical practice is dependent, from this vantage point, on the clinical reality between patient and healer—the matrix of epistemological and cultural assumptions (shared or otherwise), the interpersonal dynamics, and the cultural settings which define this relationship. Medicine should be less about understanding the phenomenon of disease from a scientific 'objective' perspective, and more about understanding 'illness' through a focus on the dynamics of social relationships and *praxis*. That distinction is most clearly put in the words of Oliver Sacks:

> to restore the human subject at the centre [of health-care provision]—the suffering, fighting, afflicted, human subject—we must deepen a case-history to a narrative or a tale; only then do we have a 'who' as well as a 'what', a real person, a patient, in relation to disease.[12]

Sacks and Kleinman, in different ways, ask us to move away from Rey's conception of the reality of sickness. Diagnosis is really about how people talk to each other.

Reading Imperial medical culture through this Kleinmanian lens allows us to move beyond the current view of diagnosis and see its

---

[9] On medical anthropology and clinical practice in a modern setting: Hunter (1991), 5–26, along with Mattingly and Garro (2000), esp. 6–9. For increasing interest in the 'experience' of illness inspired by Kleinman: Cassell (1985) on the way medicine reinforces social and economic ideologies of control and power and Frank (1995). In modern medical discourse, this has led to a focus on patient-based narratives which explain illness and the experience of symptoms in patients' own terms: Sacks (1998). For applications of this discourse to the ancient world, see (initially) Nijhuis (1995), King (2002), and, now, Israelowich (2015), esp. chapter 2. Petridou and Thumiger (2015) is explicitly framed to provide a more patient-centred account of ancient medicine (see pp. 3–4), but on the problems with their approach, see below (text to nn. 23–4).

[10] For his elaboration of the 'core clinical functions' germane to all health-care systems: Kleinman (1980), 71–2. For applications of these functions to the study of ancient medicine: Nijhuis (1995) and Israelowich (2012), 40–3.

[11] Kleinman (1980), 71–2.   [12] Sacks (1998), viii.

engagement with pain in more appropriate terms. The majority of (the limited) ancient scholarly work on diagnosis has been conducted on Galen's corpus and the limitations of current approaches might be best illustrated in that context. Jonathan Barnes, along with Luis García Ballester, has pointed out that Galen's diagnostic system combines different elements, such as the application of rationality (*logismos*), the sensorial perception of patients' bodies and symptoms (*aisthēsis*), and the process of talking and discussing past and present symptoms, treatments, and lifestyle with the patient and their attendants.[13] In this context, scholars have focused on the epistemological assumptions that Galen harnesses throughout his medical practice. This has been especially prevalent in critical analyses of Galen's clinical epistemology, where scholars have drawn attention to his combination of both experiential forms of knowledge and theoretical reasoning.[14] Barnes, for instance, argues that Galen combines the rational division of diseases and their symptoms into their various *genera* and species with the use of logical deduction to 'prove' his diagnostic conclusions (*logismos*).[15] This is precisely the type of scholarly approach to Galen's work that stands behind Rey's discussion of pain which we discussed in the Introduction. The sensorial aspects of Galen's diagnostic practices have also received some treatment: Vivian Nutton has investigated the importance of sensorial perception in the diagnosis of the ill body.[16] What has been less analysed in this climate is the intricate process of questioning and discussing the patients' conditions with them and integrating the physiological data of the body into broader narratives which allow it to be understood, managed, and treated.[17]

Kleinman's stress on narrative operations exhorts us to shift scholarly focus to the analysis of medical language and narrative. Narrative hermeneutics are important not only because the acts of diagnosis are

---

[13] García Ballester (1981) and Barnes (1991).

[14] Frede demonstrates Galen's unusual combination of both dogmatic and empiricist forms of knowledge: Frede (1981), reprinted in Frede (1987), 279–98. On this issue, see also Hankinson (2008c) and (1995). On Galen's philosophy in general: Moraux (1981).

[15] Barnes (1991). For a similar discussion of sign inference and 'indication' (*endeixis*): Kudlien (1991).

[16] Nutton (1993). This is particularly relevant in the case of diagnosis of the pulse, in which the fineness of touch allows the doctor to understand the nuances of the patient's pulse.

[17] Some work has been done on questioning the patient: Mattern (2008), 98–158, Roby (2015), and Letts (2014) and (2015).

reported in the context of broader narratives or self-aware literary accounts, but because diagnosis is itself predicated on language and narratives (of symptoms and perceptions, causal explanations, and disease chronologies both backwards and forwards in time) which provide believable accounts of the body's conditions. Questions about narrative, the nature of clear or effective speech, and the value of the patient's voice were heavily theorized by different Imperial authors. Rufus of Ephesos' second-century-CE treatise, *Medical Questions*, is dedicated to the need to ask the patient about their symptoms and previous lifestyle in order to produce a 'more accurate diagnosis'.[18] That treatise, drawing on the work of Hippocratic *Aphorisms*, lays down what questions the doctor should ask to achieve the best diagnostic and therapeutic outcomes; it also argues that particular symptoms and the experience of disease as a whole can undermine the patient's ability to communicate effectively; and that the patient's own (not always honest) agenda might influence how and what they relate.[19] The question of how the patient might translate or speak clearly about what they perceive, how disease impacts on that process, and the strategies that the doctor might employ to eradicate any doubt about the patient's honesty are explored by Rufus, Galen, and other contemporary medical figures. Diagnosis was a practice sewn into the narrative fabric of the clinical encounter; how to speak to the patient, what to ask, and what might be gleaned from the answers were hotly debated and fought over.

The second aspect to Kleinman's approach—the emphasis of the interpersonal realities of the doctor–patient relationship—is also important, allowing us to understand the ways in which different narratives within the clinical encounter might be inflected by the power relationships that exist between different individuals. If narrative is a vehicle for reifying social and cultural authority, then how do the narratives created in the clinical encounter reflect and shape those relationships? How do these factors inflect the experience of illness and pain? Kleinman's

---

[18] Ruf. Eph. *Quaest. Med.* 1 (Gärtner): ἐρωτήματα χρὴ τὸν νοσοῦντα ἐρωτᾶν, ἐξ ὧν ἂν καὶ διαγνωσθείη τι τῶν περὶ τὴν νόσον ἀκριβέστερον καὶ θεραπευθείη κάλλιον. ('it is necessary to ask the patient questions from which one might diagnose more accurately some element of the disease and provide better therapy.') On this treatise, see Letts (2014), 1005–6 and the implications of this line.

[19] Ruf. Eph. *Quaest. Med.* 2–3 (Gärtner) (on the different factors that can influence patient reportage and its interpretation) and 42–3 (on further factors, including mendacity).

Diagnosing and Treating the Pained Body   41

framework helps us to see Galen's and others' use (or rejection) of patient language not only in terms of the difference between objective and subjective accounts of pain, but also in terms of interpersonal power, discursive positioning, and social authority.[20] It also allows us to analyse the ways in which different types of medical narrative intersect and the work that has to be done to create cohesive accounts of disease within clinical encounters. A contemporary medically-orientated author, the *rhētōr* Ailios Aristeides, raises precisely these questions in his famous *diēgēsis* of his own illness in the *Sacred Tales*. Aristeides' assumption of a quasi-epic voice for his personalized account of his illness explicitly explores what type of account and which narrator might be considered as authoritative. Aristeides uses language to mediate the relationship between doctors (either divine or human) and patients as they navigate the complexities of power relationships and the interconnections between different systems of understanding.[21] Kleinman's work allows scholars to return to the analysis of diagnosis, and the treatment of pain, with a new framework. It asks us to consider the complexity of diagnosis both in terms of the application of various forms of knowledge and also in terms of how it functions as a social process, defined by the complex and complicated relationship between doctor and patient.

While Kleinman's conclusions and the recent development of medical anthropology inspire renewed focus on the complexity of doctor–patient relationships, his work is not without its problems when applied to the ancient world in general and the doctors studied in Part 1 in particular. Recently, two books have done much to draw a Kleinman-like approach into the study of ancient medicine. Susan Mattern's *Galen and the Rhetoric of Healing* has shown that Galen's accounts of patients' experiences combine different levels of narrative, including the direct and indirect quotation of patients and third-person external conclusions about an individual's condition. Mattern's work reveals the complexities of the narrative situation in Galen's case-histories and the complex social world in which his clinical practice is embedded.[22] In a similar vein, a number of the

---

[20] Discursive authority: Gal. *Loc. Aff.* viii.113K; on his authority over patients, see Chapter 3 (text to n. 6).
[21] Aristid. 47.2–3K on the impossibility of narrating his condition and his silent submission to the god 'as to a doctor'.
[22] Mattern (2008), with 27–47 for the most thorough discussion of the 'genre'. Cf. (2009), who also stresses the differing objectives of Galen's and Hippokrates' case-histories.

chapters in Georgia Petridou's and Chiara Thumiger's volume *Homo Patiens* argue that patients were often a source of diagnostic information and that they often contributed significantly to the clinical scenario.[23] These two excellent studies have provided an important stepping stone to analysing the way in which the patient might be seen as part of the history of ancient medicine. Indeed, *Homo Patiens* explicitly begins with a call for the history of medicine 'from the bottom up', in which the patient becomes a central object of study.[24]

Where they fall short, however, is their analysis of rhetorical representation in much of the ancient material. Rufus' theoretical delineation of the importance of speech is a representation of the doctor–patient relationship and the patient's contribution, not an account of it. The patient's historical role in medicine is, it seems to me, unrecoverable. Galen and Aretaios (and others such as Arkhigenes) represent a particular type of relationship which takes account of the patient. Claims to engage in patient-centred language constitute a rhetorical move; they are best seen as a polemical act of self-presentation which involves representing the patient's role in pain diagnosis. The full implications of this have not been thoroughly considered. When seen in this light, the critical question becomes not just 'How is the doctor–patient relationship figured in ancient medicine?' nor 'How are patients integrated into, or how do they contribute to, diagnostic and medical practice?' but 'Why at this particular time and place does it become important to represent that relationship in a particular way?' The answer to that question speaks to the construction of the medical authority of the doctor, the formation of the medical discourse, and to a particular way of conceptualizing the experience of pain in this culture.

---

[23] For the scholarly context of *Homo Patiens:* Petridou and Thumiger (2015), 3–4. For more detailed discussions of the work of Rufus of Ephesos, see Letts (2015) and, for Galen, Roby (2015), 304–22.

[24] Petridou and Thumiger (2015), 3–4.

2

Aretaios of Kappodokia

I start with the shadowy figure of Aretaios of Kappodokia, about whom little is known and whose works are often absent from scholarly discussions of Imperial medicine. Aretaios' four extant works—*On the Causes and Signs of Acute Diseases, On the Causes and Signs of Chronic Diseases, On the Therapy of Acute Diseases,* and *On the Therapy of Chronic Diseases*[1]—present the cultural historian with considerable difficulty. He is generally thought to be writing between the second half of the first century CE and the first half of the second, possibly in Alexandria, but such details are far from certain.[2] The lack of verifiable historical detail about his cultural context, however, does not preclude the study of this fascinating author. His works still offer us valuable clues to the medical landscape. Scholars have often

---

[1] Aretaios' works are divided across eight books: books i–ii = *On the Causes and Signs of Acute Diseases* (*SA*.); iii–iv = *On the Causes and Signs of Chronic Diseases* (*SD*.); v–vi = *On the Therapy of Acute Diseases* (*CA*.); vii–viii = *On the Therapy of Chronic Diseases* (*CD*.). On the nature of the books, and their organization into these four titles: Roselli (2004c), 164.

[2] The dating of Aretaios and his surviving works is highly problematic. The only secure references to Aretaios are from the sixth-century-CE author Aetius: *Aet.* viii.50. For discussion of the late references to Aretaios: Roselli (2004c), 163 n. 1 and Oberhelman (1994), 942. Wellman proposes a date in the third century CE on the basis that Aretaios had copied the early second-century-CE work of Arkhigenes: Wellmann (1895b), 24. A date between the second half of the first century CE and the first half of the second century CE has been generally accepted, though this is not without its problems. He is referred to in the *Euporista*, attributed to Dioskourides (ii.119.2 *Euporista*), but the critical passage is probably spurious. According to Kudlien, Aretaios can be dated because he manifests a 'pure' form of pneumatism, and therefore should be placed in the first century CE before it became 'eclectic': Kudlien (1964), 1098–9. Discussions of what constitutes a 'pure' form of pneumatism or trying to pin it down to a particular text, and mapping that onto a historical context for an author are, to my mind, highly problematic. For general discussions of the problems of dating: Oberhelman (1994).

connected Aretaios with a number of second-century doctors, especially Arkhigenes of Apamea, whose ideas about the pulse and pain and now lost work *On Affected Parts* were significant enough to warrant considerable polemical engagement from his later contemporary, Galen of Pergamon.[3] Opinion about the nature of Aretaios' connection with Arkhigenes has vacillated between viewing either Aretaios or Arkhigenes as a close copyist or a plagiarist of the other.[4] Moreover, although Galen never mentions or refers to Aretaios, it is increasingly clear that there are points at which the work of the two doctors intersects.[5] Aretaios probably contributed to, or at least engaged closely with and was embedded in, medical thought and practice during the second century CE.

Aretaios' four extant works are part of the nosological tradition. This tradition aims at providing the reader with handbooks for recognizing or diagnosing and treating the diseases patients present with.[6] Aretaios' works extensively catalogue the various symptoms which define acute and chronic conditions and link that act of classification with the provision of effective treatment for patients. Amneris Roselli has suggested that they are unusual when considered against other forms of nosological writing: unlike other texts, Aretaios' own voice and views are repeatedly expressed in the first person; the discussions of diseases and therapies are framed by *prooimia* which locate the disease within broader visions of the clinical encounter and the nature of health-care provision.[7] Aretaios' texts combine the classification of diseases and their corresponding treatments with his vision of the ongoing relationship between patient and doctor. These descriptions are, of course, rhetorical representations designed

---

[3] On Aretaios' connection with Arkhigenes, see Mavroudis (2000). Wellmann (1895b) for Arkhigenes as a member of the Pneumatic sect. For Arkhigenes' relationship with Galen, see Chapter 3 (nn. 22, 28, 37–9, with corresponding text).

[4] See, e.g., Wellmann (1895a), 669–70 and (1895b), 24 and 48–9. For the opposite view: Kudlien (1964), 1098–9.

[5] The absence of references in Galen to Aretaios has been used as evidence against a pre-Galenic date, but this absence of evidence is not sufficient reason to reject the possibility of an early Imperial context. Nutton suggests that there are lots of connections between Aretaios and Galen: Nutton (2004), 210. Cf. Gal. *Subf. Emp.* 10 (Deichgräber) and Gal. *SMT.* xii.312K with Aret. *SD.* iv.13.20 for their use of a similar story about the treatment of a leper.

[6] The tradition can be traced back to the Hippokratic *Epid.* and *Aph.*, at least. On this tradition: Langholf (1990), 150–63.

[7] For examples: Roselli (2004c), 165–6. Most of the *prooimia* are now lost (esp. at *SA.* i). For one extant example: *SD.* iii.1, discussed below (text to nn. 34–5).

to further his own agenda. But they are valuable texts for revealing pain's incorporation into medical culture precisely because they offer a rhetorical argument for a particular doctor–patient relationship and the role that pain plays in shaping it. Aretaios' texts may be generic oddities, but it is that quality of unusualness that makes them fertile ground for the archaeology of this culture's interest in pain.

Pain takes centre stage in Aretaios' diagnostic and therapeutic project: it constitutes not only an ever-present symptom which must be recognized, but also a phenomenon which impacts on all those who encounter it. Aretaios' texts resonate with sad, compelling accounts of the physical perception, the *aisthēsis*, of pain symptoms. His attendance to this particular sensation sits alongside the treatment of other symptoms to which the ill body is susceptible, but no other receives the rich, intricate analysis offered to the sensation of pain. This analysis of Aretaios starts from three related questions. What is Aretaios' understanding of pain as a sensory phenomenon? Or, put another way, what scientific or philosophical ideas stand behind how Aretaios approaches pain and its relationship to the ill body? Secondly, how does Aretaios incorporate the pain perceptions reported by his patients into his diagnostic classification? Finally, how are these two elements integrated into a broader understanding of the pain experience within the clinical encounter between doctor and patient?

1. PAIN AS A SENSORY PHENOMENON

Aretaios rarely elaborates, in detail, a theoretical or philosophical vision of what constitutes pain. Rather, in classifying different conditions and their treatment, he reveals some aspects of his understanding of the phenomenon, its genesis, and the different ways that it can be perceived within the body.[8] Aretaios distinguishes between two

---

[8] Aretaios' terminology for pain suggests that he is not determined to differentiate between pain terms: the treatises repeatedly slide between the use of *ponos, odunē*, and *algos*. While there are occasions when specific terminology is used for different types of pain, it is clear that Aretaios extracts little intellectual or classificatory mileage out of shifts in terminology: pain = pain = pain. Where different language is adopted to describe particular conditions—such as when referring to pain in the head which arises from an immediate cause (*kephalalgia*) or its chronic relation (*kephalaia*)—he

tropes of pain sensation: that which is related to internal causes and is determined by the body's humoral mixture; and that which is linked to the interaction of sensory bodies with external stimuli. These two categories figure pain as a phenomenon tied to the nature of the body and its capacity for sensory perception, grounding it in the universally consistent functions and structures of the *sōma*.

Aretaios' most telling discussion in this context is his treatment of the condition arthritis. His explanation of this condition begins from the general assertion that arthritis is a pain that exists in all parts of the body; while it often originates, or is primarily located, in a particular joint or limb, it spreads throughout the body of the patient.[9] 'The origin' of this condition, Aretaios holds, 'is the nerves, the tendons of the joints, and those things which extend from the bones and are inborn in the bones'.[10] To Aretaios' mind, the causes of this pain are confounding and, therefore, in need of specific explanation: 'the gods alone know the exact cause', but he will say what seems probable.[11] Aretaios' self-effacing caveat flags the speculative nature of the conclusions and also heightens the stakes in the explanation: if pain is prevalent throughout the body of the arthritic, then this condition is also especially telling for his theories concerning pain itself.

Although bones and teeth are subject to external trauma, such as being cut or squeezed, these processes 'do not pain' (οὐ πονέει, Aret. *SD.* iv.12.2.2) them as much as that which occurs internally; in contrast, however, if they are pained 'from themselves' (ἐξ ὡυτέων), then 'nothing else pains more powerfully than this' (οὐδὲν ἕτερον ἀλγέει τοῦδε δυνατώτερον, iv.12.2.2-3). The diverse experiences of the parts of the body and their different intensities of pain and pleasure can be explained in terms of their physiology. According to Aretaios, the densely structured parts of the body are 'insensible to

---

exchanges his general predilection for *ponos* in favour of the technical terminology for the specific ailments: see κεφαλαλγίη at Aret. *SD.* iii.2.1.2. On the importance of Aretaios' treatment of a migraine as opposed to a symptomatic headache: Didsbury (1936), 260-7 and Koehler and van de Wiel (2001), 253-61.

[9] Aret. *SD.* iv.12.1.1-2: ἁπάντων τῶν ἄρθρων πόνος ἡ ἀθρῖτις ('arthritis is a pain of all the joints'). On the specific names for various forms that this condition takes: Aret. *SD.* iv.12.1.2-3. For further insistence on its movement throughout the body: ἢν αὐξηθὲν τὸ κακὸν ἅπασι ἐπιφοιτῇ ('if the evil increases, it travels to every part', Aret. *SD.* iv.12.1.6-7).

[10] Aret. *SD.* iv.12.1.7-2.1: ἀρχὴ δὲ νεῦρα, τὰ δεσμὰ τῶν ἄθρων, καὶ ὁκόσα ἐξ ὀστέων πέφυκε καὶ ἐν ὀστέοισι ἐμφύνει.

[11] Aret. *SD.* iv.12.3.1-2.

Aretaios of Kappodokia

touch or wound' (ἀναίσθητον ψαύσιος καὶ τρώσιος, iv.12.3.3). This is because 'pain [arises] in rough perception' (ἄλγος γὰρ τρηχείᾳ ἐν αἰσθήσει), and 'that which is densely-structured is not roughened and does not feel pain because of this' (τὸ δὲ πυκινὸν ἀτρήχυντον, διὰ τόδε καὶ ἄπονον, iv.12.3.4–5). In contrast, that which is 'finely-structured is highly perceptive' (τὸ δὲ ἀραιὸν εὐαίσθητον) and, as a result, is 'roughened by wounds' (τρηχύνεται τρώματι, iv.12.3.5–6). Those parts of the body which are dense perceive in a different way since they are affected by types of internal change: 'the densely-structured parts live by an innate heat and perceive by this heat' (τὰ πυκινὰ ζῇ ἐμφύτῳ θέρμῃ καὶ αἴσθεται τῇδε τῇ θέρμῃ, iv.12.3.6–7). The delineation of these different tropes of pain causation looks towards Classical and earlier models of the structure and *phusis* of the body, particularly those developed in the Aristotelian and Hippokratic models of bodily sensation, generation, and health:

> εἰ μὲν οὐσιώδης ἡ δρῶσα αἰτίη ἔοι, οἷον ἡ μάχαιρα ἢ λίθος, τὸ οὐσιῶδες τοῦ πάσχοντος οὐκ ἀλγέει· πυκινὸν γὰρ τὴν φυήν. ἢν δὲ τῆς ἐμφύτου θέρμης δυσκρασίη λάβηται, αἰσθήσιος γίγνεται τροπή. τοῦτο ὧν ἐξ ἑωυτέης πονέει ἡ θέρμη, ἐκ τῆς κατὰ αἴσθησιν ἔσωθεν ἐγείρεται ὤσιος· φύσιος δὲ τῆς ἐς μέζω ἢ περιουσίης τὰ ἄλγεα.

> If the active cause might be substantial, such as either a sword or a stone, it does not pain the substance of the affected part because it is, by nature, densely-structured. But if *duskrasia* might seize the innate heat, a change in perception occurs. In this instance, the heat pains from itself; it is roused from within by the pressure on the sense. The pains then are from nature's being increased, or a redundancy of these.

Aret. *SD.* iv.12.3.7–4.4

The distinction between that which is densely- and that which is finely-structured points to a larger dichotomy between the ways in which different parts of the body perceive. The contrast between the 'finely-structured' (τό ἀραιόν) and that which is 'densely-structured' (τό πυκινόν) figures Aretaios' interest in pain in terms of philosophical debates about the formation and nature of matter, linking the perception of pain with the ways in which matter or *ousia* is structured in the body. The choice of τραχύς to describe the notion of pain gestures towards a number of philosophical discussions of the subject of painful perception. According to Diogenes Laertios, Aristippos, the fourth century Cyrenaic philosopher, likened the sensation of pain to a 'rough movement' (τραχεῖα κίνησις) within the body; the metaphor appears, moreover, to have been commonplace in a number of Hellenistic and later philosophical schools.[12] But it is also linked with broader discussions of sense perception in both Archaic and Classical philosophy. *Trakheia* implies a sense of violent movement or alteration within the body and, as such, it is immediately reminiscent of the discussion of perception in Plato's *Timaios*, where pain is linked to those perceptual processes that are overwhelming and violent.[13] The metaphor of rough perception is also familiar from pre-Socratic debates about sensory perception. According to Theophrastos' *On Sense Perception*, Demokritos held that the relative 'roughness' and 'smoothness' of sensory objects influence the ways in which painful or pleasurable perception arises.[14] It may be that Aretaios' use of τραχύς reflects little more than a sense of philosophical gesturing, but it does help to embed his vision of pain in scientific discussions about the nature of perception.

Aretaios' reference to 'innate heat' also directs his readers to one of the more enigmatic concepts in Greek medical and philosophical theory. The notion can be traced, at least, to references in pre-Socratic elemental philosophy.[15] It is, as is generally understood, also a fundamental aspect of Aristotelian and Hippokratic physiology. In both contexts, it is linked to the processes of nutrition and the generation of living animals.[16] A useful piece of evidence concerning the nature

---

[12] See, e.g., Aristippos, Frag. 197A (Mannebach). For Khrysippos: Frag. 411 (Usener). Cf. Gal. *PHP.* v.636–7K. For the connections, see Tsouna (1998), 9–10.

[13] Pl. *Ti.* 64d on violent and overwhelming change and perception.

[14] Thphr. *Sens.* 63–4 (= T. 135 DK) ; see 65.2, 66.11, 67.3, 67.9, and 73.3 (= T. 135 DK) for the discussion of Demokritos' views of roughness among different sensory objects and their impact on painful or pleasant perception.

[15] It is, of course, a common association to link heat, broadly conceived, with life: Parmenides associated life and death with the presence or absence of heat: Solmsen (1957), 19–20. For its association with Stoic thought: Gal. *Nat. Fac.* ii.88–92K (= Frag. 410 *SVF*).

[16] For references to the importance of heat in the body, especially in the bloodstream, in Hippokratic physiology, see Hp. *Carn.* 2–3 and 6; cf. also, *Nat. Hom.* 12. For the reference to the 'innate heat' explicitly as a cause of disease within the body: Hp. *Aph.* i.14. For the interaction of this quality with *pneuma* throughout Hippokrates: Frixione (2013). Aristotle's treatment is spread across a number of works, e.g. *Juv.* 469b1–20, with other references at *PA.* 650a–b and *de An.* 416b28–9. At *GA.* 766a16–b13, he suggests that the innate heat is fundamental to generation and nutrition and the continued existence of physiological matter. According to some scholars, he is committed to the idea that the vital heat plays an important role in the process of sensory perception. For discussion of this line of thought in Aristotle, see Solmsen (1957), Studtmann (2004), Frixione (2013), and Kleywegt (1984).

of vital heat might be taken from Galen's writings. Galen claims, at *Natural Faculties* ii.89K, that the innate heat is intricately linked with the individual's 'vital soul'. As such, its maintenance is fundamental to continuing existence, good health, and other areas of human activity; Galen explicitly attributes this notion of the vital heat to earlier Stoic thinkers, especially Khrysippos, but also claims that the Stoics adopted this idea from Aristotle and Hippokrates.[17] Those accounts do not appear to link innate heat explicitly with the process of perception, but they do see it as something fundamental to the production and continuing good functioning of the body. Aretaios appears to be operating within the boundaries of a particularly Aristotelian and Hippokratic method of thinking about the body's formation and continued functioning. One immediate consequence of this connection is its role in therapeutic activity, where it is often connected with *pneuma*. In his treatment of pleurisy, for instance, dissipation of *pneuma* and the body's heat appears to reduce the sensations of pain in patients.[18]

There are several conclusions to draw from Aretaios' speculation about arthritis. Aretaios lays claim to a particular philosophical and medical tradition. In the language of *trakheia*, he not only adopts philosophical models for conceiving pain, but adapts them to suit a medicalized understanding of sensation and pain. In doing so, he aligns himself closely with an Aristotelian and Hippokratic model of the body in which pain is linked to external causes, but also to shifts in the body's humoral nature and innate heat. Secondly, his interest in the way in which pain arises in this specific context links the emergence of pain to elemental structures of the body. In so doing, Aretaios develops an understanding of pain as connected with the body's *phusis*. At this level, pain has little to do with individual pain perception, or the idiosyncratic symptoms of the ill or pained body, or the broader emotional impact of pain on the individual.

---

[17] For the discussion in Galen: Gal. *Nat. Fac.* ii.88–92K (= Khrysippos, Frag. 410 *SVF*), where he attributes to it a role in nutrition, generation, and the coalescence of matter. See also Gal. *MM.* x.636K on innate heat and its connection with the heart.

[18] Aret. *CA.* v.10.2.1–6. See also the case of satyriasis: Aret. *CA.* vi.11. For the need to maintain the appropriate balance of *pneuma*: Wellmann (1895b), 137.

2. PAIN SYMPTOMS AND THEIR CATEGORIZATION

In this section, I turn to Aretaios' classification and organization of the various pain symptoms that the body feels during illness. I showed above that Aretaios envisages pain as a general phenomenon embedded in the *phusis* of the body; in this discussion, I investigate the ways in which he nuances various pain sensations and symptoms and how these symptoms are narrated or described in a clinical and diagnostic context. Across his four works, Aretaios repeatedly returns to the classification of diseases or conditions according to the particular concatenation of different symptoms (*ta patheia* or *ta pathēmata*) perceived by the patients. The classification and organization of symptoms plays a critical part in Aretaios' project, allowing conditions to be recognized and treated by doctors. The nuances of that process are particularly revealing because they constitute the moment at which Aretaios constructs the interaction between patients' felt perceptions, descriptions of pain, and his categorical and diagnostic aims.

Aretaios repeatedly uses the language of 'form' or 'type' (*eidos*) to designate the different diseases and conditions, symptoms, and forms of therapy.[19] In terms of the sensation of pain, he adopts three interlinked strategies which graph the *eidos* (or *eidea*) of the *aisthēsis* the patient reports in terms of its temporal qualities (short, intermittent, chronic, or acute), its intensity (bearable, intense, or sharp), and, occasionally, its quality (dull, pricking, or pulsing).[20] This process of classification is especially associated with the Hippokratic *Epidemics* and *Prorrhetics,* where *eidos* and its cognate forms repeatedly indicate the variety of different diseases, particular subcategories of larger groups of diseases, and the multitude of symptoms with which the

---

[19] For the use of 'form(s)' in relation to general symptoms, see, e.g., SA. i.7.5.8 (τάδε... εἴδεα, 'these... forms') and ii.2.9.6 (τόδε τὸ εἶδος τῆς ἀγωγῆς, 'this is the form of the movement'). For more specific references to *eidos* in relation to conditions (*nosēmata*), see SA. ii.3.5.1, SD. iv.13.8.2–3, and CA. v.praef.4. For the plethora of forms that might exist in specific instances of pain, see the discussion of headache, which has 'thousands of forms' (ἰδέαι δὲ μυρίαι, SD. iii.2.1.4–5), or the case of liver complaints, where the 'form of pain is variegated and diverse' (πόνου ἰδέη ποικίλη καὶ παντοίη, SA. ii.7.3.4–5).

[20] For the division between acute and chronic conditions in ancient medicine: Laskaris (2002); Drabkin (1950) is also informative about the important authors Soranos and Caelius Aurelianus, who also use this temporal division.

patient might present to the medical practitioner.[21] Aretaios takes up a familiar language to authorize his project of nosological cataloguing and, in so doing, locates his text within a tradition of scientific writing which seeks to order logically and to structure the possible symptoms and perceptions of the ill individual.

For all its familiarity with a Hippokratic heritage, however, Aretaios' classificatory and explanatory system is far more complex than that inherited from the pre-Hellenistic period. His methods and assumptions for delineating different symptoms have been heavily influenced by the anatomical work of Erasistratos and Herophilos. Aretaios' explanations may start from Hippokratic ideas or symptoms, but he elaborates them in ways that were impossible before the anatomical revolution. The variation in the forms of symptoms throughout the ill body presents the doctor with a variety of diagnostic and therapeutic possibilities; navigating those possibilities to ensure the proper recognition of the condition and the selection of the appropriate therapeutic path is central to the doctor's skill. As we shall see, this can only be accomplished through an assumption of the relationship between the body's inner structure, its influence on the ways in which pain is manifested in certain areas, and their connection with the nature of particular conditions.

Embedded in this process of categorization is his interest in the different ways of describing or naming particular sensations. Aretaios combines different types of names or descriptions for pain drawn from different cultural contexts. These metaphors and descriptive terms include forms that are so general as to be considered part of everyday language: pain is 'dull' (νωθής), 'strong' (καρτερός), or 'sharp' (ὀξύς); patients feel as though they had been 'struck by a club'.[22] Much of this language is traceable across different literary and epigraphic contexts from a wide range of periods. Importantly,

---

[21] Hp. *Epid.* i.2.9.29, 2.9.72, ii.1.4.5, iii.3.12.1. Types of diseases: Hp. *Prorrh.* ii.1.11, 2.11, 11.9, 11.14, 24.2. For further discussion of categorization through forms of *eidos* or *ideē* in Hippokrates, see Gillespie (1912), 179–203.

[22] For νωθής: *SD*. iii.13.6.3 (although there are many occasions when it is not applied to pain such as, e.g., *CA*. v.2.14.6). πόνοι καρτεροί: *SA*. i.6.7.5, 7.4.5–6. ὀδύνη καρτερή: *SA*. ii.7.3.9; perhaps 'strong' is used to contrast the use of βαρύτατος at *SA*. ii.7.3.7. ἐπιπόνος: *SA*. i.6.1.1, *SD*. iii.1.1.5, 4.2.3, iv.2.1.7, *CA*. vi.8.6.2, and *CD*. vii.4.1.2. ὀξύς: *SA*. i.7.2.9, ii.5.1.2–3, 12.4.3, *SD*. iv.4.5.6 (ἄλγος ὀξύ), and *CA*. vi.9.1.4. For the simile of being beaten with a club, see *SD*. iii.2.2.9–10: ὡσπερεί τινος πατάξαντος ξύλῳ ('just as when someone is beaten with a club').

this linguistic register is combined with terminology and metaphors which are traceable primarily in medical literature and appear to operate as formal technical terms for specific types of sensation. The various combinations of these terms help to map out shifts in the forms of pain and, in due course, the conditions of the internal body. They also return us directly to the ways in which the pained body feels and how medical knowledge and understanding might emerge in the clinical encounter. It substantiates a way of viewing and talking about the *aisthēsis* of pain which combines different linguistic registers and which links the understanding of anatomy to the use of formal terminology for pain. In short, it is this combination of language that represents a way of understanding pain through the combined efforts of doctor and patient.

On a number of occasions, pain is simply described as present through the ubiquitous formula 'with pain' or the straightforward statement that pain arises in a particular condition.[23] On a number of occasions this is further nuanced by the suggestion that it occurs in certain conditions and not in others or that it is circumscribed to particular areas of the body. Perhaps ironically, the absence and presence of pain are among the more telling diagnostic distinctions that Aretaios draws. Arguably, one reason for this is that understanding the presence of pain or its absence within the body entails attending closely to what patients report or claim to feel. Indeed, the relationship between being pained and not feeling pain can only emerge after a considerable degree of physical examination and/or close questioning of the pained individual. In this context, pain's presence or absence becomes explicitly revelatory about the conditions of the body because of the link between anatomical theory and patients' reportage.

In pneumonia, for instance, Aretaios claims that the condition is associated with 'painlessness, if the lung, alone, is inflamed' (ἀπονίη, ἢν μοῦνος φλεγμήνῃ πνεύμων, SA. ii.1.2.5–6). The use of the ἐάν and subjunctive figures an 'if x, then y' formula and immediately stresses the way in which pain attests to the spread of the condition into more sensitive areas of the body. As Aretaios goes on, he points out that as soon as the inflammation encroaches on more sensitive parts of the

---

[23] See, e.g., the discussion of the diseases of the bladder at Aret. SD. iv.4.8.2–3 or of epilepsy at SD. iii.4.1.4, or the repeated references to pain in the discussion of *kephalaia*: SD. iii.2.1.1–5.

body, then pain is felt immediately. The painlessness of the lungs is, furthermore, determined by their anatomical structure: they do not feel pain because they have a particular texture, small nerves, rough arteries, and no muscles.[24] Painlessness, here, appears to be a quality that requires considerable discussion with the patient in order to verify the boundaries and nature of pain perception, but is ultimately explained in terms of the physical anatomy of the body.

The presence of pain in specific locations also reveals the extent or existence of a particular disease. In the evacuation of blood, for instance, it is the perception of pain that indicates the areas from which blood is being emitted. If evacuated from the artery in the throat, the blood will be fluid, it will be brought up with a cough, and there will be 'a perception of pain as well, where the windpipe is, either just above or below it',[25] while there will be heaviness in the chest and 'freedom from pain' (ἀπονία) in that area. As he goes further into the elaboration of this condition, he stresses that 'if one brings up blood from the thorax, the pain, [stretching] through the chest to the front indicates the damaged part' (ἢν δὲ ἀπὸ θώρηκος ἐπανίῃ, ἐς τὸ πρόσθεν κατὰ τὸ στέρνον πόνος διασημαίνει τοῦ ἐρρωγότος μέρεος, SA. ii.2.16.1–2). Aretaios' one-line description resonates with the issues which are at stake in locating pain precisely within the geography of the body. Here, it is the reach of pain as far as the sternum which 'indicates' the ruptured or affected part. The choice of 'indicate' (διασημαίνει) figures the concern with the location of pain, with its movement through the spaces of the body, in terms of diagnostic semantics: pain, like other symptoms, is important because it has the capacity to reveal to the external viewer the nature and condition of that which is hidden from sight; the movement of pain through the body must be precisely mapped in order to help categorize conditions—different parts of the body are susceptible to pain under different contexts—and to indicate which parts of the body are

---

[24] Aret. SA. ii.1.2.6–9: ἄπονος γὰρ ἡ φύσις αὐτέου· μανὸς μὲν γὰρ τὴν οὐσίην, εἰρίοισιν ἴκελος· ἀρτηρίαι δὲ διελήλανται τρηχεῖαι, χονδρώδεες, καὶ αἴδε ἄπονοι· μύες δὲ οὐδαμῇ, σμικρὰ δὲ νεῦρα, λεπτά, ἐς κίνησιν ἐπίκαιρα· ἥδε τῆς ἀπονίης αὐτὴ ἡ αἰτίη. ('their nature is to be painless, because they are loose-textured in terms of substance, like wool; but rough arteries, cartilaginous ones, are extended throughout them, and these particular arteries do not feel pain; there are no muscles, and the nerves are small and fine, appropriate for movement. This fact is the cause of their painlessness.').

[25] Aret. SA. ii.2.15.3–4: αἴσθησις δὲ καὶ πόνου, ἔνθα ὁ βρόγχος, σμικρόν τι νέρθεν ἢ ὕπερθεν.

affected. Understanding the intricacies of the body's internal condition through pain's revelatory capacity requires navigating this complex oscillation between where pain is felt and where it is absent. It requires an exacting interest in where the patient reports to feel pain or where they note its absence.

If the distinction between those parts of the body which feel pain and those which do not is diagnostically revealing, so too is the distinction between differing degrees of pain. Graphing the various intensities of pain sensation helps to differentiate between subsets of particular conditions and situations in which different types of conditions are combined. In many cases, distinctions between those pains which are 'mild' or 'bearable' and those which are more difficult to handle mark a shift in the nature of the condition that the patient is suffering from. In a historical context in which scientific and instrument-based methods for tracking the progression of disease are lacking, differentiating between these modes of pain perception provides one means for mapping the evolution, intensification, and transformation of disease within the body.[26]

This diagnostic strategy is especially on show in Aretaios' discussion of ulcers near the tonsils. There are, according to the author, two broad types of inflammation related to ulcers. They are accompanied by differing pain perceptions: mild ulcers are characterized by similarly mild experiences and occur largely 'without pain' (ἀνώδυνα). In more problematic cases, pain arises 'from the veins, just as in a carbuncle' (πόνος φλεβῶν, ὡς ἐπ' ἄνθρακος, SA. i.9.1.8). In a third case—the most deadly form of ulcer, known either as Egyptian or Syrian ulcers—'there is a pitiable form of death, accompanied by sharp and hot pain, as in a carbuncle' (τρόπος δὲ θανάτου οἴκτιστος· πόνος μὲν δριμὺς καὶ θερμός, ὡς ἐπ' ἄνθρακος, i.9.5.1–2). Aretaios' explanatory model charts the increasing seriousness of the condition in terms of the evolving nature of pain perception; it maps that alteration onto shifts in the nature of language, moving from the very general and banal description 'without pain' to more technical medical terminology.[27] The way in which pain symptoms are expressed maps

---

[26] The bibliography on modern pain measurement is exhaustive; for a brief introduction to the general issues and the main problems, see the essays in Aydede (2005), Breivik et al. (2008), and Kumar and Tripathi (2014). For the McGill pain register, see Melzack (1975).

[27] For the connection between pain and the veins, see the treatment of pain at Hp. *Genit.* 55.13; further connections at *Genit.* 15.30, 44.14, and 48.13; αἱ φλέβες

the seriousness of the disease, perhaps giving the doctor clues to diagnosis of the particular condition the patient presents with; the potential of the patient to recover from, and the specific nature of, their condition are mapped onto escalating perceptions and shifts in the descriptions of pain.

In the case of pleurisy, which is 'accompanied by acute pain' (πόνος ὀξύς, SA. i.10.2.1) under the clavicles in the particular membrane located there, Aretaios' approach involves a number of different interpretive strategies. In certain circumstances, the pain can extend as far as the back: 'the pain' (ἡ ὀδύνη) 'is stretched along the whole of the connection of the membrane to the shoulders and the collarbone, and in some cases even to the back and the shoulder blade' (ἀποτέταται... ἄχρι τῆς ἁπάσης ξυναφείης τοῦ ὑμένος ἐς ὤμους καὶ κληῖδας, μετεξετέροισι δὲ καὶ ἐς νῶτα καὶ ἐς ὠμοπλάτην, i.10.2.4–6); 'earlier doctors called this dorsal pleurisy' (τὴν νωτιαίην τὴν πλευρῖτιν ἐκάλεον οἱ πρόσθεν). As the condition worsens, however, it becomes empyema, which 'is indicated' (ἐνδείκνυται) by rigors and 'pulsing pains' (πόνοι νυγματώδεες, i.10.5.2). This description of pain is built on a technical term for a 'pulsing pain'; indeed, the term is absent from non-medical contexts in earlier literature. It is, however, widely used by contemporary medical writers in association with various pain perceptions. Soranos' *Fractures* and *On the Diseases of Women* use the term to indicate forms of pain;[28] Galen refers explicitly to the pain associated with inflammation as *nugmatōdēs*. According to *On Affected Parts*, 'the pain of pleurisy is called pulsing by almost all the doctors' (τὸ τῆς πλευρίτιδος ἄλγημα νυγματῶδες εἶναι σχεδὸν ἅπασι τοῖς ἰατροῖς ὡμολόγηται, Gal. *Loc. Aff.* viii.86K). In *On the Composition of the Art of Medicine*, he elaborates more fully on the experience of pleurisy: in this condition, 'man feels pain, since he suffers from inflammation. And the form of the pain is pulsing' (ἀλγεῖ μὲν οὖν ὁ ἄνθρωπος, ὅτι φλεγμονὴ τὸ πάθος. ἡ δὲ ἰδέα τῆς ὀδύνης ἐστὶ νυγματώδης, Gal. *CAM* i.274K).[29] Galen's assumptions about the form of pain in

---

πεπονήκασιν ('the veins are pained') at Hp. *Nat. Hom.* 14.16. For Hippokratic connections between warmth and pain, see the use of θέρμη and πόνος at *Genit.* 44.14 and 48.13.

[28] Sor. *Fract.* xv.1.4, xvii.1.3 for the discussion of ἄλγημα, and xviii.1.3 with πόνος; cf. Sor. *Gyn.* iii.37.1.5.

[29] Pulsating pain as distinct from heavy pain: Gal. *Loc. Aff.* viii.108K: ὁ δὲ νυγματώδης, φησὶ, πόνος τοῦ βάθους ἐστίν· οὐκ ὀρθῶς· ὑμένος γάρ ἐστιν, οὐ βάθους ἴδιος ('the pulsing pain, they say, is a deep pain. This is not right. For the specific

cases of inflammation are linked with assertions about the nature of the particular organ affected. The form of this pain is defined by the substance of the particular organ: 'the form of the pain is pulsing, since the substance of the affected part is membranous' (ἡ δὲ ἰδέα τῆς ὀδύνης ἐστὶ νυγματώδης, ὅτι καὶ ἡ οὐσία τοῦ πεπονθότος ἐστὶν ὑμενώδης, CAM. i.274K). Aretaios, then, chooses not only a term seeded within the medical discussions of this condition, but also one whose use is predicated on the anatomical knowledge of those who use it.

Aretaios and Galen both substantiate their references to the pulsing pain on medical tradition, or at least, widespread medical practice. Importantly for this context, it plays a key role in shaping how different pain experiences might indicate internal conditions and how the leap between the sensory perception and diagnostic recognition is made. The use of *endeiknumi* by Aretaios stresses the importance of sign-based inference in his diagnosis of conditions from their apparent symptoms.[30] Ostensibly, Aretaios' discussion does little more than flag the issue through the use of the loaded term, but it taps into the intellectual work that stands behind the connection between pulsing pains (and other symptoms) and the broader condition indicated by them. That connection is built upon the assumed (or at least unexplained) anatomical principle that the membranous elements of the body must necessarily experience a certain form of painful symptom.

Aretaios' use of *endeixis* links his project with the explanatory techniques of what we might call 'locative diagnosis'. That method of interpretation was predicated on the way in which certain conditions and symptoms manifest themselves in different areas of the body; it was assumed that certain symptoms could be particular to

---

location is the membrane, not the deep [tissue]'), and *De. Cris.* ix.554K: εἰ τύχοι ἐπὶ πλευρίτιδος εἴς τε τὸ νυγματῶδες ἄλγημα τῆς πλευρᾶς ('if it leads, in the case of pleuretics, to a pulsing pain in the pleura').

[30] Kudlien (1991a) and Barnes (1991) on *endeixis*. Throughout Galen's work, at least, it is particularly associated with the capacity of the 'form' to indicate certain treatments; it is also connected with loaded terms such as 'clearly' (*saphōs*) or 'vividly' (*enargōs*) and refers to those things which are thought to provide an indication of those things which are 'unclear' or 'not apparent' (*adēla*). On *adēla* as part of the scientific vocabulary, see Hankinson (1995), 60–83. For its place in Hellenistic philosophy: Frede (1982), 4–5; see also the chapters in Brunschwig, Burnyeat, and Schofield (1982), esp. Burnyeat (1982).

locations within the body (*idiopathic conditions*); that different areas of the body could suffer different conditions or display different symptoms either as a result of differing conditions or in sympathy with primarily affected areas (*sympathic conditions*); and that symptoms and conditions could spread to various areas within the body. This form of diagnosis is commonly associated with works such as Arkhigenes' *On Affected Parts* and Galen's later work of the same title, where the authors outline the relationship between the affected parts of the body, the reported or observed symptoms, and conditions. Galen's *On Affected Parts*, at least, linked this approach to the body and its diagnosis with the anatomical work of Erasistratos.

Importantly for the purposes of this discussion, metaphors and descriptions of the spatial qualities of various symptoms become particularly telling. Aretaios' description of pleurisy traces the movement of pain throughout the spaces of the body, charting its trajectory through an internal corporeal geography. The metaphors of movement and space used in this context appear repeatedly throughout his texts. Prepositions of limit and extent of movement are habitually used to modify different symptoms: ἄχρι ('up to') and εἰς ('to', 'into') map out where pain occurs within the body; at the same time, verbs of movement are given increased significance. The use of ἀποτέταται in the paragraph above is just one example. This and other verbs characterize the way Aretaios (and others after him) conceptualize what is significant about pain sensation. We may choose, for instance, to see the significance of Aretaios' use of the eloquent metaphor διᾴσσειν ('to dart') through its connection with tragedy, especially Sophokles' *Women of Trakhis*, where the term is used to describe the way pains of madness 'dart' through Herakles' flank. Yet for all its metaphorical or tragic connotations, it seems to draw its significance from its spatial reference. Taken together, these metaphors subsume the felt sensation of pain into the way in which doctors understand the internal geography of the body.[31]

Aretaios' texts map the internal structures of the body and their perceptions of pain for diagnosis. This spatial concern links the interest in pain perception, its reportage, and anatomy. It connects an attentiveness to the *aisthēsis* of pain with an abiding interest in the anatomical structure of the *sōma*: trying to map the movement of pain through the body emphasizes the importance of understanding

---

[31] Soph. *Tr.* 1083. cf. Hp. *Morb.* i.22. *SA.* ii.6.5.3, 4.8.3 for Aretaios' use of the term.

not only how the different parts of the body intersect, but also how and why different parts of the body are susceptible in different ways to the perception of pain. This anatomical tenor to the interest in pain is, then, quite a telling factor in how descriptions and reportage of pain symptoms might be understood within Aretaios' medical practice. By incorporating the symptoms that patients feel and their reportage of their presence, intensity, and nature into anatomical explanations of the body, Aretaios shapes the way in which patients and doctors might understand disease and the experience of pain. Secondly, by combining quotidian language with increasingly technical terms and understanding, a type of relationship emerges. Aretaios' texts construct (or, at least, aim at constructing) a way of speaking between doctor and patient. This is not about subjective patient-based language for the description of pain, but rather about a type of combined language developed between patient and doctor for the effective explanation and recognition of pain symptoms and the conditions they indicate.

3. DEVELOPING MODELS OF EXPERIENCE

So far, in this chapter, I have been tracking the way in which pain is conceptualized with increasing specificity as a sensory or felt phenomenon. I have shown how Aretaios connects diagnosis to the ways in which pain might be described and to his understanding of the body's anatomy. In this section, I focus more on the emotional framework for understanding pain sensation. How does sensory perception intersect with more confronting affective and distressing elements of the doctor–patient relationship and the experience of pain that develops in that context? Turning to the question of experience involves investigating the psychological and emotional impact of pain on the individual and how that impact is navigated by patients and those around them. It is at this point that I will return explicitly to the questions raised by modern medical anthropology.[32] Aretaios represents pain as a phenomenon which influences deeply the psychological and emotional state of the individual and shapes how they

---

[32] See Chapter 1 (text to nn. 9–12).

are seen by others: pain stands at the heart of Aretaios' conception of doctor-patient rapport and how the broader community engages with those who suffer pain. Pain, on this reading, ceases to be an objective 'thing', but emerges as a psychosomatic and interpersonal experience.

The most obvious place to begin this discussion is the opening to Aretaios' *On the Causes and Signs of Chronic Diseases*. Aretaios' poignant *prooimion* reverberates with ideas about the centrality of pain to medical practice, shaping the experiences of the patient and the therapeutic process itself. He begins with a nod in the direction of the Hippokratic sentiment that life is short and the art is long: 'the pain of chronic diseases is great, the period of deterioration long, and recovery uncertain' (χρονίων νούσων πόνος μὲν πουλύς, χρόνος δὲ μακρὸς ξυντήξιος, καὶ ἀβέβαιος ἡ ἄλθεξις, SD. iii.1.1.1–2). For all its vague recollection of the famous Hippokratic *bon mot*, this depressingly macabre statement transforms the concern of the Hippokratic text from medicine to pain itself.[33] As the passage continues, pain emerges as a defining quality of the elongated process of therapy:

ἢ γὰρ οὐδ' ἐξηλάθησαν ἐς τὸ ξύμπαν, ἢ ἐπὶ σμικρῇ ἁμαρτωλῇ παλινδρομέουσι αἱ νοῦσοι. οὔτε γὰρ ἀτρεμέειν οἱ νοσέοντες τολμέουσι ἐς τέλος· ἀτὰρ ἠδὲ ἁμαρτάνουσι ἐν τῇσι μακρῇσι διαίτῃσι, κἢν ἀτρεμέωσι. ἢν δὲ καὶ πόνος ἔῃ ἐπιπόνου ἰήσιος, δίψης, λιμοῦ, φαρμάκων πικρῶν, καὶ ὀδυνέων, ἢ τομῆς, ἢ καύσιος, ὧνπερ ἐστὶ ἐν τῇσι δολιχῇσι νούσοισι χρέος, ὑποδιδρήσκουσι οἱ κάμνοντες ὡς θανάτου δῆθεν αὐτέου ὀρεγόμενοι. ἔνθα δὴ ἀρετὴ διαείδεται ἀνδρὸς ἰητροῦ, καὶ μακροθυμίης, καὶ ποικιλίης, καὶ χάριτος ἀβλαβοῦς τῶν ἡδέων, καὶ παραιφάσιος· ἀτὰρ καὶ τὸν νοσέοντα χρὴ ἄλκιμον ἔμμεναι, καὶ ξυνίστασθαι τῷ ἰητρῷ κατὰ τοῦ νοσήματος. οὐ γὰρ τοῦ σώματος μούνου ἀπρὶξ λαβόμενον ταχὺ ἀνασμύχει τε καὶ δάπτει, ἀλλ' ἐς πολλὰ καὶ τὴν αἰσθησίην ἐκτρέπει, ἀλλὰ καὶ τὴν ψυχὴν ἐκμαίνει ἀκρασίῃ τοῦ σώματος.

Either the diseases are not driven out entirely, or they return at a slight error, because the ill either do not have the courage to persevere to

---

[33] Deichgräber (1971), 8–12, esp. 8: 'In Syntax und Stil aber ist als Vorbild sofort erkennbar *Aph*. i.1..., mit anderen Worten, der erste Satz ist geformt nach dem Muster des berühmtesten Aphorismus.' ('In syntax and style, *Aphorisms* i.1. is immediately recognizable as a model... in other words, the first clause is formed according to the model of the most famous aphorism.') For the *bon mot*, see Hp. *Aph*. i.1: ὁ βίος βραχύς, ἡ δὲ τέχνη μακρή, ὁ δὲ καιρὸς ὀξύς, ἡ δὲ πεῖρα σφαλερή, ἡ δὲ κρίσις χαλεπή ('life is short, and the art long, opportunity fleeting, experience misleading, judgement difficult').

the end or, if they do persevere, they make errors over the course of a long regimen. And if there is also pain from an extremely painful remedy—from thirst, hunger, bitter and painful medicines, surgery, or cauterization—of the sort which is sometimes necessary in difficult diseases, the patients run off, since they really prefer death itself. In these circumstances, the virtue of the medical man is revealed, from his great-spiritedness, his variety [in treatment], his indulgence of pleasant things which are not damaging, and his encouragement. But the patient also needs to be courageous, and to stand with the physician against the disease. For, when it takes a firm hold, it quickly wastes and corrodes not only the body, and frequently disorders the sense perception as well, and even deranges the soul by the disorder of the body.

Aret. *SD*. iii.1.1.2–2.7

The importance of pain is flagged by the continued repetition of the language of *ponos* and *odunē*; pain emerges not only as a phenomenon which ensues from the condition itself, but also as one that is created by the therapeutic process and continues to influence the doctor–patient relationship throughout their interaction: 'the virtue' ($ἀρετή$) of the doctor lies in his 'great-spiritedness' ($μακροθυμίης$), his ability to adopt strategies to alleviate or accommodate that which is painful, and in having the grace to counter the *ponos* of some treatments with that which is *hēdus*. Aretaios' presentation of the doctor's position in relation to the pained body casts him as an almost superordinate figure with the power to alleviate pain and transform it into pleasure. Despite this superlative representation of the doctor, however, he and the patient are connected by their common interests. If pain underpins how the doctor should treat the patient, so too it underlines the quality of heroic bravery (figured, here, in the use of $ἄλκιμον$) which patients need to demonstrate;[34] the prefix $σύν$ to modify $ἵστημι$ further emphasizes the joint effort in confronting the *nosos*. Heroic language, in this context, elevates the clinical encounter with disease to an epic level—both the patient and doctor take on similar, and complementary, heroic qualities.

The account of the vagaries and vicissitudes of the therapeutic process moves beyond thinking about *nosos* solely in terms of

---

[34] For $ἄλκιμος$ as a heroic quality, see, e.g., Hom. *Il*. 5.529 (a stout heart as a heroic quality); or 6.437 (stout-hearted, son of Tydeus). For other Homeric allusions in the passage: $διαείδεται$ at *Il*. 13.277.

definitional categories and concatenations of symptoms. Pain is conceptualized as part of the elongated process of management; the patient and doctor jointly and heroically manage the individual's capacity to cope; the intricate interpersonal relationship allows that process to run smoothly. Aretaios moves, then, from a concept of pain and disease as the biological phenomenon to a vision of illness experience as the patient's and doctor's combined negotiation of a biological reality.[35] That shift is perhaps most clearly developed in the final lines of Aretaios' *prooimion*, where he suggests that disease simultaneously takes hold of the body and the mind. The verbs *lambanein* and *daptein* underscore disease's impact on the body and the *psukhē*: the use of 'disorder' (ἀκρασίη) recalls immediately the mind's dependence on the humoral balance within living organisms developed in Hippokratic humoral theory. However, for all its humoral connotations, it also carries with it the more general meaning of disorder. Disease impacts on the body (its sensory functions and structure), undermining the psychological and emotional stability of the individual.

At this point, the emotional ramifications for the patient's experience of disease are explicitly connected with the nature of chronic diseases, but they also resonate throughout Aretaios' entire project. Many of the emotional complexities that are elaborated in this *prooimion* are writ large in his treatment of the evacuation of blood, discussed at On the Causes and Signs of Acute Diseases ii.2. I have already shown that this condition—which oscillated between painless and painful situations—was particularly telling for how Aretaios understood the relationship between pain and anatomy. What interests me here is the way in which Aretaios takes this distinction a step further by theorizing the connection between pain, painlessness, and the emotional experience of disease. He begins by elaborating a paradoxical emotional reaction to evacuating blood:

θῶμα δὲ μέγα τόδε. ἐπὶ γὰρ τῇ ἀπὸ πνεύμονος φορῇ μούνῃ χαλεπωτάτῃ ἐούσῃ οὐκ ἀπογιγνώσκουσι ἑωυτῶν οἱ ἄνθρωποι, κἂν ἐν τῷ ἐσχάτῳ ἔωσι. δοκέω δὲ ἔγωγε τὴν τοῦ πνεύμονος ἀπονίην αἰτίην ἔμμεναι· πόνος γὰρ κἢν σμικρὸς ἔῃ, θάνατον ὀρρωδέει, καὶ ἔστι ἐν τοῖσι πλείστοισι φοβερώτερος ἢ κακίων· ἀπονίη δὲ καὶ ἐν τοῖσι μεγάλοισι κακοῖσι ἀφοβίη θανάτου, καὶ ἔστι κακίων ἢ φοβερωτέρη.

---

[35] For this approach to illness vs disease, see Chapter 1 (text to nn. 9–12).

But this is quite amazing. In the discharge from the lungs, which alone is very dangerous, patients do not despair of their lives, even if they are in the final stages of the condition. I, at least, think that the cause of this is the absence of pain in the lungs; for pain, even if it is slight, induces fear of death, but in the majority of instances it is more fearful than evil. But, freedom from pain, even in extreme conditions, does not induce the fear of death, and is more dangerous than fearful.

Aret. SA. ii.2.18.1–7

So Aretaios alerts his readers to the paradoxical nature of the fear of death during disease. This form of the condition is most dangerous and indicates, from an external point of view, the nearness of the patient's demise, but does not have a commensurate emotional effect on the patient due to the absence of pain. The irony of the situation is brought home by the reversal of the terminology of fear and danger in the final clause of the passage. The patient's sense of hopelessness—their confrontation with their own mortality—is allied with the experience of pain and its capacity to impact on the *psukhē* of the individual. Aretaios' passage may highlight the absurdity of particular emotional reactions in this specific condition, but his reference to pain 'in the great illnesses' suggests that this situation is relevant to much of his thinking about all diseases, incorporating it into a way of conceptualizing and explaining the psychosomatic experience of illness.

Just as the relationship between pain and fear is particularly amazing, so too Aretaios describes the intricacies of patients' reactions to bringing up blood as curious. Every discharge of blood 'is followed by dejection and despondency at the rejection of life' (ἕπεται δυσθυμίη, δυσελπιστίη ἀπογνώσει τοῦ βίου, SA. ii.2.17.6–7). Reference to the quality of dejection (*dusthumia*) reminds the reader of the central role of the doctor in providing encouragement to patients and his 'great-spiritedness' discussed in his *prooimion* to On the Causes and Signs of Chronic Diseases.[36] Rather than using this term to differentiate between patient and doctor, Aretaios uses it to elaborate more exactly the common experiences of disease and death: 'for who', Aretaios asks, 'is so well placed that, when he sees himself suffering like a sacrificial victim, does not also fear death?' (τίς γὰρ οὕτως εὐσταθὴς ὡς ὁρῆν μὲν ἑωυτὸν σφαγῇ ἴκελον πεπονθότα, μὴ ὀρρωδέῃ δὲ ἀμφὶ θανάτου, ii.2.17.7–8). The reason for this fear is that 'even the greater and more stout-hearted animals, such as bulls, die very

---

[36] Aret. SD. iii.1.

quickly from loss of blood' (γὰρ καὶ τὰ μέζω τῶν ζώων καὶ τὰ ἀλκιμώτερα, ὁκοῖον οἱ ταῦροι, αἱμορραγίῃ θνῄσκουσι ὤκιστα, ii.2.17.9–11). Here, conversely, it is the bull that demonstrates 'stout-heartedness' and, even though he does so, still falls. The term σφαγῇ, which I translated as 'sacrificial victim', is particularly eloquent in this context because of its associations with ritual forms of slaughter and especially the slaughter of animals;[37] the comparison with the bull—the sacrificial animal *par excellence*—invites further reading of this condition against the framework of ritualized slaughter.[38] For all the intimations of heroic bravery and steadfastness in the patient, the possibilities of it are dramatically undercut by the comparison drawn with the sacrificial animal which will inevitably fall.

The suggestions of ritual slaughter reverberate. They help to explain patients' reactions to the *pathos* by offering clues as to how they might conceptualize or understand their experience. The sacrificial resonances also suggest where external viewers might locate such figures on the cultural landscape. Do sufferers of this condition conceptualize themselves as somehow less than human, reduced to the status of a sacrificial animal? Are others meant to view them or their condition as one which is both sacrificial and subhuman? Can this be reconciled with the vision of the patient as one who is heroic and displays the heroic virtue of 'stout-heartedness'? Is the patient caught between a heroic status and that which appears to be particularly wretched?

The use of θῶμα throughout this discussion of bringing up blood further emphasizes the importance of viewing or spectatorship in the treatment of the pained individual. On one reading, the use of *thauma* means 'this is amazing'. But it carries implications about the process of viewing: this is an amazing sight, an amazing *thauma*. The language of amazement complicates the relationship between the pain sufferer and those who engage visually with them. The way in which disease implicates the act of viewing is developed especially in the discussion of tetanus, which incorporates questions of how the

---

[37] The term is common in tragedy, especially applied to human slaughter: σφάζοντες/ σφάζειν at Ael. NA. vii.38 (= E. Frag. 857 Nauck); A. A. 1057, 1092, 1096, and 1433 (along with similar references at 209, 1278, 1389, and 1599). Cf. LSJ s.v. σφάγη.

[38] For other examples of slaughtered bulls being used to conceptualize the experience of disease: ἐσφαγμένοισι ταύροισι at Aret. SA. i.5.4.3. For further examples in relation to epilepsy, see Porter (2014), 86. For a brief, but informative, discussion of this passage, see Porter (2014), 84–5.

viewer should sympathize or feel pity for the patient. The discussion of tetanus begins by informing readers that this condition is an 'inhuman calamity' (ἐξάνθρωπος ἡ ξυμφορή). Tetanus removes the patient to a position outside of humanity. Critical scholarship has stressed that this term is unusual within the nosological tradition: if it is a neologism created by Aretaios, then its use here points to the especial impact of the experience of tetanus.[39] As the passage continues, his elaboration of the disease is framed in telling language which assimilates the experiences not only of those who are pained, but also of those who watch them:

καὶ ἀτερπὴς μὲν ἡ ὄψις, ὀδυνηρὴ δὲ καὶ τῷ ὁρέοντι θέη· ἀνήκεστον δὲ τὸ δεινόν· ἀγνωσία δὲ ὑπὸ διαστροφῆς καὶ τοῖς φιλτάτοις ἀνθρώποις. εὐχὴ δὲ τοῖσι παρεοῦσι ἡ πρόσθεν οὐχ ὁσίη, νῦν ἀγαθὴ γίγνεται, ἀπελθέμεναι τοῦ βίου τὸν κάμνοντα ἐς ἀπαλλαγὴν ξὺν τῷ ζῆν καὶ τῶν πόνων καὶ τῶν ἀτερπέων κακῶν. ἀτὰρ οὐδὲ ἰητρὸς παρεὼν ὁρέων οὔτε ἐς ζωὴν οὔτε ἐς ἀπονίην, ἀτὰρ οὐδὲ ἐς μορφὴν ἔτι ἐπαρκέει. εἰ γὰρ καὶ ἐπευθῦναι ἐθέλοι τὰ μέλη, ζῶντα ἂν διατμήξαι καὶ κατάξαι τὸν ἄνθρωπον. τοῖσι ὦν κεκρατη μένοισι οὐκέτι ἐγχειρέων ξυνάχθεται μοῦνον. ἥδε ἐστὶ τοῦ ἰητροῦ μεγάλη ξυμφορή.

The sight is unpleasant, a painful spectacle even for the one who looks on. The terrible condition is incurable. [The victim is rendered] unrecognizable to their dearest mortals by the distortions. The prayer among the attendants—which was earlier on irreverent, but is now noble—is that the patient be released from life and for release from the pains and unpleasant evils which accompany his continued existence. Indeed, the physician, although present and looking on, cannot provide help for life nor freedom from pain, not even against deformity. For if he wishes even to straighten the limbs, it is necessary to cut and break the man. With those, then, who are overcome by the condition, no longer applying his craft, he only feels distress in common with the patient. This very fact is the great misfortune of the physician.

Aret. SA. i.6.8.6–9.7

Once again, Aretaios plays on the connection between illness and death. In this context, death is represented as a prayed-for release from all that is endured by the victims of tetanus.[40] The use of *opsis*

---

[39] For the exact phrase: SA. i.6.8.5–6; cf., ἐξάνθρωπος at SD. iii.4.3.3. On the unusualness of this term, see Pigeaud (1987), 73–4. Cf. ἄκοσμον κακόν SA. ii.12.4.4.

[40] On the theme of praying for release: Porter (2014), 57–64. Patients desiring death: Aret. SA. ii.2.17.6–7, SD. iii.2.3.6–7, iv.1.9.6.5–6, and CA. vi.5.1.10–11.

and *theaomai* recalls the reference to *thauma* in the example of bringing up blood—in both instances, Aretaios presents pain as something that must be seen. If it must be seen, then that act is itself problematic: the language of spectatorship is underpinned by the distressing emotions that the viewers feel at the sight of pain. The force of *kai* (which could be translated as 'even' or 'also') in the first line ensures that the pain of the condition reverberates among those who view the patient. Aretaios' determination to bring home the point is, perhaps, also reflected in the sudden and oblique references to pleasure (the first time he uses it in the whole extant text). The concatenation of (*a*)*terpsis* and *aponiē* with *ponos* and *odunērē* stresses not only the distance between pain and pleasure in this situation, but also the connections between patient and viewer. Just as the viewer experiences 'an unpleasant sight' which is 'painful', so too are the patients' ills 'unpleasant'. Finally, the repeated references to disaster continue to construct the experience of pain: does disaster, here, mark out this event as a type of moral tragedy? *Sumphora* is certainly reminiscent of the way in which tragedy emphasizes reversals of fortunes. Either way, its application to both the patient and doctor appears to iterate, one final time, the intersection of experiences between the two figures.

One theme that has been consistent throughout this discussion concerns the ways in which the patient and doctor develop emotional connections. As has been pointed out, there are many occasions in which Aretaios expresses pity for those who feel pain or who are ill.[41] Those who suffered certain ulcers were likely to die 'a pitiable death', for instance. Similarly, there are occasions in which he clearly believes that death will offer some degree of release from the individual's experience of suffering. It is the failure to provide 'freedom from pain' (*aponia*) which is part of the great *sumphora* of the doctor. In this instance, it is notable that the doctor claims that he 'feels distress in common' (ξυνάχθεται) with the patient. What interests me in this context is the way in which the ξυν prefix reiterates the theme of commonality between patient and doctor. The implications of this connection are reinforced because the sense of distress conveyed in the terms ἄχος and ἄχθομαι are very often attributed to the patients'

---

[41] Porter (2014), 49–88 on the general theme of emotional empathy towards certain conditions in Aretaios.

experiences of their conditions.[42] Here, its use in ξυνάχθεται reiterates the common sense of distress between the patient and those around them. The level of emotional awareness which lies behind these representations of the doctor's engagement with those who feel pain speaks directly to the ways in which Aretaios conceptualizes pain's impact and its role in social relationships.

Aretaios' interest in the diagnosis and treatment of pain, then, stretches across a number of different themes in his work. He starts from a scientific and philosophical conception of pain as a phenomenon inherently linked to the body's physiology, its anatomical structure and make-up. At a second level, the felt perceptions of patients—the symptoms of pain—are also incorporated into his approach: the felt perceptions of pain are classified, organized, and explained in terms that render them meaningful to the scientific process of recognizing the internal conditions of the body. Finally, these two processes are combined in a broader vision of the patient as someone who experiences pain at a physiological and psychological level. In revealing the ways in which pain might be managed or understood within a broader context, Aretaios elaborates the ways in which pain helps to shape the relationship between patient and doctor/viewer.

---

[42] *SA.* ii.11.1.7 and ii.12.1.10; *SD.* iii.2.3.6, iii.6.11.2–3, iii.15.11.8, iv.13.19.7, and *CA.* v.2.6.3.

3

Galen

In the last chapter, I focused on the way in which pain was incorporated into medical practice by the important, but often undiscussed, figure of Aretaios of Kappodokia. In this chapter, I continue to pursue some of the issues which were raised in that discussion by turning to one of the most significant polymaths of the Imperial period—Galen of Pergamon.[1] Across his voluminous corpus, Galen develops a complex understanding of pain and its role in clinical practice: arguably, no other single author from the ancient world spends as much time elaborating a theory of pain and its role in medical practice as Galen. The approach to pain and its clinical importance which emerged from Aretaios' nosological texts is phrased in very different terms in Galen's explicitly theoretical diagnostic and didactic works. What remains constant across these two authors, however, is pain's importance in the relationships which define the clinical encounter. Galen, like Aretaios, moves from a biological conception of pain, in which it is seen as a phenomenon linked to the body's natural process of alteration and sensation, to an approach in which he is concerned with navigating the affective and social elements of pain experience. Galen's concern for pain's impact on the individual and its centrality to the dynamic relationship between doctor and patient

---

[1] On Galen's life and importance to Imperial culture: Nutton (1973), Schlange-Schöningen (2003), Boudon-Millot (2012), and Mattern (2013). Brief introductions on his life and career can be found in Nutton (2004), 222–53 and Hankinson (2008b). For Galen's own views about the importance of his practice at Rome, see *Praen.* xiv.612–13K. His status at Rome was questioned by Scarborough (1981), although there seems to be plenty of evidence to confirm the main details of Galen's opinion of his own importance. See *Praen.* xiv.606–16K for his interactions with other doctors and his own catalogues of his literary output in, e.g., *Ord. Lib. Prop.* On these works: Boudon (2000).

is particularly telling when mapped against Aretaios' approach: pain experience emerges as one of the key discursive battlegrounds of Imperial medicine.

Galen's approach to medicine was robustly aetiological. Galen's affiliation with what he saw as the rationalist sect advocated the process of seeking out the specific causes of the disease that patients presented with.[2] Three related implications emerge from this rationalist theme. As was touched on in Chapter 1, Galen's diagnostic and clinical practice was based on three levels of interpretation: the application of the rational understanding of the body developed through anatomical knowledge (*logismos*), and often enhanced by anatomical training or experience; the sensory perception of the patient's symptoms (*aisthēsis*); and, finally, the process of close questioning of, and discussion with, the patient, which elaborated past and current symptoms and their trajectory through time (*logos*).[3] These elements allowed the *aition* of a particular disease to be recognized, its future course to be foretold, and (very occasionally) for it to be successfully treated. Pain is integrated into Galen's practices at all of these diagnostic levels—it is defined by the anatomical structure of the body; it is perceived by the patient, and both they and doctors spend a considerable amount of time discussing, reporting, and naming pain sensations that might arise during illness.

Galen predicated diagnosis on anatomical knowledge and an Aristotelian approach to the definition and classification of relevant physiological, nosological, and symptomatic information. His literary output provides a large part of what Galen sees as the critical information about the body and disease which underpins the practice of medicine. Works on anatomy—*On the Usefulness of Parts* and *On Anatomical Procedures*, for example—form a type of anatomical

---

[2] Galen's connection with 'rationalist medicine' is well established: for broad descriptions of his medical philosophy, see Frede (1981), esp. 66 and (1987), 279–98, and Moraux (1981). On Galen's views of the differing medical 'sects': Gal. *Sect. Int.* i.64–6K; and on his own place within them: *Opt. Med.* i.53–63K.

[3] For his diagnostic reasoning in general: Riese (1968). For the three categories listed here: García Ballester (1981) and Barnes (1991). *Logismos*: Barnes (1991), esp. 65–6; on the application of taxonomical division to disease, see Johnston (2006), 65–80 for a discussion in relation to *On the Differences of Symptoms* and *On the Differences of Diseases*. *Aisthēsis*: Nutton (1993) and Boudon (2003b). *Logos*: Roby (2015) and Mattern (2008), 40–2 and 138–54. For a view of Galen's diagnostic and prognostic practices in connection with less 'rational' or 'empirically based' 'science': Barton (1994), 133–68, van Nuffelen (2014), and Hankinson (2005).

overview of the structure of the human body. *On the Causes of Symptoms* and *On the Differences of Symptoms*, along with the complementary works *On the Differences of Diseases* and *On the Causes of Diseases*, provide a bedrock of classificatory material and substantiate his rational understanding of the different areas of disease, symptoms, and their relationships to the anatomical structure of the body. This knowledge could then be applied in the diagnostic and practical contexts recounted in *On Affected Parts* or *On Method of Healing*. Mario Vegetti has suggested that the image of the body (and by implication Galen's vision of himself) developed in natural and physiological treatises contradicts the view which emerges from the medical treatises.[4] From the perspective of Galen's complex diagnostic practices, however, these different texts are mutually constitutive, each supporting and building on the work of others. One of the reasons the anatomical level of thinking is important is that the treatment of pain is embedded in the general truths that anatomical knowledge provided. Galen constantly negotiates between the general anatomical reality of the body and the specific individual's perception and experience. That process is bound up with how Galen conceptualizes and controls the relationship between anatomical reality, pain symptoms, and their description or narration.

This brings me to the final implication raised by Galen's approach to diagnosis, which concerns how scholars understand his relationship with patients. Galen's own view of his importance is a common theme among modern critics.[5] Galen is determined to stress his own authority over both other doctors and, in many circumstances, the patients themselves.[6] At the same time, however, the way in which

---

[4] Vegetti (1981). For refutation of this particular argument, see Singer (1997), which stresses the consistency of explanation for disease causation across different generic contexts. A brief reading of Gal. *Loc. Aff.* viii.14K or 69–70K removes any doubt that anatomico-physiological and biological texts were fundamentally relevant to diagnosis.

[5] See the various case-histories in Gal. *Praen.* for Galen's own view of his status and rise at Rome, especially the case of Eudemos: *Praen.* xiv.605–19K and 625–6K for explicit statements of his fame. For scholarly treatments of his self-aggrandizing habit, see Hankinson (2008b), 5–7, with further references to cases in *Praen.*, and Mattern (2008), 2–4, with some sensible caveats about the 'man himself'. For accounts of his time as doctor to the gladiators, see chapter 5 of Schlange-Schöningen (2003), along with, e.g., Gal. *UP.* iii.286–7K for his official position at Pergamon.

[6] Galen's case-histories and their (non-Hippocratic) objectives: Lloyd (2009). Mattern (2008), 80–91 for 'amazement' as a strategy of control and power within

he represents pain's influence on the relationship between doctor and patient suggests that a more nuanced approach is necessary. As with Aretaios, pain stands at the heart of both Galen's epistemological concerns and his sense of the evolving connection between patient and doctor. He oscillates between activities and ideas that present a positive, close affiliation and those that solidify his rational authority over the patient. He stresses, at times, the way in which perceptions reported by patients can only be understood because the doctors have experienced similar phenomena themselves; at the same time, however, he uses narrative practices to reinforce his intellectual and diagnostic superiority over patients and his discursive position against other practitioners. The patient's voice is, ultimately, incorporated into the clinical encounter on Galen's terms. Medical anthropology has attempted to revalidate subjective, personalized accounts of the body's condition and symptoms. That critical effort has been undertaken in response to the ways in which subjective patient narratives have traditionally been disempowered in relation to those of the rational, objective, and authoritative doctor. Despite his rational approach to medicine and his intense concern with his own social and discursive status, Galen's diagnostic practices do not fit into these binary categories consistently or universally. Indeed, they demand that the medical historian return to, and re-evaluate, the nuances of the categories of patient subjectivity vs medical/scientific/rational objectivity.

1. PAIN AND THE BODY

Galen's interest in anatomy and physiology formed the bedrock of his interest in pain perception and how it might be useful for health care.

clinical encounters, with Gal. *Loc. Aff.* viii.363–5K and also *Praen.* xiv.656–7K. For competing with other doctors: Gal. *MM.* x.382K, 676K, *Cris.* ix.682–3K, and *Praen.* xiv.657–61K (for the treatment of Marcus Aurelius). For the practice of dominating the patient, see the famous case of the wife of Justus: Gal. *Praen.* xiv.631–3K. For more positive relationships with the patient, see, e.g., the case of Eudemos: *Praen.* xiv.605–19K. For challenges and interaction with 'standers around', who question Galen and are (often) rival medical figures, see *e.g. Aff. Dig.* v.19K. For further discussion, see Mattern (2008), 69–88, esp. 76–83 on the agonistic context of medical practice, particularly when conducted at the bedside, and 233 nn. 19–20 and 28–9 for further references. For relationships with the patients: Mattern (2008), 145–9. For competition in anatomical contexts: Gleason (2009), esp. 86 n. 3.

Galen makes statements about how he understands pain throughout his corpus, but his approach is outlined most elaborately in *On the Causes of Symptoms* and *On the Differences of Symptoms*. In these works, Galen presents pain as a quality which is fundamental to the human body's propensity for alteration or change and its capacity for sensory perception. For my purposes, this has two immediate consequences: it develops a carefully situated relationship between disease and pain; more significantly, Galen develops a view in which pain is embedded in a consistent natural physiology in which the phenomenon is common to all bodies and dependent on the formation and structure of matter within the *sōma*.

In an important passage in *On the Causes of Symptoms,* Galen argues that pain is the perception of overwhelming change. According to *On the Causes of Symptoms* vii.115K, 'pleasure and pain occur in all senses, although clearly not in the same way'.[7] Galen expands his general contention by turning explicitly to his two great authorities, Plato and Hippokrates, who both held, he claims, that pain arises when an overwhelming or violent and contrary-to-nature experience occurs in us.[8] Pain is presented as a pastiche of Hippokratic and Platonic views, combining a sense of 'overwhelming change' in the body and its natural state. The connection is elaborated a number of times across his corpus, particularly in book 6 of his *According to the Opinions of Plato and Hippokrates*. In that text, he stresses that for pleasure or pain to occur, 'smooth' or 'rough' movements within the body must be connected to the perception of each movement.[9] Galen's choice of 'smooth or rough . . . movement' (λείαν ἢ τραχεῖαν . . . κίνησιν) immediately returns readers to the

---

[7] Gal. *Caus. Symp.* vii.115K: ἥδεσθαι δὲ καὶ ἀλγεῖν ἁπάσαις μὲν ἐγγίγνεται ταῖς αἰσθήσεσιν, οὐχ ὁμοίως δὲ ἐναργῶς.

[8] Gal. *Caus. Symp.* vii.115K. Galen's language, at this point, paraphrases Pl. *Ti.* 64d. The reference to Hippokrates is more problematic: ὁ δὲ Ἱπποκράτης ἔτι παλαιότερος ὤν, τοῖς τὴν φύσιν, ἔφη, διαλλαττομένοισι καὶ διαφθειρομένοισιν αἱ ὀδύναι γίγνονται ('and Hippokrates, who is even more ancient, said pains occur in those who are changed and corrupted in relation to nature'). There is no passage in the Hippokratic corpus that corresponds precisely to this statement.

[9] Gal. *PHP.* v.636K: οὐδ᾽ ἀρκεῖ λείαν ἢ τραχεῖαν ἐν τῷ σώματι γενέσθαι κίνησιν εἰς ἡδονῆς ἢ πόνου γένεσιν, ἀλλὰ χρὴ προσελθεῖν αἴσθησιν ἑκατέρᾳ τῶν τοιούτων κινήσεων ('it is not sufficient for a soft or rough movement to arise in the body for pain or pleasure to occur, but it is necessary to connect perception with each of the particular movements').

medico-philosophical representations of pain that I discussed in relation to Aretaios.

This particular understanding of pain is allied to Galen's theory of disease. Galen's view of disease fluctuates slightly across his corpus, although there are some oft-repeated themes in his various definitions. In the treatise *On the Differences of Symptoms*, he adopts a simultaneously structural and functional definition: 'disease is...any constitution [*diathesis*] contrary to nature by which function is harmed, primarily'.[10] For Galen, a *nosos* or a *nosēma* exists when either a constitution or an enduring state of the body has arisen which is contrary to, or has undermined, the natural structure or condition of the body or undermines the normal functioning of the body or one of its parts. The focus on both the condition of the body—that is, a situation in which the structure of the body has been changed—and the functional—when processes or activities can no longer operate normally—shapes the way that Galen approaches pain generation. In a telling passage in *On Affected Parts*, Galen tells us that it is appropriate to differentiate between two different kinds of movement within the body or its parts: 'activities' or 'functions' (*energeiai*) which occur 'from themselves' and 'passive experiences' or 'affections' (*pathē*) which denote movement caused 'from outside'.[11] This movement, Galen continues, can be defined in two ways, as either a 'metabolic alteration' (ἀλλοίωσις) or as a 'spatial transition' (φορά):[12] 'when such metabolic change results in a conditioned state' (ὅταν εἰς μόνιμον ἀφίκηται διάθεσιν ἡ ἀλλοίωσις), 'it is called a disease' (ὀνομάζεται νόσημα), for 'it is clear that there is a condition which is contrary to nature' (παρὰ φύσιν οὖσα δηλονότι διάθεσις).[13] There is a clear

---

[10] *Symp. Diff.* vii.43K. Cf. *Morb. Diff.* vi.837–8K, and *MM*. x.71–5K and 78–80K. For further discussion of the essential unity of ostensibly different definitions of disease in Galen: Singer (1997). For this definition of disease: Hankinson (2008d), 230–1. For a good introduction to the whole issue: Johnston (2006), 21–4.

[11] Gal. *Loc. Aff.* viii.32K: ἐνεργεῖν μὲν λεγομένου τοῦ τὴν κίνησιν ἔχοντος ἐξ ἑαυτοῦ, πάσχειν δὲ τοῦ τὴν κίνησιν ἔχοντος ἐξ ἑτέρου ('activity is said of a thing which has movement from itself, but affection of a thing which has movement from another source').

[12] For this sense of movement, see Arist. *Ph.* 226a–b and Thphr. *CP*. iv.5.5. Galen's descriptions often collapse the three divisions of Aristotle's model of movement (i.e. metabolic, quantitative, and locomotive) into two: Gal. *Nat. Fac.* ii.3K, where Galen focuses on metabolic and locomotive movement. The sense of metabolic movement discussed here is seeded in Platonic thought: Pl. *Prm.* 138b–c and *Tht.* 182d–e. See Urmson (1990), 18–9 for further discussion of the term *alloiōsis*.

[13] Gal. *Loc. Aff.* viii.32K. For discussion, see Johnston (2006), 38.

relationship between the notion of change that leads to the condition of disease and that which causes pain within the body. Despite this similarity, however, Galen insists on a definite distinction between the two phenomena. Galen's model of disease allows for the possibility that changes within the body could occur imperceptibly or be such that they damage the capacity for perception. In both of these cases, Galen holds that pain cannot occur. Pain arises at a specific level and degree of change, somewhere between the types of alteration that do not impair the perceptive capacity and those that are so slight as to be gradual and unnoticed. The processes that lead to disease are also those that produce pain, but while they are closely linked, it is clear that they are not coterminous.

As well as linking pain with his understanding of disease, Galen's thinking taps into two broader issues within the Galenic corpus: the physical nature of the material body and the process of sensory perception. This connection is elaborated at a number of points, but is most explicitly developed in *The Elements According to Hippokrates*. Here, he goes to great lengths to defeat a number of atomist views about the elements, the structure and nature of the body, and sensory perception itself. In this context, Galen is determined to place his understanding of nature on an Aristotelian footing, explicitly arguing against the elemental theories of Demokritos and Epikouros.[14] As Galen reports it, atomist views of sense perception were predicated on the subjective interpretation of the arrangement of unchanging primary atoms within the body or in different sensory objects; although these primary bodies themselves did not change, they could be arranged in multiple ways which, depending on the perceiver, might be interpreted as 'cold', 'wet', 'dry', etc. Epikouros and Demokritos, on Galen's reading, held that the experience of pain relied on subjective interpretations of the various ways that such atoms were arranged or rearranged within the body in response to various stimuli. While the correctness of Galen's reading of these philosophical interpretations does not concern me, the engagement with these philosophies does reveal some aspects of how he sees the relationship between pain and the body. In response to Epikouros'

---

[14] Kupreeva (2014) for the discussion against atomism. For Galen's Aristotelian notion of nature, see Hankinson (2008d), 210–14. For Aristotelian biology and its relation to medicine: von Staden (1997b). For the Hippokratic connections developed in *Hipp. Elem.*: Singer (1997).

statement that primary elements are unbreakable and unchangeable due to their hardness (*Hipp. Elem.* i.418–9K), Galen argues that we would not feel pain if this were, in fact, the case. If our bodies were constructed in this way, we would not feel pain (οὐκ ἂν ἠλγοῦμεν), he announces, but 'we do feel pain' (ἀλγοῦμεν, *Hipp. Elem.* i.420K). Galen goes on to argue that since even the smallest needle prick causes pain, it must effect changes in the smallest parts of the human body. Because we are capable of being changed—that is, because we are not constructed from unchangeable primary bodies—we are susceptible to pain.

This interest in change and perception is reiterated at other points in Galen's corpus, most notably in the discussion of pain in *On the Causes of Symptoms*. Galen's initial discussion at vii.115K was designed to elaborate what is 'common' to pain; as well as doing this, it initiates a prolonged disquisition on the ways in which pain arises in specific sensory functions or organs throughout the body. Galen argues that each sensory function, except for touch, experiences pain in a manner specific to its functional activity. In contrast, the sense of touch has acquired a particular relationship with the experience of pain over and above the others.[15] Touch's distinctiveness is based on the ways in which sensory organs interact with external and internal stimuli. Whereas sight, sound, smell, and taste are all affected by external objects, pain arises in the sense of touch from both external and internal stimuli: pain arises from external stimuli such as those things which 'warm' or 'cool', 'cut', 'stretch', or 'bruise' the sensory organ; as well as from internal ones such as humoral change, especially the emergence of *anomalous duskrasia*.[16] When other organs experience pain from external sources, it is really because they are being affected in relation to their connection with the sense of touch. The organ of taste, for instance, is affected both by the processes that affect touch—by the organ's capacity to be warmed or cooled, or to be crushed, cut, stretched, or eroded—and by those things which affect taste specifically, such as sharp, bitter, sour, and pungent tastes.[17] The distinction speaks to a nuanced conception of

---

[15] Gal. *Caus. Symp.* vii.116–7K. Cf Gal. *Symp. Diff.* vii.56–7K. For discussions of the importance of touch in Galen's medicine as a reflection of philosophical interest in the subject, see Le Blay (2006).

[16] Gal. *Caus. Symp.* vii.116K. For further discussion of *anomalous duskrasia*: Gal. *Caus. Symp.* vii.175–7K.

[17] Gal. *Caus. Symp.* vii.117K.

how pain arises in various sensory functions of the body, allowing Galen to develop both structural and functional definitions of pain sensation. Pain in non-tactile sensory functions arises in relation to their sensory activities—that is, they experience overwhelming and violent change in terms of their interaction with their various specific sensory objects.

In turning to an explanation of what sensory objects cause specific forms of pain, Galen explores the ways in which the body interacts with the world around it. A particularly good example of this is the act of vision, which is pained or pleased by different forms of light: 'the most painful is that [light] which is both bright and simultaneously white, such as the sun' (ὀδυνηρότατον τό τε λαμπρὸν ἅμα καὶ λευκὸν, οἷον ὁ ἥλιος, Caus. Symp. vii.118K), whereas blue is the most pleasant and black is less painful than others. Galen's explanation of this odd assumption is embedded in his understanding of the nature of the substance of the sensory organ and its sense object.[18] The organ of sight is 'light-like' (αὐγοειδές, vii.119K) and 'every ray is fine-particled in relation to substance' (αὐγὴ δὲ πᾶσα λεπτομερὴς οὐσία), whereas black is 'always dense' (ἀεὶ παχυμερές). It is invariable, Galen claims, that something that is 'fine-particled' (τό λεπτομερές) is more capable of acting than that which is 'densely-particled' (τοῦ παχυμεροῦς). As a result, the fine-particled is able to effect overwhelming changes on its opposite. Galen closes his discussion by stressing that the fine-particled is more likely to separate the organ than its opposite:

> οὕτως οὖν καὶ ὁ ἥλιος ἀνιᾷ τὴν ὄψιν, ὅτι λεπτομερέστερος ὢν ἑτοίμως αὐτὴν διακρίνει. τῇ μὲν οὖν οἰκειότητι τῆς οὐσίας ἧττόν ἐστι τῶν ἐναντίων ἀνιαρός, τῷ δὲ ἰσχυρῷ τῆς ἐνεργείας βιαιότερος ὑπάρχων, τούτῳ καὶ τὸ τάχος ἴσχει τῆς εἰς τὴν ὄψιν βλάβης.

In this way then, the sun distresses vision, because, being more fine-particled, it immediately separates it. Therefore, because of the similarity of substance, the distress is less than with opposites, but, because of the force of the activity it is more violent, and in this lies the speed of the damage to vision.

Gal. *Caus. Symp.* vii.119–20K

---

[18] For the connection between theories of vision: Boudon-Millot (2012b). This passage is discussed by Siegel (1970), 10–126.

Galen's explanation provides a highly functional account of the way in which particular sensory objects interact with, and influence, the body and cause painful sensation. The language of *phusis* embeds that functional explanation in the natural qualities of the body and its place within the natural elemental world. Pain, on this reading, emerges not only as a consequence of damage to function and structure, but also as part of the body's embeddedness within, and sensory perception of, the world around it and its capacity to be acted upon by the stimuli of that external world. That physiological account denies, to a large extent, the possibility of a subjective, personalized perception of pain. As with Aretaios, the nature of pain sensation, at the most fundamental level, is conceptualized in terms of the way in which the body functions and is structured as a natural, consistent organism.

The view of pain that I have been tracking over this discussion emerges, then, through a consideration of the body's fundamental nature and its capacity for change and alteration. Pain arises because of the ways in which the primary atoms which comprise all human bodies are susceptible to change. One of the implications of this process is that pain is closely allied with, but distinct from, disease or illness. A second implication of this view is that pain is seen, at this level, as an almost universal experience—all human bodies are susceptible to pain in exactly the same ways.[19] Negotiating that level of common experience is one of the key challenges of Galen's corpus and it relates directly to how he sees the individual and the possibility of subjective, personalized pain perceptions within the clinical encounter.

2. PATIENT SENSATIONS AND REPORTAGE

The treatment of pain as a biological or physiological phenomenon seems to leave little room for the consideration of specific perceptions of pain among patients. Such pain sensations, however, are a critical part of Galen's diagnostic and therapeutic system. In this section, I turn to one of Galen's most thorough explorations of the perception of pain, contained in the second book of his *On Affected Parts*. Here,

---

[19] Gal. *Loc. Aff.* viii.87K for the discussion of common or universal symptoms.

Galen offers an extended discussion of the rational diagnosis of the patient through recognizing those parts of the body that are affected in illness and the differences in symptoms which arise in those parts. There are two complementary lines of argument developed in this context: that pain's role as a sign is dependent on the correct understanding of the differences between symptoms and their relationship to areas of the body and its anatomy; and, secondly, that the description of such symptoms is critical to their capacity to reveal the inner workings of the body. Galen's interest in the description of pain sensations constructs a close relationship between language and the body's perceptions. It also underpins a nuanced multivalent connection between doctor and patient, their shared understandings of various pain sensations, and how they communicate.

Galen's engagement with the language of pain sensation is focalized largely through his polemical discussion with the now lost *On Affected Parts* of his predecessor, Arkhigenes of Apamea.[20] Arkhigenes' primary works are preserved only in fragments, of which his rival Galen is an important (if unreliable or, perhaps, disingenuous) mine.[21] He is thought to be a member of the pneumatic sect, and, to judge by the fragments of his work contained in Galen's *On the Differences of Pulses* and *On Affected Parts,* his theories about the pulses and about diagnosis show signs of pneumatic influence.[22] It is clear from Galen's *On Affected Parts* that Arkhigenes' treatment of the sensation of pain was substantial. The nature of pain perceptions and the way they were integrated into medical practice were controversial issues; debates about them were rife with theoretical and sectorial difference and conflict. Galen's debate with him is particularly telling because it sets out some of the polemical and ideological background against which Galen's notion of pain perception and reportage was formed. Galen continually attempts to defeat Arkhigenes' approach to pain terminology and his understanding of pain's relationship with anatomy. Both authors attempt to control the types of language and descriptive terminology used by patients and doctors about their symptoms; both are caught in a battle for discursive authority which is fought

---

[20] On Arkhigenes' life: Mavroudis (2000).
[21] For the fragments of these works, see the editions of Brescia and Larizza Calabrò. For Galen as a source of Arkhigenes' writing: Schäffer (1941) and Tsoukanelis (1988) Arkhigenes is perhaps most famous for his work on the pulses: see Schäffer (1941), Ihm (1996) and Lewis (2015).
[22] Wellmann (1895b) and Kudlien (1974).

over the relationship between the body, language, and diagnostic recognition. The dispute starts from the question of what constitutes appropriate terminology for particular pain symptoms. It expands, however, into broader issues which are relevant to medical practice as a whole: the value of objective, scientific descriptions of the body and subjective, patient-based understanding; as well as the significatory value of various cultural metaphors and linguistic registers for pain. The perception is, then, afforded a central place in both the doctor–patient relationship and the doctors' conception of their medical practice.

According to the opening lines of the second book of Galen's *On Affected Parts*, the rational approach to diagnosis requires the individual 'to train the reasoning faculty' (γυμνάζειν τὸν λογισμόν) in the recognition of those parts of the body that are diseased. One must understand the parts or 'places' (τόποι) of the body, 'the causes and conditions' (αἰτίας τε καὶ διαθέσεις) to which they are susceptible, and the 'differences' (διαφοραί) between symptoms.[23] Galen explicitly links this approach to diagnosis with the figure of Erasistratos and his anatomical work: for all that recognizing what occurs in different areas of the body is attested in pre-Hellenistic medicine, the focus on anatomical structure and the nature of the body ensures that pain's incorporation into medical thinking takes on a particular hue in this context. Certain pains become indicative of a particular part of the body, or a particular condition.[24] Throughout the treatise, Galen's use of adjectives like *dēlōtikos* ('indicative') and verbs such as *sēmainein* ('to indicate') underscores pain's capacity to reveal the inner condition of the body because of its foundation in anatomical structure.

This indicative capacity, however, is finely nuanced by how Galen conceptualizes the intricacies of locative diagnosis and its dependence on the differences of various symptoms. Particular pain sensations can be divided in terms of their temporal qualities (short, long-term, intermittent), their strength (violent, weak, bearable), and their

---

[23] Gal. *Loc. Aff.* viii.69K for the connection with Erasistratos; cf. viii.1K and viii.14K.
[24] Gal. *Loc. Aff.* viii.70K: τὸ μὲν ἄλγημα τόδε τῶνδε τῶν διαθέσεών ἐστι δηλωτικὸν ἢ τῶνδε τῶν τόπων ('this particular pain is indicative of this condition or this place'). The indicative capacity of any symptom is underpinned by Galen's understanding of *endeixis*. For a discussion of Galen's use of this term: Durling (1991) and Kudlien (1991).

character (what form or manner they might take).[25] These perceptions are further differentiated by the complex nature of the body in which they arise. Galen claims that certain symptoms are 'specific' or 'particular' (*idios*) either to places within the body or to particular conditions. Consequently, they can reveal or indicate in a straightforward manner the presence of a particular condition or its location.[26] To make matters more difficult, pain—under the influence of various factors such as the qualities of a part of the body, the characteristics of certain conditions, or patient behaviour while ill— can spread through the body, evolving as it moves, changing in form depending on the parts of the body it affects and their relationship with surrounding anatomical structures. Pain sensations are further shaped by the concatenation of sensations (*aisthēseis*) with particular conditions (*diatheseis*) which affect sensory perceptions throughout the body.[27] This complex nexus of interpretative possibilities can be summed up effectively as understanding the *diaphorai* of pain symptoms. Diagnosis by these differences is fundamental to Galen's (as well as Arkhigenes') medical practice, but capitalizing on the revelatory power of the symptom involves understanding the nuanced changes in, and relationships between, different pain perceptions, conditions, and physiological contexts which constitute a fragile and complex body.[28]

---

[25] For a substantial list of the pain types used by Arkhigenes and Galen: Gärtner (2014), 599–601. For Arkhigenes' various pain terms: Gärtner (2014), 606–7 and Pigeaud (2004). Throughout *On Affected Parts*, Galen generally rejects the use of *eidos* in favour of *tropē*, though there are times when he refers to 'types' of pain, such as at *Sim. Morb.* xix.5K.

[26] For a general discussion of the various elements which comprise locative diagnosis: Gärtner (2014), 592–3, which gives greater emphasis to the different epistemological strands of diagnosis. For specific symptoms linked either with specific causes or parts of the body: ἴδια συμπτώματα ('specific symptoms') at *Loc. Aff.* viii.69–70K. Some perceptions can occur in a uniform manner in different locations of the body: *Loc. Aff.* viii.100–1K. For the association of certain parts of the body with specific symptoms in specific conditions: *Loc. Aff.* viii.79–80K (the kidneys), 83K (the small intestine), and 85K (the large intestine).

[27] On the influence of bodily structure on symptom perception: e.g. *Loc. Aff.* viii.103–4K (the membranes, their location within the body, and their relationship with surrounding areas of the body). Pain moving through the body: *Loc. Aff.* viii.101K. For Arkhigenes' habit of 'running together' or confusion of a condition with *aisthēsis*: Gal. *Loc. Aff.* viii.72K and 120K.

[28] The use of revelation is repeated in Galen's characterization of Arkhigenes' approach to pain: ὁ Ἀρχιγένης ἐκ τῆς τῶν ἀλγημάτων διαφορᾶς ἡγούμενος δηλοῦσθαι

Anatomical justification is allied with Galen's interest in the names that patients and doctors use to describe these pain sensations. The names given to certain pain types correspond, in Galen's mind, to natural realities—divisions in language correspond to apparent divisions and differences in the real world. Like the pain sensations themselves, pain names can be explained and justified through a rational division of the body's anatomy.[29] The intricate, delicate relationship between language and anatomy raises two important points. Firstly, it points to the issue of diagnostic recognition. What is at stake in this connection is Galen's construction of language's capacity to indicate or to reveal both the felt sensations of the patients he encounters and the internal conditions of the body. Secondly, it argues for a particularly nuanced relationship between patient and doctor. Language's capacity to indicate involves fitting together common experiences and familiar understandings through the use of common language. Put another way, despite Galen's rationalist approach to the body, and realist approach to language, patients' descriptions and doctors' terminology matter because they help to develop a sense of common experience between patient and doctor, albeit one that is managed and controlled by Galen.

Let us begin with a particularly telling passage in which Galen constructs the authority of the patient's and the doctor's respective voices. According to *On Affected Parts* viii.88–9K, it is appropriate to eschew the use of unclear names for diseases and it is better to discuss them with clear terminology. One of the problems that arises from this approach is that it means communication, diagnostic recognition, and medical knowledge are ultimately contingent:

χαλεπὸν δὲ τὸ τοιοῦτον κριτήριον, ὡς ἂν ἑτέροις πολλάκις ἀναγκαζομένων ἡμῶν πιστεύειν οὔτε παρακολουθοῦσι σαφῶς, οἷς πάσχουσι, διὰ μαλακίαν ψυχῆς, οὔτ', εἰ καὶ παρακολουθοῖεν, ἑρμηνεῦσαι δυναμένοις, ἢ τῷ μηδ' ὅλως οἵους τ' εἶναι λόγῳ δηλῶσαι περὶ ὧν πάσχουσιν—οὐ γὰρ μικρᾶς δυνάμεως τὸ τοιοῦτον—, ἢ τῷ μηδ' εἶναι ῥητὸν αὐτό. καταλείπεται τοίνυν

τὰ πεπονθότα μόρια ('Arkhigenes thinks [it is possible] to reveal the affected parts from the differences in pain'), Gal. *Loc. Aff.* viii.70K.

[29] Hankinson (1994a) and von Staden (1995a) are both seminal in this discussion. For further treatments of Galen's general interest in language: Morison (2008). For the connection between Galen's medical aims and commentaries on Hippokrates, see, in addition to von Staden (1995a), Sluiter (1995a) and (1995b) and Manetti (2009). For Galen's own views on language: *Med. Nam.* and *Soph.* xiv.582K.

αὐτὸν πεπονθέναι τὸν μέλλοντα γράφειν ἑκάστου τῶν ἀλγημάτων τὴν ἰδέαν ἰατρόν τε ὄντα καὶ ἄλλοις ἑρμηνεῦσαι δυνατὸν ἑαυτῷ τε παρηκολουθηκότα μετὰ φρονήσεως, ἡνίκ᾽ ἔπασχεν ἄνευ μαλακίας ψυχῆς.

Such a criterion is difficult, as often we are forced to trust others, who either do not understand clearly the experiences they endure because of a weakness of their soul, or, if they do understand, are unable to express it clearly since they are not able to reveal in words [or rational discourse] what they suffer, since this requires not a small amount of ability, or it is inexpressible. It is appropriate that the one who is intending to write about each of the forms of pain has suffered and, being a doctor, is able to speak clearly to others, since he has understood for himself in his mind what he has suffered, without weakness of soul.

Gal. Loc. Aff. viii.88–9K

Galen's passage speaks immediately to the ways in which a doctor and patient relate to each other. On one level, medical knowledge and diagnosis require an intimate trust-based connection. The suggestion of a close affiliation, however, is ultimately undermined by the unreliability of the patient's voice. It always threatens to fail. As the passage continues, Galen's determination to construct and solidify the narrative authority of the doctor becomes more apparent: for all its emphasis on the patient, this passage is actually about the validity of the doctor's voice. This arrogation of authority is dependent on the relationship between language and experience. Doctor and patient are both evaluated on their capacity to transform the sensations of the body into effective public discourse. The patient's voice is, however, superseded by the authority attributed to the doctor, who has firsthand knowledge of a particular condition, superior mental abilities or understanding, and greater linguistic capacity.[30] Of course, the doctor's own voice is not without its problems. The suggestion that the doctor is in the best place to write about pains that he has himself experienced raises some immediate questions because, as Galen acknowledges, no doctor has experienced all forms of pain.[31] The force of this argument is, ultimately, to defeat Arkhigenes' treatment of pain language, since he writes about these symptoms 'as if he has experienced all forms of pain'.[32] Nevertheless, such caveats about

---

[30] For an alternative view of this passage, see Roby (2015), 314–15.
[31] Gal. Loc. Aff. viii.89K. For the pointed jibe that Arkhigenes could not have experienced certain pains unique to women: Gal. Loc. Aff. viii.117K.
[32] Gal. Loc. Aff. viii.89–90 and 117K.

the ideal form of description (arguably marked by καταλειπέται) do not undermine the broader point of the passage: Galen arrogates authority to a particular kind of doctor on the basis of his capacity to speak effectively concerning what he has experienced.

As Courtney Roby has pointed out, Galen's discussion of this issue is embedded in his general theories of language. The passage hinges on Galen's choice of the term ἑρμηνεύειν ('to speak clearly' or 'to translate') to designate different speaking abilities. The root meaning of the term looks towards the translation or transformation of information. Galen consistently uses it to designate the process of transforming unclear phenomena into clear, effective discourse in the public realm. The term often occurs with explicit statements of Galen's capacity either to speak with a 'rational *logos*' or to speak 'clearly' (*saphōs*) about matters which are precisely the opposite. As Galen proceeds through this passage, he elaborates on the need for a clear linguistic register in a number of ways. In the first instance, pain resists easy explanation—discourse that is 'clear' or 'indicates clearly' requires a high level of ability. His suggestion that at times 'it is inexpressible' (τῷ μηδ' εἶναι ῥητὸν αὐτό) goes further by recalling references throughout his corpus to things which are 'unspeakable' (ἄρρητα). Galen often describes individual pain sensations as *arrētos*, as well as other sensory perceptions or bodily conditions.[33] Tobias Reinhardt and others have pointed out that those things which are *arrēta* in Galenic thought are particularly important for conceptualizing the individual's ability to perceive and to communicate that perception in language.[34] Pain, like many other sensory perceptions, sits at the boundary of that which can and cannot be communicated publicly. It is at this juncture that the capacity to describe things in a rational discourse becomes vitally important. Heinrich von Staden has shown that 'rational discourse' or *logos* becomes relevant in situations in which phenomena appear to have no immediately apparent name; when the individual encounters phenomena which are anonymous, it is necessary to explain and define them with rational discourse, and, in more extreme circumstances, to use a metaphor to

---

[33] E.g. Gal. *MM*. x.604K, 731K, and 810K.
[34] Reinhardt (2011) for the connection between *arrēta* and Stoic theories of language, especially the notion of the *lekton*, along with Frede (1994), 109–28 and Roby (2015), 316.

help communicate what is felt.[35] Galen's suggestion that the experience could not be put into language appears to be connected to his engagement with the inherently resistant qualities of pain experiences, but it is also figured in the intellectual capacities of understanding and linguistic ability. The construction of an authoritative voice for the description of pain (and other conditions) hinges on precisely the point where language fails to relate effectively to experience: authority in this context is predicated on the management of an effective relationship between first-hand experience and language or descriptive ability. The contexts in which *hermēneuein* is adopted throughout Galen's corpus suggest that Galen's passage in *On Affected Parts* is far from an innocent discussion. It relates, in a large part, to Galen's desire to control language and to reinforce the conditions under which language might be seen as either revelatory or useful in a diagnostic context. It is not elaborated explicitly, but the discussion hinges on qualities that he repeatedly attributes to his own narrative practices and his own capacity for clear transmission of physiological and pathogenic information.

Some of the themes which cut across Galen's arrogation of his own narrative authority are reiterated in his later polemical discussions of pain terminology. According to *On Affected Parts* viii.110K, Arkhigenes had held that pain in the abdomen could take on various forms:

ὁ δὲ τοῦ ἥπατος ὅλκιμος ἐμπεφυκὼς καὶ ναρκώδης ἐστὶ καὶ ἀτειρέστερον ἐγκείμενος. ὁ δὲ τοῦ σπληνὸς οὐκ ὀξύς, βάρος δ' ἅμα καὶ διάτασιν ἔχει ἀντεντεινομένῳ πρὸς ἔνθλιψιν καὶ ἀποπίεσίν τινα ἔξωθεν ἐπικειμένην ἐοικώς. νεφροὶ δὲ αὐστηρούς τε τοὺς πόνους ἐπιφέρουσι καὶ μετ' ἐμμόνου σφίγξεως ἐπινύσσοντας. κύστις δὲ στύφουσι σφόδρα χρῆται τοῖς ἀλγήμασι καὶ σὺν διατάσεσιν νυγματώδεσιν, ὑστέρα δὲ ὀξέσι, διαΐσσουσι, νυγματώδεσι, διατείνουσιν, ἐμπίπτουσι στροφωδῶς. τοιούτῳ μίγματι πέφυκε πονεῖν, καθ' ὃ καὶ ἀπορίαν τοῦ ἰδιώματος ἐμποιεῖ.

The pain in the liver is dragging, fixed, numbing, and exerts pressure more stubbornly. The pain in the spleen is not sharp, but heavy and simultaneously has tension, like being stretched against a certain

---

[35] Von Staden (1995a) on the methods to overcome the difficulty of ineffability. References to matters which are 'without a name' (ἀνώνυμος) occur throughout Galen's corpus, but are particularly closely associated with the different types of pulse: Gal. *Diff. Puls.* viii.508K, 525K, 680K, and 692K. For further references, see von Staden (1995a), 511.

pressure or squeezing which lies against it from outside. The kidneys provide harsh pains and pricking ones, along with a lasting constriction. The bladder inflicts astringent pains combined with pulsing distension. The uterus gives sharp, shooting, pulsing, stretching pains, which occur during colic. One can feel such a mixture of pains that it even leads to some difficulty of expression.

Gal. *Loc. Aff.* viii.110K

The quotation from Arkhigenes' text outlines the earlier doctor's understanding of the forms of pain which arise in various internal organs in the abdomen. This passage taps into the process which he and Galen share of diagnosing the body through the *diaphorai* of pain symptoms and attempting to give names to them. Galen tells his readers in the preceding lines that this was taken from a section where Arkhigenes and his followers used the differences in pain types to diagnose his patients.[36] The passage looks directly to the polemical debate between Galen and Arkhigenes in which the capacity to differentiate and communicate different pain sensations is highly contested discursive turf.

Arkhigenes' description of pain symptoms is remarkably specific. He outlines pains in terms not only of their quality, strength, and spatial movement, but also links multiple types of descriptor to each sensation in order to give a more nuanced differentiation of certain pain perceptions. A pain in the spleen is both 'heavy' and 'distending' and feels as if something is being applied to the organ from the outside. The complexity of this particular vision of pain raises, for Arkhigenes, a combined epistemological and linguistic problem: the variety or mixture of pains produces 'difficulty of expression' (ἀπορίαν τοῦ ἰδιώματος ἐμποιεῖ). The phrase τοῦ ἰδιώματος, used to emphasize the difficulty felt by the patient, seems brilliantly chosen for its ambiguity, pointing simultaneously to the difficulty of 'specific parts' of the body or, in its allusion to idiom, to patient expression and language. Arkhigenes represents, at the level of his own language, the linguistic and sensory ambiguities created by pain.

Galen's engagement with the passage is multifaceted. Although he clearly accepts some of the types of perception that Arkhigenes lists, such as the pulsating and distending pain, there are also, in his view,

---

[36] Gal. *Loc. Aff.* viii.110K: διδάσκουσαν καὶ αὐτὴν ἐκ τῆς τῶν πόνων διαφορᾶς διάγνωσιν τῶν πεπονθότων μορίων ('[another part of Arkhigenes' work] which also teaches diagnosis of the affected parts from the differences of pains').

numerous problems with Arkhigenes' description. He argues that Arkhigenes confuses the boundaries between different forms of sensory perception and their linguistic representation. Arkhigenes' use of the terms 'rough' and 'astringent' are particularly problematic because they produce what Galen sees as a confusion of sensory categories: 'for these are the names of humours, which are recognized from perceptions of taste through the organ of tongue' (ἔστι γὰρ ταῦτα χυμῶν ὀνόματα, δι' ὀργάνου μὲν τῆς γλώττης, αἰσθήσεως δὲ τῆς γευστικῆς διαγινωσκόμενα, *Loc. Aff.* viii.113K). Galen holds that Arkhigenes has failed to understand that each quality of touch and taste has a specific name. As a result, his attempt to 'speak clearly about specific forms of pain' (τὰς ἰδιότητας τῶν πόνων ἑρμηνεύειν) ended in unintelligibility (ἀρρήτους, *Loc. Aff.* viii.114K).[37] The implications of Galen's terminology are hard to miss. Galen's choice of ἑρμηνεύειν returns the reader immediately to the debate about authoritative voices at viii.88–9K; the reference to 'unintelligibility' (here translating ἀρρήτους) stresses, in conjunction with that earlier passage, the distance between these individual sensations and the capacity for meaningful speech.

Galen's criticism is more biting than this, however. His dismissal of Arkhigenes taps into the concept of 'common' or 'habitual' language; it also raises further questions about how language indicates and reveals and who uses it within the clinical encounter. The word 'drawing' (ὅλκιμος), Galen claims, is 'not customary' (ἄηθες) among Greeks and it is, thus, 'not easy to discover exactly what it signifies' (οὐδὲ τί σημαίνει ῥᾴδιον εὑρεῖν), 'since it is only by widespread usage that terms gain significance' (ἐκ γὰρ πολλῆς χρήσεως ἡ τῶν σημαινομένων εὕρεσις γίνεται, *Loc. Aff.* viii.111K). The repetition of forms of *sēmainein* looks directly to the capacities of the body to indicate internal conditions. Revelation of the body's parts and conditions is replayed on the linguistic plane and, consequently, the linguistic unclarity of Arkhigenes is likened to those parts of the body which fail to provide a diagnostic sign: unclear terminology simply fails to indicate the conditions being discussed by doctors and patients. The problems with Arkhigenes' language have an immediate impact on discussions between patient and doctor. In the first instance, 'all specific forms of

---

[37] For further discussion of his linguistic failings, see Galen's criticism of Arkhigenes as a ψευδοδιαλεκτικός ('pseudo-dialectician') at Gal. *Diff. Puls.* viii.629K (in specific reference to his failed use of names for different types of pulse).

pain are inexpressible even by the patients themselves' (ἄρρητός ἐστιν ἰδιότης πᾶσα καὶ κατ' αὐτούς, Gal. *Loc. Aff.* viii.117).[38] The repeated references to *ta arrēta* or that which is *arrētos* continue to disconnect language from the sensations it is meant to indicate: such specific terminology adopted by Arkhigenes actually destroys the referential qualities of language.

Galen continues by stressing the point that one should employ terminology dictated by Hellenic custom to describe different perceptions. All the previous doctors 'who wrote about the differences of pains' (τὰς διαφορὰς τῶν πόνων γράψαντες, *Loc. Aff.* viii.116K) 'did not dare' (οὐκ ἐτόλμησαν) to use 'names other than the customary ones' (ἑτέροις ὀνόμασι χρήσασθαι τῶν συνηθῶν) which it was 'possible to hear from the patients themselves' (παρ' αὐτῶν τῶν καμνόντων ἐστὶν ἀκοῦσαι, viii.116K).[39] In contrast to Arkhigenes' specific terminology, what one hears from a patient is that they feel as if they are being 'pierced by a needle', or 'pierced by a trepan, bruised, torn apart, drawn or pulled up or down'.[40] Galen's passage attributes to patients a fascinating combination of different types of pain descriptions. In the first instance, it seems that a number of their descriptions do in fact map onto Arkhigenes' descriptions. Secondly, it strikes me as odd that being 'pierced by a trepan' might be seen as common or habitual language. On the one hand, this might be seen as a type of common or easily imaginable metaphor for pain sensation, but at the same time, it seems to me, it is relevant that it is also the metaphor used at *Odyssey* 9.385 to describe the blinding of the Kyklops. It is not always clear where everyday and common patient language begins and marked literary metaphor ends. Galen's ostensible focus on what can be heard from patients has often lent itself to scholarly claims that he

---

[38] Galen's use of ἄρρητος ('unspeakable'), here, recalls his suggestion that pain is sometimes inexpressible at 88–9K. In this context, however, he appears to be referring to specific forms of pain, apparently documented by Arkhigenes, rather than making a general statement about the ineffability of the experience.

[39] NB also his reference to Hellenic custom at Gal. *Loc. Aff.* viii.116K: ὡς ἔθος ἐστὶ τοῖς Ἕλλησι ('as is the custom among Greeks').

[40] Gal. *Loc. Aff.* viii.116K: ὡς ὑπὸ τρυπάνου τιτρᾶσθαι καὶ θλᾶσθαι δοκεῖν καὶ διασπᾶσθαι καὶ τείνεσθαι καὶ ἀνασπᾶσθαι καὶ κατασπᾶσθαι καὶ βάρους τινὸς αἴσθησιν ἔχειν ἐνίοτε μὲν ἐκκρεμαμένου τῶν ὑπερκειμένων, ἐνίοτε δ' ἐγκειμένου τοῖς περιέχουσιν ('[the patients say that] they seem to be pierced by a trepan, bruised, torn apart, distended, or pulled up or pulled down, and they have the perception of a kind of heaviness, at times, from something which hangs from things which lie above them, and at other times, from being pressed against things which surround them').

favours a patient-centred language over the theoretically-driven scientific language of Arkhigenes.[41] This has led some to suggest that Galen privileges subjective knowledge over the objective theoretical knowledge of the doctor.[42] While this may be right in some cases, I think that what Galen is stressing is best conceptualized in slightly different terms.

There are several reasons why pain terminology is best left at the level of the ways in which patients describe that sensation. In the first instance, he suggests that we are ignorant of any type of suffering that we have not experienced ourselves. A disease, Galen argues, should be 'common' (κοινός) and the meaning of the terms to describe its symptoms 'familiar to the listener' (συνήθη τοῖς ἀκούουσιν, viii.118K). It is this sense of familiarity between patient and doctor that underpins the capacity of language to effectively communicate pain symptoms. Using terminology such as 'being ill at ease' (τό ἀλύειν) is easily understood and 'clear' (δῆλος) since we have 'suffered in this way' (τῷ πεπονθέναι, viii.118K). But it is 'not possible to recognize' (οὐδ'... νοῆσαι δύναται) the 'harsh' (αὐστηρός) pain since one does 'not know to what this name refers' (οὐκ εἰδὼς, καθ' ὅτου ποτε πράγματος ἐπιφέρει τοὔνομα, viii.118K), even if we have experienced it. We all know the pricking pain, or the tearing pain, as well as understanding other aspects such as its strength, severity, violence, or its continuous or intermittent nature. We know these because 'they have been related clearly by common names and they arise daily among everyone' (ὡς ἂν ὑπὸ συνηθῶν τε τῶν ὀνομάτων ἑρμηνευομένους αὐτούς τε γινομένους ὁσημέραι παμπόλλοις, viii.118K). Galen's argument plays up the way in which language refers to, and is based on his notion of, shared physiological experience. Instead of conceptualizing this process as one in which Galen favours a patient-centred language rather than the overly theoretical, it seems that Galen holds that language mediates between shared subjective experiences and commonly held perceptive awareness, often between doctor and patient. The categories of subjective vs objective or patient-centred vs objective and theoretical do not map onto either his vision of language use or his vision of the commonality of symptoms across different people.

---

[41] Pigeaud (2004), 46–7, for a 'communal language'. For Galen favouring a slightly nuanced version of the patient-based language of modern medicine: Mattern (2008), 125. The most developed discussion of 'patient-based language' is Roby (2015), 312–17.

[42] E.g. Temkin (1971), 37.

Ostensibly, Galen's approach focuses on the ways in which patient language can be incorporated into the clinical scenario and is ultimately rendered useful for diagnosis. One point that is not analysed sufficiently in the scholarly analysis of this issue is the way in which Galen's approach aligns with his vision of himself as a gatekeeper of the medical tradition and proper linguistic usage. Galen's interest in what constitutes legitimate language is underpinned by a number of strategies. It is worth pointing out that some of his central examples of pain terminology are those which are very well established in the Greek literary tradition, especially in Hippokratic texts.[43] This does not mean that they were not used by patients themselves or were not habitual ways of describing pain, but it does imply that Galen's vision of effective or legitimate language often aligns with the language of the medical tradition. As we have seen, Galen often validates language by reference to all the earlier doctors who dared to write about pain or to usage which is the custom among the Greeks. Such ascriptions immediately raise problematic questions. Who has the power to define what 'the custom' among the Greeks is? Who is able to define what all the earlier doctors said? It is exceptionally difficult to divorce Galen's authorizing strategies from his identity as a commentator and a scholar who sees himself, in a large part, as responsible for determining, protecting, and managing the medical tradition.[44] Standing behind Galen's interest in what is habitual or linguistic custom is his combined identity as a doctor, a linguistic theorist, and a textual commentator: the patient's voice is incorporated into medicine in precisely the terms that stress Galen's own authority.

3. NARRATING AND EXPERIENCING PAIN

In the previous discussion, I showed that Galen saw the description of pain symptoms as predicated on a sense of common experience and understanding: pain descriptions were indicative and contributed to

---

[43] For the problematic use of τό ἀλύειν ('ill at ease') in poets, see Plut. *Quomodo Adulesc.* 22e. The term is ubiquitous throughout the Hippokratic corpus, especially to refer to the general weakening of the body: e.g. Hp. *Epid.* i.3.13(11).4, iii.3.17(7).4, and v.1.64.5.

[44] On Galen's self-appointed status as a linguistic, literary, and intellectual gatekeeper: Sluiter (1995a), along with von Staden (1995a).

diagnosis because they were predicated on common usage and knowledge. I turn towards Galen's understanding of pain experience by investigating some of the ways in which Galen represents the impact of pain on the individual patient and the negotiation of that impact within a number of clinical scenarios. Galen's vision of the experience of pain draws on questions about how patients understand or organize their perceptions of pain, some of the emotive and psychological factors that underpin that process, and the patient's navigation of health care.

Galen's medical practice presents a multifaceted interest in pain's impact on patients in either psychological and emotional ways or intellectual ones. Emotional experiences, such as 'distress' (λύπη) and 'anxiety' (ἀνία), are common throughout Galen's corpus.[45] As a physician, Galen attends to both the physical and emotional problems which patients present.[46] As well as dealing with emotional or psychological difficulties in their own right, Galen views these mental experiences as linked to the emergence and progression of physiological diseases: 'distress' and many other *pathē* (anger, fear, desire) are both antecedent causes of diseases and caused by them, so much so that to talk of the categories of psychological and emotional distress as separate from the experience or perception of physiological pain is highly problematic.[47] The boundary between the physiological aspects of pain (or disease in general) and its emotional or psychological elements was always fluid in Galen's work.

This close relationship between *pathē* and physical disease must also be seen in relation to the fact that Galen is not often concerned to display emotional sympathy with, or empathy for, his patients. Compassionate emotions—and their implications for how one

---

[45] There is, of course, a large bibliography on these various issues. I give only an outline: Mattern (2008), 203–24, Gill (2010), 243–329, esp. 316–22, and King (2015), with further bibliography at n. 47, below.

[46] *Hipp. Epid. VI.* 485.5–487.17 (Pfaff) for a number of telling case-histories. The original Greek of much of *Commentary on Hippokrates' Epidemics VI* has been lost. I have used here the German translation by Pfaff of Wenkebach's edition of the extant Arabic. Cf. the cases at Gal. *Praen.* xiv.631–4K and also *Loc. Aff.* viii.301–2K.

[47] This collocation is bound up with Galen's humoral views of the body and emotional states expressed in a number of treatises. For important and influential discussions of Galen's approach to this combined mind-body problem, see García Ballester (1988), Sorabji (2000), esp. chapter 17, Hankinson (2006), and Gill (2010), 243–329. For Galen's approach to the soul and psychology, in general: Hankinson (1991), von Staden (2000), and Tieleman (2003).

conceptualizes the experience of disease and health care—are excised from much of Galen's work: unlike Aretaios, pity is absent from Galen's representation of himself as a doctor and his representation of his interaction with the patient. When quasi-emotional reactions, such as 'amazement' or 'wonder' (figured through forms of *thaumazein*), do play a part in the doctor–patient relationship, they are closely connected to the substantiation of Galen's authoritative interpretation of the patient's condition; when Galen is interested in such emotions, he very often connects them with the capacity to produce effective outcomes or to astound his onlookers.[48] This absence should be read against the backdrop of other writers' attempts to emphasize the emotional aspects of the doctor–patient relationship. Galen deliberately excises the emotive aspects of that relationship and the compassionate aspects of his engagement with patients in order to position himself against figures such as Aretaios (and others such as Ailios Aristeides) within a highly competitive discursive landscape.

One way in which it is possible to think about pain's impact on the patient and Galen's interest in the broader aspects of pain experience is to examine the way in which he represents its narration within the clinical encounter. How patients and doctors talk about pain symptoms—and how the process of narration is connected with diagnostic recognition—is central to the way in which Galen constructs pain experience. A fundamental tenet of modern medical anthropology has been that the ways in which patients and doctors tell stories about their pain symptoms or their medical history are important for the shaping of illness experience. We have already learnt from Oliver Sacks (among others) that the movement from a case-history to a 'story' is critical to our ability to see more than just a disease in the clinical encounter and to engage with a person instead.[49] Galen's management of that process of narration and explanation is central to his ability to shape and control patient experience.

This focus on stories and narration looks immediately to the examples of clinical practice found in the case-histories and accounts of clinical practice placed throughout Galen's corpus.[50] Mattern sees

---

[48] For the importance of *thaumazein* to figure audiences' sense of amazement at Galen's cures: Mattern (2008), 85–6, with further examples.

[49] Chapter 1 (text to nn. 9–12).

[50] For the case-history 'genre', see Mattern (2008), 28–31. For discussion of the status of Hippokratic case-histories in Galen: Lloyd (2009) and Mattern (2008), 40–3. The accounts studied below draw on a long tradition which can be traced back

these case-histories as narratives which emphasize the alternative perspectives of patient and doctor: '[e]ven though', she claims, 'direct speech is rare, these stories resemble a dialogue: a back-and-forth negotiation between Galen and the patient'.[51] This negotiation plays into what Mattern sees as a 'patient-centred narrative' within the case-histories. She is undoubtedly right that there are some examples which take on the appearance of a dialogue between doctor and patient.[52] To my mind, however, Mattern does not place enough emphasis on these accounts as rhetorical representations of the historical situation. It is hard to see these narratives as anything other than Galen's incorporation of the patient's voice into his reports: patients are asked questions, quoted, paraphrased, and allowed to tell some of their story in a process that is controlled by Galen. That process is not only a consequence of his creation of an effective diagnostic narrative in a given text, but also a situation that he represents as having taken place in the real world—this is how Galen represents the practice of diagnosis. It seems to me that this representational element should not be seen as distinct from Galen's agonistic relationship either with the patient or with other doctors. The doctor–patient relationship and the broader aspects of the experience of pain are worked out in a highly discursive context in which Galen seeks to defeat his patients and his rivals and substantiate his own authority.[53]

The first area of discussion that I want to turn to in this investigation concerns the way in which pain and disease are communicated in

---

to the Hippocratic corpus at least: *Epidemics*, for instance, was read, commented on, and contributed to medical practice throughout the Imperial period. The work of Rufus of Ephesos from the early second century CE contains a number of accounts of clinical encounters which may have circulated as a discrete collection of therapeutic case notes: Mattern (2008), 33 with Ullman (1978). For a description of this work, now preserved in Arabic, containing approximately 20 accounts of patient treatment: Mattern (2008), 33–4 and 216 nn. 107–8, with further bibliography. According to Galen, reading case-histories formed an important part of the training of Empiricist doctors, who were able to increase their 'experience' by incorporating the knowledge gained by reading the accounts of therapy provided by other doctors. On *historia* and the development of medical experience, see pages 298–301 in Deichgräber. Arguably, some case-histories were used as notes to assist in rhetorical medical displays at different points throughout the first and second centuries CE: Ullman (1978), 24–5.

[51] Mattern (2008), 125.
[52] E.g. Proteus the rhetor: Gal. *Alim. Fac.* vi.598–601K. Antiper: *Loc. Aff.* viii.293–96K. Eudemos: *Praen.* xiv.606–7K, 621–4K.
[53] I have very much been influenced in this reading of the case-histories by the work of Lloyd (2009). See also, on this issue, Barton (1994), 133–66.

fragmented or incomplete stories. In the last section, I discussed a telling passage at *On Affected Parts* viii.88–9K, where Galen was particularly interested in the ways in which medical diagnosis was contingent upon the various capacities for narrative demonstrated by the doctor and patient. In that particular scenario, what was at stake was pain's resistance to transformation into effective and clear language either because of its inherent qualities or because of the patient's failure to understand it through a 'psychical weakness' (μαλακία ψυχῆς); in contrast, the doctor was able to 'go along with' the things that he suffered 'without psychical weakness' (ἄνευ μαλακίας ψυχῆς). The differing abilities of patient and doctor to understand and narrate their respective experiences were mapped onto a moral order.[54] Galen's conception of different people's reactions to their experience is figured, in a large part, in terms of their moral or ethical qualities.[55] Importantly for Galen, that process has an immediate impact on the nature of the narrative-based relationship that defines the clinical scenario. In that case, it underpins their failure to communicate it effectively to others, to translate what they feel into the public world of language and clinical recognition.

Many of the issues present in that discussion are also at work in a similar example of the failure of the patient's voice during an epileptic attack at *On Affected Parts* viii.194K.[56] In this example, Galen emphasizes the inability of the particular sufferer to relate his experience of epilepsy effectively. Galen begins this scenario by telling us that a boy began by 'narrating the beginning of his condition' (διηγουμένου τὴν ἀρχὴν τῆς διαθέσεως, *Loc. Aff.* viii.194K). The case-history starts with a standard diagnostic opening, i.e. the patient describing the beginning and course of the illness throughout his body. The choice of *diēgēsis* intimates an interest in how this individual patient might shape his experience through the construction of a story. As Galen's account continues, however, it emerges that the boy is unable to describe the final stages of his condition effectively:

---

[54] Particularly striking are the references to those with weak souls in Plato and Xenophon. Importantly, those figures are set in opposition to the legitimate citizens of the *polis* in Pl. *Grg.* 491b4; cf. the use of πονηρότατοι and πονηρίαν at X. *Oec.* i.19.4.

[55] Gal. *Loc. Aff.* viii.301–2K on the role of strong souls in overcoming the dangers of gastric *sunkopē* and King (2015), 265–7.

[56] For a discussion of this passage from a slightly different angle: Roby (2015), 304–6.

ἐπειδὰν δὲ πρῶτον ἐκείνης ψαύσῃ, μηκέτι παρακολουθεῖν ἑαυτῷ. τὴν μέντοι ποιότητα τοῦ φερομένου πρὸς τὴν κεφαλὴν ἐρωτώμενος ὑπὸ τῶν ἰατρῶν ὁποία τις εἴη, λέγειν οὐκ εἶχεν ὁ παῖς· ἀλλ' ἕτερός γέ τις ἐκείνου νεανίσκος, οὐκ ἄφρων, ἀλλ' ἱκανῶς αἰσθάνεσθαι τοῦ γιγνομένου δυνάμενος, ἑρμηνεῦσαί θ' ἑτέρου δυνατώτερος, οἷον αὔραν τινὰ ψυχρὰν ἔφασκεν εἶναι τὴν ἀνερχομένην.

When the condition first took hold of that part of him, he was no longer able to go along with it. When he was asked what sort of thing the transference to his head might be, the boy was unable to say. But, a certain other youth, not without his wits, but perhaps better able to perceive the events, and more able to speak clearly than the other one, said that it was like a kind of cool breeze going upwards.

Gal. *Loc. Aff.* viii.194K

The account begins, then, by simultaneously intimating the possibility of a narrative in which the patient can represent their own experiences, only to then deny that possibility. The dynamics of speech and description look back to his earlier treatment of the patient's voice at viii.88–9K. As in the earlier passage, the difficulty of dealing with the descriptions of the patient is emphasized. The passage is characterized by the fragmentary narrative of the epileptic sufferer. This incapacity appears deliberately set against the ability of the 'other youth' (ἕτερος ... νεανίσκος) to 'speak clearly' about (ἑρμηνεῦσαί) the experience based on his possession of a different level of mental acuity, figured here by the tag οὐκ ἄφρων. The division between *pais* and *neaniskos* perhaps marks out differing stages in the ancient conception of young life and certainly flags the differing experiences of the two individuals. Galen appears to be aware of the possibility of two different narratives and he manages this potential diversity of experience through the narrative strategy of incorporating one story into the gaps contained in another.

A number of scholars have suggested that the 'other youth' is, in fact, a different figure who also suffers from the disease and is, therefore, describing his own symptoms. For Mattern, this passage constitutes two distinct case-histories.[57] Galen shows little concern for this ambiguity or the difficulties raised by this passage. The questions

---

[57] Mattern (2008), 181. It is arguable that he may just be one of the habitual 'observers' who are present at many medical diagnoses: e.g. at Gal. *Praen.* xiv.609K and 659K. The use of *aisthanomai* suggests that he may be one who has also perceived the symptoms. For further discussion, see Mattern (2008), 84–7.

which might occur to a modern reader—did the two figures have the same experience? Can one person's account stand in for another's?—are simply not discussed. Galen is, to my mind, largely uninterested in the potential problems involved in exploring and resolving some of the complications created by these questions. The second patient's account is inserted at precisely the point where the child's experience resists effective transformation into language. Galen's strategy subsumes one experience into another, one which is more fecund and worthwhile in narrative and diagnostic terms. Galen's desire to create a single coherent narrative of the experience of this form of epilepsy downplays any possibility of variety or difference across these two individuals. The potential richness of a variety of experiences is undermined by the creation of a single unified narrative concerning the body's physical symptoms from multiple (potentially) heterogeneous accounts.

The second issue raised by this passage concerns the language with which the second youth describes the experience and its relationship to Galen's theory of epilepsy. On initial glance, the terms used to describe the event—'a kind of cool breeze' (αὔραν τινὰ ψυχράν)—reflect Galen's desire to hear symptoms in the everyday terminology of patients. Supporting this reading, Temkin suggests that this is one scene in which the terminology later adopted by medical science—notably, the 'epileptic breeze'—is introduced into medical discourse by a patient.[58] In fact, however, the reference appears to be knowingly discursive: the metaphor of the 'cool breeze' is already seeded in the literary and medical traditions of Greek culture. The term 'cool breeze' (αὔρα ψυχρά) appears in, for instance, the description of vapours rising from the sea in Aristotle or 'cooling breezes' in Hippocratic texts such as *Airs, Waters, and Places*.[59] In these texts, the phrase is not used to describe the progression of epilepsy through the body. The idea of a cool breeze or wind was, however, a common metaphor for the onset of the disease: the Hippocratic text *On Breaths* attributed the onset of epileptic attacks to the winds and vapours moving through the body.[60] There is further evidence that the terminology adopted by the *neaniskos* reflects the language and

---

[58] Temkin (1971), 37.   [59] Arist. *Mu.* 394b and Hp. *Aër.* 6.7.
[60] See the use of πνεῦμα ('breath') and ἀήρ ('air') at Hp. *Flat.* 14, where their ability to mix with, and cool, the blood is linked with epilepsy. NB also the common theme of cooling and breaths (φῦσαι) at *Flat.* 12.

phraseology of earlier medical texts. A fragment of Erasistratos describes the symptoms which occur among epileptics in remarkably similar terms: 'a certain cool breeze which travels up about the brain' (αὔρας τινὸς ἀνερχομένης κατὰ τὸν ἐγκέφαλον).[61] The confluence of metaphorical descriptions between case-history and medico-literary tradition could be due to a number of factors involving the circulation of narratives and literature concerning epilepsy throughout elite culture in the second century CE. Nevertheless, it is significant that, in a narrative context in which speaking with clear language for the purposes of teaching and diagnosis is mired in the close relationship between the language of patients and the habitual language of the literary tradition, gaps in patient language are overcome with passages which reflect Greek culture's habitual way of speaking about an experience and its symptoms. The fragmentary story of this patient is translated into clear, effective narrative through the strategic insertion of language already seeded in the discourse. Galen overcomes the gaps in the patient's narrative, fills in the missing information, with the language of the literary tradition.

A second aspect to Galen's engagement with patient narratives is his reaction to patients' misrepresentation of their pain experiences. In his treatise *How One Might Spot a Malingerer*, Galen presents a number of scenarios in which he manages to discover, through the process of discussion and therapy, occasions in which he believes patients to be misrepresenting their pain. This type of discussion is particularly important because, in elaborating how it is that he is able to catch them at their dishonesty, Galen reveals his understanding of the relationship between pain, the psychological and intellectual experiences of being pained, and the individual's engagement with therapy and health care. Put another way, thinking about the ways in which pain is deceitfully narrated leads Galen to reflect on the relationship between narrative, experiences of pain, and the doctor–patient interaction.

The case that I am interested in concerns a slave who, Galen claims, is lying about pain in his knee. The case begins with Galen's didactic assertion that through experience and good fortune it is possible 'to discover those who pretend to suffer pain violently' (εὑρίσκει δὲ καὶ τοὺς ἀλγεῖν προσποιουμένους σφοδρῶς, Gal. *Sim. Morb.* xix.4K): as is

---

[61] Erasistratos Frag. 293 (Garafalo). NB also the use of ἀνέρχεσθαι ('go up') at Hp. *Flat.* 14.

often the case, Galen's account is presented as an example of good practice and a model to follow. The reference to *heuriskein* suggests that Galen sees the process as equivalent to more traditional forms of diagnosis in which he 'discovers' or 'seeks out' the cause of a patient's illnesses. Galen begins by assessing his character and behaviour by asking both the slave's master and other slaves about his condition and personality. He then threatens to apply a number of harsh treatments to the wound, which the patient explicitly begs him not to apply. Finally, he questions the man himself about his pain sensations: '[b]ut when I also asked him what the form of the pain was, he did not answer me immediately, willingly, nor consistently' (ἀλλὰ καὶ τὸ τῆς ὀδύνης εἶδος ἐρωτῶσιν ἡμῖν, ὁποῖόν ἐστιν, οὐκ εὐθέως οὐδ' ἑτοίμως οὐδ' ἑαυτῷ συμφώνως ἀπεκρίνατο, Gal. Sim. Morb. xix.5K). Galen's request to know 'the form of pain' immediately returns readers to the ways in which Galen and others diagnosed pain on the basis of graphing the *eidos* of a particular symptom against their understanding of the anatomy of the body. Galen's assertion that the patient did not answer immediately, willingly, or consistently reveals his methods for evaluating patient speech. Galen asks questions that aim at facilitating diagnosis by revealing the type of pain. The failure to produce this information in the way that Galen thinks it should be supplied reveals (or at least helps to reveal) that the patient's claimed perceptions are not genuine. In the ensuing lines, Galen offers the patient a placebo and the patient reports that this drug has eased, and then removed, his pain. It may be, of course, that Galen is quite correct in his assertion that the patient is not being honest. The falsity of the patient's claims are, however, less interesting than Galen's strategy for revealing them. The failure to speak as Galen believes one should reveals deceit. Language that does not fit with Galen's expectations or understanding of the ways in which the experience should be communicated results only in the moral and ethical rejection of the patient and the validity of his reported condition.

In this case, Galen is able to make these interpretative leaps because of his assumptions about people's reaction to pain. There are, he claims, certain physiological signs, such as pallor and changes in pulse, which attest to real pain. Importantly, people also react to the possibilities of medical treatment in certain ways:

ἔτι δὲ ἐὰν μὲν σφοδρῶς ὀδυνῶνται, πᾶν ὑπομένειν ἕτοιμοι γίνονται βοήθημα καὶ πρότερον αὐτοὶ παρακαλοῦσι τοὺς ἰατρούς, ὅ τί περ ἂν βουληθεῖεν, πράττειν ἕνεκα τοῦ θεραπευθῆναι τὸ πάθος. ἐὰν δὲ μετρίως ἢ μηδ' ὅλως ὀδυνῶνται, τὰ τοιαῦτα τῶν βοηθημάτων ἀποδιδράσκουσιν οὔτ' ἀσιτίας μακρὰς ὑπομένοντες οὔτε δριμέων φαρμάκων προσαγωγήν, ἃ χρὴ λέγειν ἡμᾶς αὐτοῖς ὡς ἰασόμενα μόνα τὰς τοιαύτας διαθέσεις, ἡνίκα φασὶν ὀδυνᾶσθαι σφοδρῶς, καὶ πρὸς τούτοις ἐκτομὰς καὶ καύσεις καὶ παντὸς ἀποχὴν πόματός τε καὶ ἐδέσματος, οὗπερ ἂν ἴδωμεν αὐτοὺς ἡττημένους.

And if they are pained violently, they are willing to endure every assistance, and they call eagerly upon the doctor to do on account of the therapy of the condition whatever might be able to help. If they are pained to a moderate degree or not at all, they flee such helpful things, enduring neither lengthy fasting nor the application of bitter drugs which, it is necessary for us to tell them, will alone heal these types of conditions, when they claim to be pained violently, and in addition to these, amputations and burnings, and ligatures and bonds, on account of which we might see them controlled.

Gal. *Sim. Morb.* xix.6K

Galen's passage is fascinating on a number of levels. The reference to those who will not endure certain forms of pain returns us to the commonly recognized point that medical treatment in the ancient world was itself often a cause of pain. The choice of ἀποδιδράσκουσιν (which I translated as 'they flee') recalls Aretaios of Kappodokia's similar description of some patients who scarper at the prospect of a painful regimen.[62] Yet there could be no greater contrast with Aretaios' description in his *prooimion* to *On the Causes and Signs of Chronic Diseases*. In that context, harsh therapy and the extreme experiences of patients motivated the doctor to engage sympathetically with the patient in the confrontation of disease. In Galen's hands, the suggestion is driven towards an evaluation of the truth content of patients' claims. Readiness to undergo prolonged painful treatment reveals that patients' experiences might be genuine; alternative reactions reveal something else. Galen's distinction straitjackets patient behaviour into a framework focused on evaluating their genuineness, rather than engaging explicitly with the possibility of how the patient might feel about certain events, perceptions, or therapeutic activities. There is much in this passage that suggests a particularly combative relationship between doctor and patient. In the first instance, the constant reference to doctors as 'us' appears to widen any emotive or

---

[62] Aret. *SD.* iii.1.

intellectual gaps that exist between the two. More significantly, the description turns on a particularly forceful effort of narrative control on the part of the doctor: when patients say that they suffer pain violently, the doctor must lie to them about the prospect for treatment. This is to be done so that 'we might see them controlled' (ἴδωμεν αὐτοὺς ἡττημένους). This scenario is controlled and managed by Galen's forceful relationship with the patient, developed through (his own) use of deceitful language.

The third aspect of Galen's diagnostic practice which I want to discuss concerns the patient's past experiences and their narration. It is necessary, he claims in *On Affected Parts*, 'to examine everything closely' (πάντ' ἐπισκέψασθαι), including 'both present symptoms and those which occurred before' (τά τε παρόντα καὶ τὰ προγεγονότα συμπτώματα, viii.8K).[63] This process of learning about what has passed involves questioning not only the patient, but those around him.[64] Galen's diagnostic practice includes, on this level, an interest in the stories that patients might tell about their past. Rather than the patient narrating their past experiences on their own terms in a manner which allows them to elaborate the significance of their own experiences, Galen controls the relationship between narration and past events very closely.

In one particular instance, after viewing a patient, Galen immediately enquires about the individual's previous experiences: 'once I had examined him, I asked about everything that had happened previously' (ἐγὼ θεασάμενος αὐτὸν ἠρώτων τε τὰ προγεγονότα πάντα, *Loc. Aff.* viii.213K). The use of ἐρωτᾶν reflects a formula used throughout Galen's corpus to enquire about his patients' lifestyles, earlier medical treatments, or their illness histories. In this case, the story is limited to those details of the patient that recount how he hit the upper part of his back when he fell from a chariot and that this contusion was then immediately treated by other doctors; this treatment proved unsuccessful (in Galen's account) because the doctors

---

[63] For the importance of questioning the patient, see the work of Rufus of Ephesos: Ruf. Eph. *Quaest. Med.* 1 (Gärtner). The idea of asking questions of the patient was well established within the case-history genre. I have been very much influenced in my reading of these processes of questioning by the study of modern clinical case-histories in Hunter (1991) and Mattingly and Garro (2000).

[64] Gal. *Loc. Aff.* viii.8K: ὅσα δ' ἔμπροσθεν ἐγένετο διαπυνθανόμενον οὐ τοῦ κάμνοντος μόνον, ἀλλὰ καὶ τῶν οἰκείων ('such things which arose before can be discovered not only from the patient, but also from those who live with him').

did not have sufficient knowledge of the anatomy of the nerves, which he has learnt from Eudemos and Herophilos (*Loc. Aff.* viii.212–4K). Galen's decision to include the phrase 'about everything that had happened previously' is particularly telling in this context. It suggests the narration of a much larger story than that which is included in the case-history account in Galen's text. Medical anthropologists, as I discussed in Chapter 1, see such situations as ones in which patients have the opportunity to define the meaning of illness on their own personal terms. Yet, in this case, the process of diagnostic recognition involves Galen's considerable editorial control over this narrative: what emerges from this case-history is less an expansive subjective (or personalized) account of experiences and more a shaped, telling narrative or structure that moulds the account (and the experiences) to the requirements of diagnosis. I do not say this to suggest that Galen uses the process of close questioning to deny or downplay experience, but rather that experience is moulded to fit its role within the diagnosis and the narrative arc of his text.

Much earlier in *On Affected Parts,* Galen recounts a similar scenario. The patient comes to Galen with a loss of sensation in his hand which has, up to this point, remained resistant to various treatments over the last thirty days.[65] This example of diagnosis has two important parts. In the first half, Galen attempts to discover the cause of the patient's problems through a structured process of close questioning of the patient and others around him. Galen begins by asking (ἠρώτησα) the patient's former doctor what medicaments he had applied; when he discovered (εὗρον) that they were appropriate, he sought (ἐζήτουν) the cause of their ineffectiveness by asking about his previous symptoms (ἠρώτων τε τὰ προηγησάμενα συμπτώματα); when the patient tells him that he did not have 'inflammation' (φλεγμονή), 'a chill' (ψῦξις), nor that he suffered a 'blow' (πληγή), Galen was 'amazed' by his answer and consequently 'asked again' (θαυμάζων πάλιν ἠρόμην) if he had been struck on any part of his body; finally, 'when he told [Galen] that [he had been struck] on the top of his back, [Galen] at once asked him how and where the blow had occurred' (ἐν ἀρχῇ δὲ τοῦ μεταφρένου πληγῆναι φάσκοντος αὖθις ἠρόμην, ὅπως τε καὶ ὁπότ᾽ ἐπλήγη, *Loc. Aff.* viii.57K). Galen's narrative presents the doctor as a type of medical sleuth seeking out the answers to his

---

[65] Gal. *Loc. Aff.* viii.56–7K.

present situation in the past experiences of the patient. What is interesting about this case is the relationship between the depth of enquiry and the questions which elicit information from the subject. Galen's questions control the information and the order of its release; one answer induces the next question by eliminating diagnostic possibilities and thus driving the search for more information; the patient is allowed to proceed to the next level of description only because his answers have failed to provide diagnostic satisfaction or because they amaze Galen. The patient's previous experiences contribute to the recognition of his current problems, in this situation, but they do so only through the structured arrangement of their narration. Perhaps the easiest way to conceptualize Galen's strategy is to imagine what could have been if he had allowed the patient to engage in a broader narrative of all of his past experiences: if the patient had related his fall from his chariot initially, would Galen's investigative technique have proceeded along the same lines? Galen's method for investigating the past experiences of the patient offers a way of structuring historical narrative so that its information can be incorporated into the process of medical recognition at the appropriate moment.

This particular instance is not explicitly about pain, but it does show how Galen shoehorns what could be expansive personal accounts of illness into a very specific delineation of what is relevant and what he feels is significant within the patient's history. As the case develops, Galen's strategy evolves to include a slightly different element which stresses the narrative fit between recounting past experiences and Galen's anatomical knowledge of the body. After hearing that the patient had fallen from the chariot onto the upper part of his back, Galen explains how he came to his conclusions about the patient's condition:

καὶ μέντοι καὶ ἀποκρινομένου . . . ἐτεκμηράμην ἐν τῇ πρώτῃ τοῦ μετὰ τὸν ἕβδομον σπόνδυλον νεύρου διεκπτώσει μόριόν τι φλεγμῆναν ἐπὶ τῇ πληγῇ σκιρώδη διάθεσιν ἐσχηκέναι. τοῦτο δ᾽ ἐνόησα μεμαθηκὼς διὰ τῆς ἀνατομῆς, ὅτι τὰ νεῦρα κατὰ περιγραφὴν μὲν ἰδίαν, ὡς αἱ φλέβες, ἐκφυόμενα φαίνονται, καὶ δόξαις ἂν ἀκριβῶς ἓν ἕκαστον αὐτῶν ὑπάρχειν, ὥσπερ καὶ τὴν φλέβα·

And when this had been determined, . . . I reckoned a certain part of the nerve at the first starting point at the seventh vertebra, having been inflamed by the blow, had become calloused. I knew this, since I had learnt through anatomy that the nerves appear to grow out in a particular circumference, just like veins, and you would know precisely where each one of them begins, just like the veins.

Gal. *Loc. Aff.* viii.57K

Galen's ability to determine what the affected parts of the body are—to diagnose and eventually treat the patient—is dependent upon the information supplied by the patient's narrative—note the genitive absolute ἀποκριναμένου. But his description of the interpretive process privileges the importance of the understanding of the body's nature: the participle μεμαθηκὼς implies, arguably, a causal relationship between understanding the significance of the patient's narrative and medical theory. Galen's technique attributes a critical role to the patient's account of his symptoms. Diagnosis is ultimately built on a constructed link between the way that the body is described by the patient and Galen's rational knowledge of the *sōma*. In so doing, Galen creates the impression that the patient's language has led to the discovery of the physical ailment. Yet, for all this focus on the patient's language, it is also clear that for the patient's story to be understood—to be given significance and meaning—within the clinical scenario, it must be submitted to, and be made to accord with, Galen's theoretical understanding of the body. Certain answers that the patient provided 'amaze' Galen because they do not fit with his anatomically-driven assumptions about the body; diagnosis takes place when a fit is created between what Galen knows of the body and the patient's descriptions, their account of their experiences and perceptions. Galen's structuring and ordering of the patient's language and narrative, his *diēgēsis*, ensures that there is never an innocent patient-based description of their pain experiences or illness experiences.

We can see that, like Aretaios, Galen is particularly interested in how a doctor and patient relate to each other throughout the diagnostic engagement. It is clear, however, that Galen's view of the relationship is far more combative than that of Aretaios. Whereas Aretaios emphasized both the impact of pain on the emotional state of the individual and the doctor's sympathetic or empathetic engagement with the individual's experience, Galen approaches the situation in robustly agonistic terms: the impact of pain on the individual is something to be closely controlled and managed through Galen's control of language and ability to manage, interpret, and shape patients' experiences. Aretaios and Galen demonstrate different approaches to the pain. But both authors are systematically interested in, feel they need to negotiate, the anatomical perception and the emotional/psychological experience of it. The discursive battleground between Aretaios and Galen is how one manages those varying elements of the physiological experience. That matters because of its capacity to help each doctor construct their discursive and medical authority, as well as establish the boundaries of pain experience.

4

Diagnosis and Pain

A central objective of this chapter has been to elaborate the way that pain and diagnosis interact in Imperial medicine. Pain's centrality to diagnosis (and the experience of disease) is recognizable in the earliest examples of Greek medical writing. The relationship takes on a particular form, however, in the specific cultural conditions of the Imperial period. Diagnosis, as it is represented by different doctors, involves attending not only to the realities of the body and its structure, and the nature of various diseases, but also engaging closely with the patient. Diagnosis is continually represented as an interpersonal process. It is in this context that pain takes on a range of meanings and is treated in a variety of ways.

Diagnosis was the *sine qua non* of rational medical practice. In the first instance, diagnosing the body involved attending to the ways in which the structure and anatomy of the body underpins the perception of certain kinds of pain types and symptoms. Both Aretaios and Galen, interestingly, suggest that the broad consistencies of anatomy ensure that pain symptoms are consistent across different individuals: all other factors being equal, we all perceive the same types of pain in the same ways.

Diagnosis also involved engaging with the ways in which patients described their symptoms. Although it is often an undiscussed element of ancient diagnosis, the process of talking to, and with, patients about their pain perception was a vitally important part of the diagnostic process. That process allowed not only pain symptoms to be differentiated and located within the various spaces of the body, but the different types of disease to be recognized and their progression or evolution tracked. This interest in language constituted an important element of linguistic thought in the Imperial period. Doctors theorized a particularly intricate relationship between the body and language: patient terminology and descriptions of symptoms could indicate hidden internal states because of an assumed connection between pain, language, and the anatomy of the body. It underpinned medical ideas about the way in which a doctor and patient should interact in the context of a clinical scenario. Finally, it underpinned questions about what constituted effective and legitimate language within clinical scenarios: what types of linguistic register allow for effective recognition of pain? And, how does certain terminology effectively share or socialize pain perceptions between the pained individual and the other? The process of diagnosis (and, in some cases treatment) was also important for the ways in which a doctor and patient navigated the social and affective impact of pain. How one feels, in this context, about pain, how one navigates its significance for one's own life matters. Indeed, it appears that navigating the broader ramifications of being in pain is one challenge and an important polemical fault line throughout the first three centuries CE.

Part 2

Representing Pain

5

Refiguring Pain Symptoms

So far, I have been tracing the way in which pain experience was thought about in some key texts of rational medicine. In the next two parts of this book, I investigate how pain is elaborated in different cultural contexts: in Part 2, I turn to the treatment of pain in a number of rhetorical, dramatic, and philosophical texts from across the first two centuries CE; in Part 3, I will focus on the treatment of pain in a culture of pictorial description and viewing. My objective, in Part 2, is to trace the ways in which the approach to pain which developed in Imperial medicine are (re)formulated in different contexts. My primary focus is on Lucian's *Podagra*, Plutarch's *That It Is Not Possible to Live According to Epikouros,* and the *Sacred Tales* of Ailios Aristeides. All these texts bring to bear on the question of pain some of the assumptions and ideas that were in play in a medical context. Importantly, however, their rhetorical, literary, and philosophical objectives ensure that this view of pain is developed in a number of telling directions. That development can be traced along three different axes: they reformulate the anatomical approach to pain symptoms, combining this understanding with a sense of physical hardship and difficulty; they underscore this broader notion of pain's impact on the individual's life, their social and affective connections with others; and, in so doing, they construct particular ways of presenting the pain-perceiver, which draw on and manipulate the status of the pained as a quasi-heroic figure and a valuable member of the community.

The diverse range of texts immediately invites questions about the ways in which they operate as part of coherent cultural discourse. Ailios Aristeides' rhetorical texts draw connections with epic, religious forms of writing, and, as we shall see, the Greek romance. Other texts are no less complicated. *Podagra* engages with tragedy at both a textual and thematic level, new and old Comedy, and other forms of literature more common in the Imperial context, such as adoxography and parody.[1] Plutarch's *That It Is Not Possible to Live According to Epikouros* is a piece of polemically driven Platonic philosophy. Their interest in pain, consequently, is expressed through different tropes and directed towards different objectives. As is well known, Aristeides' *Sacred Tales*' treatment of pain is inseparable from his interest in the power and authority of his personal rhetorical and quasi-epic voice, as well as his aretological objective of honouring and thanking his divine protector and healer, Asklepios; Lucian, in contrast, represents the experience of pain through the humourous (and ultimately parodic) treatment of a literary form synonymous with the depiction of mortal suffering and hardship. Despite these differences, however, these texts point to a common interest in the way in which pain might be negotiated, how the pained individual navigates their experience, and how they might relate to those around them.

The diverse generic and literary traditions in which these texts embed themselves are an important interpretive crux of this investigation. These texts recall, quote, and allude to literary forms that are concerned with pain, hardship, and its endurance or negotiation, especially Attic tragedy and epic. This is not the place to rehearse the complex and vast history of the reception of these two genres in Imperial Greek culture.[2] What does interest me, however, is their importance for the ways in which individuals understood and navigated experience. Pelling has suggested that tragedy, for instance, was bound up with Greek culture's habitual ways of thinking. On Pelling's reading, the use of tragic themes, motifs, and texts in the literature of the Imperial period is not a process of 'generic enrichment', but is rather reflective of the way in which this society and its individuals thought about the world.[3] For these writers, the representation of pain experience is bound up with the reception of this literature.

---

[1] For the connection with tragedy, see Karavas (2005), 235–333; for its status as an *adoxon*, Anderson (1979a), 150. For further discussion, see Whitmarsh (2013), 182–5.
[2] For the reception of Homer, see Kindstrand (1973), who is seminal, along with other important studies in Kim (2010), Zeitlin (2001), and Hunter (2004). For the reception of tragedy, I have been very much influenced by a number of studies on individual authors. For Lucian: Karavas (2005); for Plutarch: Papadi (2007) and Pelling (2016). For the reception of Philoktetes, see Bowersock (1994), 55–76.
[3] Pelling (2016), 114–16.

1. REWRITING PAIN SYMPTOMS

The connection with tragic and epic works and themes helps to broaden the notion of pain that is found in medical contexts. Plutarch, Lucian, and Aristeides start from a conception of pain that is connected with medical visions of illness and painful perception. This is particularly true in terms of the representation of gout and other 'arthritic' conditions, but also applies to the more nebulous (and undefinable?) illnesses described by Ailios Aristeides in the *Sacred Tales*. Across these texts, the terminology for pain remains remarkably consistent—all three authors use medical terminology for different types of symptoms and they adopt metaphors familiar from medical literature for different perceptions of pain. They link the perception of symptoms with the fundamental structure of the human body. They, like medical writers discussed in Part 1, ask readers to gaze at, and inside, the pained *sōma*.

This anatomical vision of pain is, however, consistently linked with broader understandings of, and approaches to, it inherited from other cultural and literary traditions. In the hands of these writers, pain is increasingly treated as a hardship or trial to be endured and navigated. Pain is caused both by certain processes within the body and by the individual's (wrong-headed) confrontation with the gods. The frameworks for understanding its meaning and importance for the individual's life are developed in connection with concepts of one's endurance and perseverance in the face of long-term hardship and difficulty. Of course, there are times in strictly medical literature when the description of pain appears to draw on ideas from other literary traditions, especially tragedy, and figures pain experience in terms of 'disaster' (*sumphora*) or some 'evil' (*kakon*).[4] In this context, however, the implications of this language are given far greater and more explicit emphasis than they are in medical writing. In moving from a focus on bodily anatomy to a broader sense of pain, hardship, and endurance, these texts situate themselves in a context that connects the works of rational medicine with the reception of tragedy and epic, and the types of narrative of hardship and 'grim experiences' (*ta skuthrōpa*) that define the Greco-Roman

---

[4] Disaster (*sumphora*): e.g. Aret. SA. i.6.8.6–9.7. Evil (*kakon*): e.g. Aret. SA. ii. 2.18.1–7.

romances.[5] This is one moment when pain perception and symptoms move close to what some scholars have designated as 'suffering'.

There are three immediate implications to this broadening of the sense of pain: that which is related to the heroism of the pain-perceiver, that which is related to their relationships with others, and that which is related to the religious aspects of pain experience. All of the authors discussed in Chapters 6 and 7 frame their treatment of the individual's pain perceptions against tragic or epic heroes. I showed, in Chapter 2, that Aretaios saw the patient as a type of heroic individual who needed to be 'stout-hearted' (*alkimos*) and show endurance in the face of disease.[6] In Galen, this lionization of the patient was less emphatic, but was still present at some points. The suggestion that some patients' experiences of pain are defined by their 'weakness of soul' (*malakia tēs psukhēs*) and others by their 'greatness of soul' (*megalapsukhia*) connects the experience of pain and management of therapy with the psychological and moral qualities with which the individual confronts it.[7] That heroic quality and ascription of social value to certain patients is given greater emphasis in this context through the explicit and repeated engagements with paradigms of pain experience and endurance.

This emphasis on the heroic aspect of the pain-perceiver's status is allied to the interest in various heroic figures throughout the Imperial period. As we shall see (in both Part 2 and Part 3), different figures drawn from mythic and epic, historical and tragic, and iconographic traditions play an important role in providing context for an individual's navigation and understanding of pain and the status of the pain-perceiver. Within this general context, the figures of Odysseus and Philoktetes are particularly important. Odysseus, as is well known, has a conspicuous influence on Imperial literature in a number of different ways, especially in relation to his wanderings and his capacity for deceitful speech.[8] In terms of his relevance for suffering and endurance, it is worth pointing out that Odysseus—as he is presented in the *Odyssey*—does not perceive physical pain and negotiate it in the way that other heroic figures from the literary canon do. More

---

[5] For the representation of pain in the novels: Chariton viii.1.4 for one (famous) example of *skuthrōpos*. On this issue, see König (2008).
[6] Aret. *SA*. ii.2.17.7–11.   [7] Gal. *Loc. Aff.* viii.88–89K.
[8] For deceitful speech, see below, n. 11. For his status as a paradigmatic wanderer: Montiglio (2005).

commonly, he is seen in this context as a figure who navigates the emotional, psychological, and physical complications of a life of hardship and woe; he is a man that is long-suffering on the basis of his physical difficulties, his troubles (*kēdea*). Odysseus, in this context, operates as a vehicle for discussing questions of extended hardship and physical difficulty, what it means to be 'long-suffering'. Philoktetes is, of course, represented in the number of tragedies—both Roman and Greek—and is the subject of a considerable amount of artistic representation and poetic and literary output.[9] Each of these representations presents Philoktetes' pain in slightly different terms: there is no one model of Philoktetes or his pain for writers of this period to engage with. What is clear is that he becomes a figure, in this context, for exploring the intensity, longevity, and the loneliness of the experience of pain. By picking and choosing certain aspects of these complex multilayered traditions, these texts are able to explore different aspects of the pain experience.

A second major implication of the representation of pain in this context concerns the ways in which the perception intersects with language. This interest is embedded in a general concern with tragic and epic language and narrative form. Lucian and Aristeides continually ask questions about what it means to express pain in a particular literary or linguistic form. For Lucian, the use of tragic forms of language—especially the expressions for distress, such as the groan or wail—helps to position both the individual's experience of pain and to shape the reactions of readers. Aristeides interrogates whether or not the epic mode of narration or sacred, mystical registers are a more appropriate, effective, or compelling form to communicate pain. How do these different kinds of linguistic registers or narrative forms help to build relationships by facilitating understanding or other affective connections between those who feel pain and others? What does it mean, in other words, to tell a (painful?) story about pain?

This interest in language is also explored through the use of Philoktetes and Odysseus. These two heroes are, in themselves, famous for their capacity to manipulate langauge and speech. Importantly, for the purposes of this argument, they are also figures who

---

[9] Bowersock (1994), 55–76 is excellent for the collection of further material on this subject. Two texts in his reception which are not discussed in Part 2 are D. Chrys. 52 and 59. There seems to be little explicit discussion of the theme of pain in these two texts.

rehearse the complex relationship between pain and language. I have already shown how Philoktetes' screams have continued to operate as a paradigm of pain's capacity to destroy language.[10] Odysseus is famous for his capacity for sophistic speech, for *doloi*, and for deceitful communication.[11] As I shall show, both figures are used to help explore how pain affects and effects the language of the pain-perceiver. They are also used, however, to explore the effects of painful stories on others. Philoktetes and Odysseus dramatize the questions of language's capacity to socialize pain perceptions and share pain experience.

This concern with language leads me to my third point: how the pained individual interacts with the other. In the medical context, I traced the pain experience by unpacking the representation of a very specific relationship between the ill individual and the other. In most instances, that relationship between doctor and patient was largely internal to the texts being discussed. In this instance, this sense of interpersonal relationship is presented in a more complex way. The representational process combines multiple types of intra-diegetic relationships as well as extra-diegetic ones. These texts often represent relationships between the pain-perceiver and others within the text. At this level, they dramatize the linguistic, emotional and psychological, and cognitive relationships between those in pain and those who engage with them. At the same time, they speak to a relationship between the pain-perceiver and external other: the reader or listener. Readers of these texts are constantly asked to develop intellectual and affective reactions to the pain perceptions, the pained individuals, and the types of internal relationships represented in these texts. Consequently, authors allow readers outside the text to navigate and then self-consciously to question their viewing or reading position. Pain experience is caught between the ways in which these different relationships and reactions are constructed and deconstructed in these texts.

This relationship with the reader—the external other—inflects a very specific Imperial-period interest in the way that the reader is distanced from the subject matter discussed in various media. An important part of this is the way in which the process of representing

---

[10] See Introduction (text to nn. 1–5 and n. 10). See also: Scarry (1985), 5–10. For the importance of the scream in the ancient reception of Philoktetes: Bowersock (1994), 55–75.

[11] The *locus classicus* is, of course, Hom. *Od.* 9.19–20. For his capacity for sophistic speech: S. *Ph*. For Imperial treatment of his lying, see, e.g., Luc. *VH.* 3.

pain proceeds through known or recognizable representational strategies, familiar literary forms, and well-troped literary *clichés*. Readers are asked to negotiate their relationship with the pain felt by different individuals through their recognition of the experience and the meanings carried by different forms of representation. Allusions to tragedy or epic, for instance, help to provide contexts which shape readers' various intellectual and affective responses to pain. They are also asked to do so in a manner that must be entirely conscious of the troped, *clichéd* nature of particular representational forms. The relationship of the external reader is constantly thought about in terms of these two interlocking levels of engagement with the material. This second level, in particular, is characteristic of the Imperial period's interest in the endless process of exposing the reader to, and distancing him or her from, the subject matter of representation. The relationships between the pain, pained, and other are developed through this practice of a self-conscious and self-aware act of distancing; imagining another's pain, and navigating the interpersonal and affective aspects of pain experience, requires negotiating this problematic relationship between the subject matter, medium, and other.

A final implication of this approach to pain experience is the importance of religious belief and practice in shaping the individual's negotiation of pain. It is abundantly clear that there existed no hard division between the fields of medicine and religion throughout the ancient world. Critics have consistently pointed to the osmosis between these two areas of activity and belief, especially in relation to religious forms of healing and health care.[12] This interaction is, perhaps, especially clear in cultural settings such as healing sanctuaries, where both medical professionals and lay individuals engaged with religiously-driven health care. As I mentioned in Chapter 1, votive offerings, as well as literary and epigraphic testimonies to the healing god Asklepios, attest to the importance of the divine in alleviating pain symptoms and curing painful conditions.[13] What interests me in this context, however, is the way in which religious practice shapes both the

---

[12] For the relationship between medicine and religion, see, e.g., Israelowich (2012), chapters 2–3 and (2015), chapter 1. Petsalis-Diomidis (2005) and (2010) for specific discussions of Ailios Aristeides. For healing-cult votives, see Edelstein (1967) and Chaniotis (1995).

[13] See Chapter 1 (n. 3 with corresponding text).

language of pain and the types of relationship that individuals foster. If religious experience provides one context for thinking about pain experience, then that context inflects the types of connections that people make with other pain-perceivers and those who are not pained. Lucian and Aristeides, in particular, underscore the ways in which pain facilitates initiation into, and participation in, a religious cult or practice. Religious activity operates as a way into certain kinds of relationships with communities of other sufferers on the basis of joint or shared experience.

6

Sore Feet and Tragedy in Plutarch and Lucian

Let us turn to some of the ways in which pain was rewritten in two literary contexts from the Imperial period. I focus on two very different types of text. The first, *That It Is Not Possible to Live According to Epikouros*, is a philosophical tract by Plutarch of Khaironea and is specifically designed to argue against different aspects of Epicurean doctrine. The second, *Podagra*, is a comical paratragic drama by the author Lucian of Samosata which pokes fun at those who suffer gout. In both of these contexts, the discussion of pain is incorporated into agenda which extend beyond the discussion of physical symptoms. Nevertheless, pain plays an important role in both of the texts. The pain symptoms that the individual feels are presented in this context in a range of different ways. Symptoms that have much in common with contemporary (or near-contemporary) medical writing are reformulated within and against tragic and heroic frameworks. As a consequence, what pain means for the individual—its impact on their life and understanding of their body—and the positioning of the sufferer and their experience of pain is renegotiated.

These two representations tap into, I hold, the significance of gout, or *podagra*, in the ancient world generally and the Imperial period specifically. The condition is a ubiquitous feature of the medical and literary landscape of the second and third centuries CE. Rufus of Ephesos composed a (now lost) Greek treatise on the condition.[1]

---

[1] Ruf. Eph. *de Podagra* (Daremberg); it is preserved through a Latin translation in Daremberg. For a brief (and superficial) survey of the different ancient treatments of gout, including that of Rufus of Ephesos, see Gritzalis, Karamanou, and Androutsos (2011).

Similarly, Aretaios of Kappodokia's theories of pain were elaborated most explicitly in the context of an analysis of arthritis, but also in discussion of gout in different joints and ligaments of the body.[2] Gout, also, was a subject for discussion outside strictly medical literature. Fronto's and Marcus Aurelius' letters continually discuss their various physical ailments, many of which correspond to gout.[3] Lucian's *Podagra* is only one example of a number of comedic works written about this condition. The similar text, *Swift Foot*, which is attributed to Lucian, but probably written by a later author, takes up the same theme.[4] There is also considerable epigraphic evidence for individuals who sought cures for the gout from across the eastern Mediterranean.[5] In focusing on gout, these two writers take up, from a literary perspective, an experience which was remarkably common across the ancient world.

1. PLUTARCH, PAIN, AND THE FRAGILE BODY

In the opening lines of his treatise, *That It Is Not Possible to Live According to Epikouros*, Plutarch takes issue with the Epicurean position that pleasure is the highest good. It is wrong-headed, he holds, because they place their faith in a body which is profoundly susceptible to pain, which lets in pleasure through a 'few entrances', but allows entrance to pain through every part:

ποία γὰρ ἡδονὴ περὶ ἄρθρα καὶ νεῦρα καὶ πόδας καὶ χεῖρας, οἷς ἐνοικίζεται τὰ δεινὰ πάθη καὶ σχέτλια, ποδαγρικὰ καὶ ῥευματικὰ καὶ φαγεδαινικὰ καὶ διαβρώσεις καὶ ἀποσήψεις;

For how much pleasure is found in the joints, the tendons, the feet, and the hands, in which live terrible and wretched affections—gout, rheumatism, ulcers, things which consume the flesh, and things which make it rot?

Plut. *Non Posse.* 1087e

---

[2] Aret. *SD.* ii.12.
[3] On Fronto's gout, see Gel. 2.26.1; cf. Fronto *Amic.* 20, 34, 50.
[4] Anderson (1979a), 149 n. 1 and Karavas (2005), 237–9 on the question of the authenticity of these two works. For further literary treatments: *AP.* xi.414.
[5] *IG* IV. 1.122.XLIII (fourth century BCE from Epidauros) and *IG* II. 4514 (second century CE from Athens).

And, moments later, he continues to present the body in a stark light:

οὐκ ὀλισθηρὰ γὰρ ἀλγηδὼν[6] οὐδὲ ἕτερα τοιαῦτα κινοῦσα καὶ γαργαλίζουσα τοῦ σώματος· ἀλλ' ὥσπερ τὸ τῆς μηδικῆς σπέρμα πολυκαμπὲς καὶ σκαληνὸν ἐμφύεται τῇ γῇ καὶ διαμένει πολὺν χρόνον ὑπὸ τραχύτητος, οὕτως ὁ πόνος ἄγκιστρα καὶ ῥίζας διασπείρων καὶ συμπλεκόμενος τῇ σαρκὶ καὶ παραμένων οὐχ ἡμέρας οὐδὲ νύκτας μόνον ἀλλὰ καὶ ὥρας ἐτῶν ἐνίοις καὶ περιόδους ὀλυμπιακὰς μόλις ὑπ' ἄλλων πόνων ὥσπερ ἥλων σφοδροτέρων ἐκκρουόμενος ἀπαλλάττεται.

For there is nothing smooth in pain, nor in moving or tickling does it provide other such things for the body. Just as the seed of lucerne, which has many twists and is rough, is planted in the ground and remains there a long time because of its roughness, in this way pain, dispersing and entwining its hooks and roots in the flesh also remains there not for days or nights only, but in some instances even seasons of the year and Olympiads and is barely released by other pains, as when the stud is driven in more violently.

Plut. *Non Posse*. 1088a

Plutarch's passage is designed to defeat specific points of Epicurean doctrine about the duration of pain and its intensity in relation to pleasure. The vision of physical pain that he develops has close links, at the same time, with medical treatments of the condition of gout and other arthritic diseases. The presence of pain in the body's internal structures—the nerves, the joints, and the hands—recalls descriptions of gout in Aretaios and other medically-orientated writers.[7] Plutarch's discussion, however, also takes us further into the types of anatomical experience of pain that I documented in Chapters 2 and 3. The comparison between pain and the seed of lucerne, which plants itself inside the ground and remains 'because of its roughness' (ὑπὸ τραχύτητος), forces the reader to imagine pain's course through the internal spaces of the body: pain, like the plant, spreads its roots and hooks, dispersing through the unseen cavities of the body. It is no accident that Plutarch applies to the *comparandum* for pain the very term (τραχύς) that stands at the heart of philosophical and medical discussions of

---

[6] The text at this point appears to be irredeemably corrupt: Westman's 1959 Teubner edition reads ὀλισθῆ...ἀλγηδὼν. I follow Einarson and De Lacy's Loeb edition of 1959 in reading Emperius' emendation of the manuscript X on the basis of the connections with the surrounding text. In other instances in this passage, I follow the Teubner as read. For further references to the quality of slipperiness, see Plut. *Quaest. Conviv.* 699b for its connection with the quality of *trakhutēs*.

[7] Aret. *SD*. iv.12.1.1–2.

pain sensation. This theme of imagining the path of pain's metaphorical roots in the body is reiterated moments later when he turns to the question of pain's removal. Pain, according to Plutarch, is often only driven out by more extreme pains. This account returns readers to the ways in which Aretaios and Galen described the act of treatment as painful: for those writers, too, pain required removal through the application of greater, more painful cures.

If Plutarch's passage starts from a highly medical view of pain symptoms, it also transforms that vision into a broader sense of hardship. The initial suggestion that the body's afflictions are 'terrible and wretched' (δεινὰ καὶ σχέτλια) frames the entire presentation in metaphorical terms. Arguably, it links specific symptoms with a broader moral view of the body's sufferings and hardship because it speaks to the ways in which the pained individual might be conceptualized: δεινός can be used to describe particularly difficult pains, but both terms also carry a significant amount of moral weight. The sense of 'miserable' or 'wretched' contained in σχέτλιος is certainly evocative of a physical, social, and moral condition—it is often linked with tragic or heroic figures who are either morally wretched or contemptuous.[8] At the same time, it also refers to those who have been rendered particularly wretched by their experience of pain and hardship.[9]

The suggestion of its chronic nature—that in some cases it extends beyond Olympiads—moves the description of precise medical symptoms into a broader understanding of what pain means for the life of the individual. 'Chronic' and 'acute' are typical categories for understanding both conditions and their attendant symptoms throughout ancient medicine.[10] Plutarch's vision of pain is also, in part, defined by the polemical nature of the treatise. Plutarch's insistence on the length of pain in this context is no doubt energized by his desire not only to contrast pain with the feeling of pleasure, which he claims is temporary and fleeting, but to emphasize that intense pains are often permanent and constitute long-standing states of the body. There is little doubt that such a sentiment is designed to counter directly the Epicurean assumption that pain is either short-lived, when it is extreme, or insignificant if it lasts a long time. Plutarch's answer to

---

[8] S. Ph. 369 and 930 for reference to those who are morally wretched. Cf. LSJ s.v. σχέτλιος i3 for the moral and degrading implications of the term.
[9] E. Hec. 783, where Hecuba is 'wretched because of her hardships' (ponōn).
[10] Laskaris (2002) and Drabkin (1950).

this point is twofold. The problem with the Epicurean focus on pleasure, he claims, is that it is both intense and, in many cases, long-lived. Plutarch's polemical position is familiar from other philosophical texts which deal with this aspect of Epicurean thought, such as Cicero's *On Ends* ii.29. What is interesting, however, is how Plutarch's vision of this wretched body, beset by the physical symptoms of pain, figures what pain means for the individual's continuing life. The individual's life, Plutarch argues, is navigated through lengthy, intense bouts of pain because it is linked to a body that is fundamentally susceptible to pains that cannot be easily or quickly removed.

Moments before this presentation of pain's long-term effect on the individual, Plutarch turns to Euripides' presentation of Philoktetes, who offers sufficient testimony (*martus*) to the nature of pain, 'for the snake, he [i.e. Philoktetes] says, has not left, but the terrible shoots from its mouth dwell in and seize my foot' (οὐ γὰρ ὁ δράκων, φησίν, ἀνῆκεν / ἀλλ' ἐνῴκισε δεινὴν στομάτων ἔκφυσιν, ποδὸς λαβεῖν, *Non Posse*. 1087f). The permanence of pain, its ability to find root in the body, and its continuing implications for the individual are emphasized by reference to the heroic figure's own experience. On one level, this quotation of Euripides can be seen to reiterate his broad argument through a poetic quotation. Recourse to Philoktetes and Euripides, here, provides a substantiating poetic paradigm. At the same time, however, there are suggestions that Plutarch's choice of Philoktetes is marked. There is an internal consistency between the vision of the body elaborated by Plutarch and the figure of Philoktetes. Recall the arguably tragic frame to the passage created by the use of *skhetlia* and *deina* and note his references to devouring diseases. Note also the references to the verb 'dwell in' in both the quotation from Euripides and the description of the disease (ἐνοικίζεται and ἐνῴκισε) and the repetition of the adjective *deinos* in both contexts. Philoktetes becomes a model for thinking about a certain kind of life and its connection with a particular type of pained body.

The use of Philoktetes to underscore Plutarch's model of the body and the navigation of long-term pain taps into a widespread interest in the figure of Philoktetes. Bowersock, in particular, has seen this interest in terms of ancient culture's fascination with what he terms 'the wounded saviour'.[11] Bowersock is right to point out that interest

[11] Bowersock (1994).

in Philoktetes was considerable, spanning a wide range of poetic, rhetorical, and literary-critical material in Greek and Latin, as well as iconographic and artistic representation throughout the Imperial period.[12] I turn briefly to one example of the interest in Philoktetes in the works of Ailios Aristeides. In the context of an oration about Smyrna (Oration 17), Aristeides turns to the figure of Philoktetes to conceptualize his task. Speaking about Smyrna is difficult, he claims, for 'just as, they say, the one who was bitten by the serpent did not wish to speak to another, but only that man who has experienced it, so also having seen the beauty of the city [I wish] to make it common only to one who has seen it' (ὥσπερ τὸν ὑπὸ τῆς ἐχίδνης φασὶ πληγέντα μὴ ἐθέλειν ἑτέρῳ λέγειν ἀλλ' ἢ ὅστις πεπείραται, οὕτω καὶ τῶν περὶ τῆς πόλεως καλῶν ἰδόντα ἰδόντι μόνον κοινοῦσθαι, Aristid. 17.18K).[13] Aristeides' allusion to Philoktetes (as well as the oblique nod to Plato's *Symposium*) looks immediately to Aristeides' pained life: although there is no direct connection here with the *Sacred Tales*, it is hard not to see references to speaking about painful experience as bringing to mind his prolonged accounts of his pained existence. The allusion to Philoktetes not only helps to (re)inforce Aristeides' view of himself as a type of heroic pain sufferer, but also positions the experience of pain through its relationship with language, beauty, and religion. Aristeides contrasts phenomena from the opposites ends of the aesthetic spectrum—the difficulty of narrating beauty is itself explained by the difficulty of narrating pain; a point brought home by his following suggestion that it would not be easy to deliver (ἐκφερεῖν) the *logos* to others (εἰς ἑτέρους), as if narrating 'holy things to the profane' (εἰς βεβήλους ἱερά). Pain, beauty, and religious experience are connected by their capacity to strain at the boundaries of language and common experience. Aristeides' use of κοινοῦσθαι also flags the question of narrative and its capacity to socialize experiences. Aristeides' reluctance 'to communicate' (or 'to make common / share') to those who do not have first-hand experience of what is being discussed is significant. Language's capacity to communicate pain is underpinned by the experiential connections and common ground between

---

[12] Literary-critical and rhetorical: Dio. Chr. 52 and 59. Poetic: *AP*. xvi.111 and 112 for poems about the hero. For further literary references to artistic representation, see Plut. *Quomodo Adulesc.* 18c and discussion in Chapter 9 (nn. 1–5 with text). For further references to the Latin material, see Bowersock (1994), 55–76.

[13] Bowersock (1994), 55–76 on Aristides and this passage, esp. 68. For the *cliché*: Pl. *Smp.* 217e. For other references in Aristeides, see 28.130K.

speaker and listener. The narrative of pain (and beauty and initiation) strains at the boundaries of linguistic communication and the ability of *logos* to make experiences public and common. Plutarch and Aristeides use Philoktetes to make different points about pain. What is common to them both, and the tradition that they both utilize, is Philoktetes' role in shaping individuals' understanding of pain experience.

2. LUCIAN'S *PODAGRA*

There is little in Plutarch's treatise that is specifically devoted to either language or religious activity to provide a context for the experience of pain. This aspect of experience is, however, given more explicit treatment in *Podagra*.[14] As has been acknowledged, it is one example of the Second Sophistic penchant for *adoxon* and is clearly intended as a humorous parody of both tragedy and gout sufferers.[15] Nevertheless, the text has a serious contribution to make to the discussion of pain experience because of its combination of religious and medical approaches to pain.

In the context of this chapter, I want to make two arguments. Firstly, that the text dramatizes the individual's negotiation of pain symptoms against a background of heroic suffering and tragic-style lamentation and woe. A number of scholars have pointed out that the text's connection with tragedy should be seen on two levels. There is a considerable amount of material—language and terminology—that is tragic in form. Indeed, the play quotes heavily from tragic texts.[16] It is also clear that *Podagra* is not a tragedy: it takes on some aspects of the plot and structure of a tragedy, but it does not develop these in a meaningful way.[17] To my mind, the connection with tragedy should be seen in the way in which certain forms of language and tragic motifs are used to help position the pain-perceiver and represent his experience. Secondly, I show that by setting up this tragic framework for understanding the pained individual's experiences, Lucian is able to undermine the legitimacy of this type of contextualizing

---

[14] On the title of the treatise: Karavas (2005), 235.
[15] Anderson (1979a), 150 for 'adoxon' and 153 for its relationship to tragedy. See also Whitmarsh (2013), 182–5. For its framing of its humorous teasing of sufferers: Luc. *Podagra*. 332–5. For the tradition of adoxography: Phil. *VA*. 4.30 (77K), *VS*. 487–8 (205–6K).
[16] On the tragic language throughout the play: Karavas (2005), 243–99.
[17] Anderson (1979a), 153.

framework. Lucian uses tragedy, then, as a framework for investigating (and ultimately deconstructing) a certain way of approaching pain.

The text is structured around the experiences of a gout sufferer, his relationship with the personified deity, Gout, and the (hubristic?) claims of doctors that they can overcome pain and cure the patient. There is much in this work that corresponds to historical aspects of both religious and medical activity: the deification of the goddess Gout and the prayers offered for the alleviation of the condition strike a chord with similar prayers to different gods for pain relief (including gout) from healing sanctuaries across the Mediterranean.[18] There is also considerable correspondence between the representation of medical activity and historical practice—both the doctors themselves and the cures listed throughout the play intersect with some known therapeutic activities.[19] For all its parodic nature, this text reveals much about pain experience in Imperial culture because the plot always has the potential to bite with contemporary medical practice, pain experience, and religious therapy.

Interpretations of the play's interest in medicine have centred on the confrontation between two Syrian doctors and the goddess, Gout. Gout's (inevitable) victory in this *agōn* and the subsequent willingness of the play's different characters to accept the power of Gout might be read as a particular comment on the relationship between medical and religious approaches to healing. In terms of pain, however, I want to focus on a more subtle incorporation of painful physical symptoms into the play. Lucian's paratragedy opens with a highly medicalized account of his symptoms. According to the protagonist, it would be far better for mortals who sin, such as Sisyphos, to feel Gout's pains (πόνοι) in their 'joints' (ἀρθροκηδέσιν, 15), rather than their familiar post-mortem punishments. As the initial description of gout continues, the speaker constructs a vision of the body which combines both medical readings of the condition with more tragic visions of the body's hardships and susceptibility:

> ὥς μου τὸ λυπρὸν καὶ ταλαίπωρον δέμας
> χειρῶν ἀπ' ἄκρων εἰς ἄκρας ποδῶν βάσεις
> ἰχῶρι φαύλῳ καὶ πικρῷ χυμῷ χολῆς
> πνεύματι βιαίῳ τόδε διασφίγγον πόρους
> ἔστηκε καὶ μεμυκὸς ἐπιτείνει πόνους.
> σπλάγχνων δ' ἐπ' αὐτῶν διάπυρον τρέχει κακόν.

---

[18] Paz de Hoz (2014), 187–9.
[19] Paz de Hoz (2014), 179–80, with further references at her n. 8.

> as this pained and wretched frame of mine
> from the fingertips to the ends of my feet
> by a wretched ichor and bitter humour of bile
> And a strong pneuma, its pores blocked,
> is locked and this closed state exacerbates the pain.
> And the feverish evil runs through my intestines.
>
> Luc. *Podagra* 16–21[20]

There is much in this passage that combines medical readings with a broader sense of pain experience. The list of symptoms recalls medical accounts of this condition: 'bitter humour' and a 'strong pneuma', which means that the condition courses through his inflamed body, resonate with medical accounts of gout in the Hippokratic tradition, especially those of Aretaios of Kappodokia and Rufus of Ephesos.[21] These conditions, however, are presented in ways that transcend the specific focus on medical symptomology. The reference to his 'wretched frame' suggests that the symptoms are best seen as part of a broader corporeal susceptibility and wretchedness. His disease is like 'the swell' (κλύδων, 26) which sweeps over him (κυματούμενος, 25). The passage is bookended, moreover, by the way in which pain relates to death. Immediately before this description, he compares what he feels to the types of sufferings Ixion and Sisyphos endured after death (9–14). A few lines later, the man claims that his symptoms are such that those who suffer gout maintain foolish and vain hopes for relief in death:

> ὦ δυστέκμαρτον πᾶσιν ἀνθρώποις τέλος,
> ὡς εἰς μάτην σε πάντες ἀμφιθάλπομεν
> ἐλπίδι ματαίᾳ μωρὰ βουκολούμενοι.
>
> Oh death, hard to understand for all mankind,
> how we all cherish you vainly,
> cheating ourselves, foolishly, with vain hopes.
>
> Luc. *Podagra* 27–9.

Lucian's words explicitly emphasize the hopes and desires for relief that individuals might have during disease. In looking to death, Lucian also recalls suggestions in Aretaios that certain conditions and experiences

---

[20] Translation adjusted from Macleod's Loeb edition of *Podagra*. Other instances where I have followed Macleod are recorded in the notes.

[21] Aret. *SD*. iv.10. Ruf. Eph. *de Podagra praef.* (pp. 250–1 Daremberg).

of pain mean that the patients (or those around them) actually desire death. In Lucian's context, the futility of that desire is made apparent by the nature of heroic sufferings that occur after death.[22] The references to Ixion and Sisyphos figure his disease as a form post-mortem heroic punishment (literally, a *tisis*) and are, in part, underpinned by Lucian's use of the tragic genre.[23] At the same time, however, that heroic context has further implications: it is precisely the gouty man's sense of heroic post-mortem retribution that convinces him that the (widespread?) desire for death is a foolish one.

As the text continues, the gouty man's experience of his symptoms and condition continues to oscillate between quotidian aspects of experience and those which intimate a slightly different context for the navigation of pain symptoms. In one scenario, when the gouty man meets the chorus, which is composed of fellow gouty men, the symptoms of pain are described in particularly telling terms. The gouty man begins by asking the chorus what rites initiates must perform to become members of their band.[24] The men respond that they do not perform a range of expected initiation rites, including spilling their own blood, growing their hair, or tearing wild animals apart, but that every spring:

> τότε διὰ μελέων ὀξὺ βέλος πέπηγε μύσταις,
> ἀφανές, κρύφιον, δεδυκὸς ὑπὸ μυχοῖσι γυίων,
> πόδα, γόνυ, κοτύλην, ἀστραγάλους, ἰσχία, μηρούς,
> χέρας, ὠμοπλάτας, βραχίονας, κόρωνα, καρποὺς
> ἔσθει, νέμεται, φλέγει, κρατεῖ, πυροῖ, μαλάσσει,
> μέχρις ἂν ἡ θεὸς τὸν πόνον ἀποφυγεῖν κελεύσῃ.
>
> Then limbs of acolytes are pierced by weapon sharp,
> unseen, concealed, sinking to the innermost part of the limbs;
> The foot, the knee, hip-joint, the ankles, groins and thighs,
> Hands, shoulder-blades, and arms, the elbows and the wrists
> It eats, devours, burns, dominates, inflames and softens,
> Until the goddess bids the pain to flee away.
>
> Luc. *Podagra* 119–24[25]

There are a number of points to note about their response to the gouty man's enquiries. As with the initial description of gout symptoms, the

---

[22] Aret. *SA*. ii.2.17 and ii.5.1.10–11, *SD*. iii.2.3.6–7, and *SD*. iv.1.9.6.
[23] NB the use of τίσις (9) and κολάζειν (13).   [24] Luc. *Podagra* 112.
[25] Translation developed from Macleod's Loeb edition.

intricacies of the body's engagement with pain are stressed. If the passage describes medicalized symptoms, it does so in language and metaphors which are less common in medical contexts. The suggestion that pain eats and devours, for instance, is evocative of the experiences of tragic heroes like Philoktetes and Herakles.[26] Furthermore, the suggestion that these experiences should be seen alongside the traditional activities of initiates intimates a religious or mystery context for the experience of pain. This sense of initiation is strengthened by the chorus' own use of μύσταις to describe sufferers at line 119. The term also picks up references to initiation and mystery cult throughout the scene. The passage is introduced by the question 'what rites are performed by the initiates?'[27] Once he has heard the description of their rites, the gouty man proclaims that he was one of the initiates all along (κατωργιασμένων, 125) and that he will praise the goddess along with the other acolytes.[28] The repetition of references to cult, mysteries, and initiation creates a religious context for navigating the experience of gout. On one level, this connection with mystery religion is hardly surprising: the whole play hinges on this theme. The goddess Gout is consistently constructed in religious terms, and described in language that is reminiscent of mystery cults;[29] the prayers that the initiates offer for release from pain are also familiar from historical votive offerings and inscriptions.[30] Behind some of the religious themes of the play lies a considerable amount of religious practice and belief which shapes how individuals engage with pain.

This scene, then, combines tragic and religious aspects to construct a context for navigating pain symptoms associated with gout. There are a number of aspects of this process, but I want to focus on the description and communication of pain symptoms. The play makes considerable mileage out of using different types of language.[31] The afflicted individuals, the gouty men, engage in a

---

[26] Paz de Hoz (2014), 187 on the cultic implications of much of this language.
[27] Luc. *Podagra* 112: τίσιν δὲ τελεταῖς ὀργιάζει προσπόλους; ('with what sort of rites do initiates honour her?').
[28] Luc. *Podagra* 128: ὕμνων κατάρξω τὸ ποδαγρῶν ᾄδων μέλος ('I shall raise up hymns, singing the song of gout').
[29] Paz de Hoz (2014), 187–9.   [30] Paz de Hoz (2014), 187–9.
[31] For the discussion of language from the perspective of self-conscious manipulation of the literary tradition, see Whitmarsh (2013), 176–85. For the general theme, Karavas (2005), with his n. 18.

type of tragic wailing.[32] These screams are also claimed by the initiates themselves: 'we initiates pay to you, Podagra, in the first days of spring / wailing lamentation' (ἡμεῖς δὲ σοί, Ποδάγρα, / πρώταις ἔαρος ἐν ὥραις / μύσται τελοῦμεν οἴκτους, 42–4). The initiates' description points to the ways in which the language of pained individuals might be conceptualized. On this reading, the reference to such wailing emphasizes the effect that pain has on language: pain, here, appears to undermine the linguistic capacities of the individual, but also locates it in a tragic context.

The concern with language is further enhanced by the ways in which the goddess conceptualizes the language of her devotees. In her first major appearance in the play, Gout describes her effect on those who incur her wrath:

> ὁ γὰρ μεταλαβὼν τῶν ἐμῶν μυστηρίων
> πρῶτον μὲν εὐθὺς εὐστομεῖν διδάσκεται
> τέρπων ἅπαντας, εὐτραπέλους λέγων λόγους·
>
> For when he, sharing in my mystic rites,
> Is taught first and immediately to speak well,
> Delighting all by speaking well-formed words.
>
> Luc. *Podagra* 180–2

Gout's view of those who feel her pain is particularly evocative. In the first instance, her representation of pain language appears to reinforce the religious connotations of the experience of Gout. How are we to read the use of εὐστομεῖν in this passage? On one level, the sense of 'to speak well' suggests that gout plays a positive role in facilitating the individual's capacity for language: the term can mean 'to praise'. It shares with these implications a range of religious connotations. It recalls the injunction in mystery cults to maintain a reverent silence both in the face of the deity and towards those outside the cultic context.[33] On one level, the use of the term implies the way in which language (and more specifically, silence) helps to deny to an uninitiated audience effective access to the experiences of others. At the same time, however, the suggestion that gout sufferers speak witty words or 'well-formed words' (εὐτραπέλους ... λόγους) seems to reinforce the positive sense of εὐστομεῖν. Tim Whitmarsh reads this reference as a

---

[32] At 289, 'the wretched' are said to be left 'shrieking loudly' (βοῶντες οἱ ταλαίπωροι μέγα). At 175, Gout tells those who cure themselves 'to wail' (οἰμώζειν).

[33] See LSJ s.v. εὐστομέω and εὐφημέω for the connections with religious and well-omened silence.

type of meta-literary marker for Lucian's own text: Gout teaches Lucian how to speak the language of his own literary work.[34] We might also read this statement as an ironic twist on the screams and shouts of those who feel pain: Gout does not teach you to speak well or develop witty discourse, it teaches you to groan and to shout. However scholars read this line, what is clear is that a connection between the experience of gout and its capacity to induce a certain linguistic register is clear. Experiencing pain induces a certain kind of language.

There are further questions raised by the allusion to pleasure as well, particularly in relation to how the pain sufferer is conceptualized by others. What kind of pleasure does the language of gout induce? One can, of course, gain pleasure from being derisive as well as taking enjoyment from the witty qualities of another's dexterous language. Perhaps one clue lies in the final lines of the play itself, where Lucian appears to speak directly to those who feel gout. 'Let', Lucian's chorus is made to say, every one of those who suffer 'bear up' (ἀνεχέσθω, 332) 'when he is teased and scoffed at' (ἐμπαιζόμενος καὶ σκωπτόμενος, 333), 'since this is what this thing is' (τοῖον γὰρ ἔφυ τόδε πρᾶγμα, 334). There is much to unpack in these three lines. In the first instance, Lucian's final words suggest that the pleasure he envisages in these lines is to be interpreted as playful and perhaps derisive. At the same time, the final lines speak to the ways in which the gouty men might be viewed by those around them: are they a source of derision? Finally, the self-reflexive comment on Lucian's play speaks directly to the external reader. It reinforces for them that the text has been a playful mocking of those who feel gout, raising further questions about the ways in which pain has been presented throughout. In a typically Lucianic move, the author undercuts the security of what he has been developing over the work: is the text a playful mocking because it plays upon the tragic and religious contexts for a quotidian experience? Does the pleasure come from the incongruities of the claims made to particular cultural traditions, practices, and ideas and the realities of the condition? Lucian's text finishes by asking the reader to return to exactly where we position, how we understand, those who feel the pain of gout.

---

[34] Whitmarsh (2013), 183–4.

7

Sacred Pain in Ailios Aristeides

Ailios Aristeides was one of the *supernovae* of Imperial Greek culture. Although he is perhaps most well known for his six *Tales*, his corpus is among the most substantial to survive from the period.[1] According to him, he met the Imperial family and was responsible for eliciting their benefaction for Smyrna when it was destroyed by earthquake in 177 CE; like Galen, he is an imposing figure in the crowded galaxy of stars in second-century-CE Greek culture.[2] The *Tales* were famous in antiquity for both their literary qualities and the picture of Aristeides they present.[3] They were probably composed in the mid-170s CE and within a generation were praised by Philostratos the Elder as examples of excellent rhetoric; Libanios, in the fourth century CE, marvels at the way in which these texts present their author.[4] The *Tales* have, however, divided scholarly opinion over the last century: they have been seen as nauseatingly self-obsessed texts, the products of a vainglorious hypochondriac, and masterful pieces of rhetoric which are embedded in a culture concerned with the body.[5]

---

[1] Throughout this discussion, I will refer to the *Tales* as plural: although they constitute a cohesive body of work, it is worth remembering that they comprise six discrete texts, which have some distinct literary aims.

[2] On their composition: Behr (1968), 11–2, with Gasco (1989) for further discussion. For references in Aristeides to his connection with the emperors, see, e.g., 42.14K.

[3] Libanios: Cribiore (2007), 22–44. Philostratos: Phil. *VS*. 581–2 (252–3K). Jones (2008) on Aristeides' reception in Byzantium.

[4] For the most recent survey of the issues of dating, see Israelowich (2012), 14. The general consensus is that they were composed in the first half of the 170s CE on the basis of the reference to Salvius as 'the present consul' at Aristid. 48.9K.

[5] Hypochondriac: Brown (1978), 41 and Misch (1950), 506. Master rhetorician: Downie (2013). On his importance to rhetorical culture, see, e.g., Boulanger (1968). On his significance within the history of biography: Misch (1950).

The *logoi* recount the *minutiae* of their author's pained existence throughout his extended illness and recovery at the hands of the healing god Asklepios. As with the medical narratives that I investigated in Part 1, Aristeides' representation of his pain experience begins from a precise physiological perspective. His pain symptoms and perceptions demonstrate connections with the world of anatomically-informed contemporary medical culture. However, Aristeides integrates this approach to pain symptoms into a much broader and nebulous sense of physical disorder and hardship—what he terms the 'tidal waves' of his body. This sense of hardship helps to provide a framework for understanding the significance of Aristeides' pain symptoms: it locates his pain within the context of his own life and his relationship with others.

This formulation of pain is allied to Aristeides' self-conscious exploration of the rhetorical representation of his pain. Aristeides probes the relationship between pain and language and in so doing shapes the way in which pain is integrated into different types of relationship and different frameworks of understanding. Aristeides adopts a number of different modes of narration throughout the *Tales* which simultaneously undermine the security of medical readings of his body, stress the amazing, unbelievable qualities of his experiences, and present him as a type of enduring heroic figure. In exploring the ways in which that experience of pain is communicated, Aristeides locates pain at the boundaries of the incredible, testing the limits of belief and certain knowledge or understanding. This representation of the body's pain combines a medically-informed approach to pain with models and ideas that occur at other points in Greek Imperial culture, especially the Greek romances and the *Odyssey*.

This approach to Aristeides' conception of his illness and pain will be familiar from recent discussions of Aristeides' *Tales*. Since the publication of Lee Pearcy's seminal article, 'Theme, Dream, and Narrative: reading the *Sacred Tales* of Aelius Aristeides', scholars have been particularly awake to the sophistication of the form and structure of the *logoi*.[6] Pearcy suggests that this sophistication should be seen in terms of the *Tales*' self-conscious narration of their own

---

[6] Pearcy (1988), which has inspired a number of (re)readings of various passages throughout the *Tales*. For further readings of the *Tales* within the context of self-conscious narrative, see Whitmarsh (2004), Harrison (2000), King (2002), and Tagliabue (2016).

creation and their exploration of their status as an artful translation of the physical experiences of their author. For Pearcy, they narrate the creation of two texts: the *Tales* themselves and the body upon which Aristeides' experiences can be read.[7] In a nuanced evolution to this argument, Brooke Holmes has suggested that rather than constructing a body upon which his experiences can be read, the *Tales* fashion an illegible *sōma* which helps Aristeides maintain a type of heroic identity.[8] There is much to take from Holmes's approach to his body, with which I largely agree. In what follows, I contribute to the debate about Aristeides by contextualizing his engagement with language and pain alongside the themes that I have discussed in Part 1. Aristeides contests creatively and consciously the ways in which medicine and anatomy manage the relationship between language, narrative, and pain: if the clinical encounter, with its interest in diagnostic recognition, was defined by the ways in which doctor and patient spoke to each other, Aristeides co-opts that interest in language and directs it towards the construction of very different types of recognition and understanding. This interest in language is directed so as to shape the way different communities, people, or readers understand or recognize his painful symptoms. Aristeides' text posits different kinds of reader, all of whom understand his body in different ways.

1. PHYSIOLOGICAL PAIN SYMPTOMS

Aristeides never outlines a coherent theory of pain perception in the manner of Aretaios or Galen. He does not demonstrate a consistent interest in the ways in which pain operates at an atomic level. It is hard, however, not to see the *Tales,* with their lingering descriptions of the physical trauma and symptoms of the pained body, as texts deeply concerned with the perception of pain. (Indeed, their focus on the destroyed body has traditionally been taken as an important marker of the author's profound self-obsession and the unpleasantness of the

---

[7] Pearcy (1988), 390–1, for the notion of 'two texts'. For their sophisticated method of composition: Israelowich (2012), 15–19. For Holmes's reaction to (and extension of) Pearcy: Holmes (2008), 82–4. For further discussions of his body and narrative: Perkins (1995), 187 and King (2001), 282.

[8] For Holmes, the body is 'metonymic' of all that lies beyond the text: Holmes (2008), 85.

works.⁹) However Aristeides' body might offend modern scholarly sensibilities, it is less out of place when considered alongside the descriptions of symptoms in the work of contemporary medical writers or the votive offerings of the Pergamene Asklepieion.¹⁰ Aristeides' way of approaching the body drew on very familiar methods for conceptualizing pain and other symptoms associated with his illness.

In describing various episodes that occurred throughout his long illness, he details physical symptoms—fever, shivering, swellings, and his inability to eat, vomit, or even breathe—as well as his reactions to the treatment of physicians and his regimen. In many instances, pain emerges as an important perception that accompanies disease or treatment: 'terrible pains' (*deinai odunai*) or 'strong pains' (*odunai iskhurai*) which were 'difficult to bear' or 'impossible to bear' are continually referred to throughout the first three *logoi*.¹¹ The reference to 'terrible pains' seems to be fairly common throughout a range of cultural and literary traditions, but the use of *iskhuros* to modify *odunē* is particularly common in medical contexts. Indeed, references to *odunai iskhurai* pervade the Hippokratic and Galenic corpora.¹² I do not want to suggest that this vocabulary for pain is solely medical. Rather, that for readers of Greek medical texts, Aristeides' descriptions of his physical pain could be read through a medical framework which uses certain types of description to define the intensity and the diagnostic relevance of pain sensations. Given the connections with rational medical practice and Aristeides' context of the Pergamene Asklepieion, it does not seem particularly surprising that Aristeides incorporated significant amounts of medical literature—and their ways of thinking about the body's perception of pain—into his own ways of understanding and discussing his symptoms.¹³

This concern with pain is given sharper focus at a range of points throughout different *logoi*. In the second *logos*, Aristeides turns to an episode which includes a substantial number of symptoms. He experiences difficulties breathing as well as 'every kind of symptom' (παντοῖα συμπτώματα, 48.57K) in his teeth and ears; there was, he

---

⁹ For the texts as 'brainsick' and 'unpleasant': Dodds (1965), 43–4.
¹⁰ For the connections with votive offerings, see Petsalis-Diomidis (2010), 221–75, Misch (1950), 499–500, and Israelowich (2012).
¹¹ See., e.g., ὀδύναι . . . δειναί at 47.62K and ἀλγήματα ἰσχυρὰ καὶ δεινὰ at 49.16K.
¹² See, e.g., Hp. *Epid.* i.3.13(9).1, ii.2.10.1, and iii.3.17(2).14; also *Loc. Hom.* 14.13. For Galen, see, e.g., *Loc. Aff.* viii.403K, and *MM.* x.431K, 814K, 841K, and 854K.
¹³ For the connections, see Israelowich (2012), esp. 40–105.

recalls, 'distension... of the veins' (τάσιν... τῶν φλεβῶν) and it was both impossible to eat and to vomit; there was a 'fiery pain which extended into [his] brain' (ὀδύνη δὲ εἰς ἐγκέφαλον διάπυρος, 48.57K). The reference to 'fiery pain' helps to position Aristeides' pain perceptions. The connection between pain and its inflamed or fiery nature is, of course, habitual to Greek medicine. The insistence on such a perception throughout Greek medicine relates, partly, to the connection between pain and fever: where fever occurs, Greek doctors, especially within the Hippokratic tradition, very often assume there is also pain.[14] The description is also reminiscent of the description of *kephalalgia* in Aretaios and in Galen, especially in its reference to fiery pains which travel inside the head.[15]

Moments after describing this painful episode, Aristeides turns to a more pervasive perception of pain. He begins by telling his readers that a particular *nosos* afflicted him: he perceived (*aisthanomai*) a tightness of breath about the chest, strong fevers overtook him, and 'other unspeakable things' (ἄλλα ἀμύθητα, 48.62K) occurred. Not long after this, his stomach swelled, 'the nerves trembled and were chilled and there was shivering throughout the whole body' (τὰ νεῦρα κατέψυκτο καὶ φρίκη διέθει διὰ παντὸς τοῦ σώματος, 48.62K), and his breath left him. In response, his doctors make an incision from the chest all the way down to the bladder, a process Aristeides represents in less than positive terms:

καὶ διῆλθεν ὀδύνη ναρκώδης καὶ ἄπορος φέρειν, καὶ πάντα αἵματι ἐπέφυρτο καὶ γίγνομαι ὑπεραλγεινός,[16] καὶ τῶν σπλάγχνων ᾐσθανόμην οἷον ψυχρῶν τε καὶ ἐκκρεμαμένων, καὶ τὸ τῆς ἀμηχανίας τῆς περὶ τὴν ἀναπνοὴν ἐπετάθη.

And a numbing pain went through me and it was difficult to bear, and everything was stained with blood and I felt extreme pain, and I perceived that my intestines were cold and hanging out, and this was exacerbated by my inability to breathe.

Aristid. 48.63K

[14] Cf. Hp. *Progn*: 22.1.
[15] Aret. *SD*. iii.2.1.1–3. Cf. Gal. *Cris*. ix.756K (where he is quoting Hippokrates).
[16] ὑπεραλγεινός is Willamowitz's correction for ὑπέργεινος, found in a number of the manuscripts (A, SDTA) and several marginal corrections in other manuscripts. Keil reads ὑπέρινος. Both terms seem difficult to justify on the basis of common usage throughout the *Tales*, as neither is repeated. I follow Dindorf, Jebb, and Willamowitz's reading on the basis that it seems to fit the context far more effectively than 'excessively purged'.

There can be few more powerful statements of the patient's reaction to the trauma of medical care than Aristeides' recollection that his intestines began to feel cold and felt as though they had been left hanging out of his body. The use of ὑπεραλγεινός is disputed (and is chosen in favour of ὑπέρινος in Keil's edition), but if it is correct, it emphasizes the extreme forms of pain that Aristeides is being subjected to at this point. The use of *aisthanomai* throughout this entire discussion emphasizes his interest in the perception of his symptoms: Aristeides' experience is defined by his hyper-awareness of what is being done to his body and how it changes during the operation. This interest in perception takes readers deep inside Aristeides' *sōma*; it is not just his body which feels cold, but the nerves which are chilled; he can feel not only his body being cut, but the changes in temperature which ensue; he perceives the fundamental disordering of the body in which that which is normally closed off, sealed from view, is left 'hanging out'.

The suggestion that pain is 'impossible to bear' (ἄπορος φέρειν) reflects a common theme throughout Aristeides' *Tales*, to which I will return in a moment. The use of the adjective 'numbing' (ναρκώδης) returns readers to contemporary debates about pain forms or types found in the medical authors of Part 1. It is especially reminiscent of Galen's discussion of the use of 'numbing' as a pain 'name' in the second book of *On Affected Parts*. There Galen attacks his earlier contemporary, Arkhigenes, for his use of the adjective *narkōdēs* to refer to pain as inaccurate for a number of reasons.[17] Galen's primary point, in that context, is that it should not be considered an effective name for a type of pain because the process of being dulled or numbed reduces one's sensory capacity, which Galen sees as necessary for the perception of pain: a numb pain can only arise when the condition of being numbed or cooled is coincidental with the perception of pain. Whatever their differences, both Galen and Arkhigenes associate this particular sensation with the process of cooling the body. If we are to believe Galen's reportage of his predecessor's views, then it seems likely that it combined a sense of coolness in the nerves with painful sensation. Aristeides' use of the term is marked within contemporary medical discourse. His symptoms—the cooling of his nerves, shivering and chilling in other parts of his body—chime with contexts in which this form of pain is thought to arise. Aristeides' choice of

---

[17] See Gal. *Loc. Aff.* viii.71–2K.

language locates his perceptions squarely in the middle of a second-century debate about the ways in which pain arises in the body; it pulls into Aristeides' account critical assumptions about how his body works, under what conditions we perceive, and how one understands pain types.

If the types of pain sensations which Aristeides perceives can be mapped onto medical visions of the body familiar in Galen and other contemporary writers, so too can his interest in his own sensory awareness and the authority of his own understanding of his condition. In a telling account of his experience of the plague in Pergamon, Aristeides describes how he felt about his experience of the disease:

τὸ μέντοι τοῦ Ὁμήρου κἂν τούτοις εἶπες ἂν τὸ 'νόος γε μὲν ἔμπεδος ἦεν·'
οὕτω παρηκολούθουν ἐμαυτῷ, ὥσπερ ἂν ἄλλῳ τινί, καὶ ᾐσθανόμην
ὑπολείποντος ἀεὶ τοῦ σώματος, ἕως εἰς τοὔσχατον ἦλθον.

However, even in these circumstances, you would have said the Homeric phrase, 'his mind was steadfast'. So in this way, I went along with my symptoms, just as one would observe someone else, and I perceived my body always failing, until I came to the end.

Aristid. 48.39K

Aristeides' description returns readers to discussions of the ways in which individuals are affected by disease and their capacity to understand what they suffer. Aristeides focuses, in this context, on the complex relationship between subjective and objective perception and his own mental abilities. I will return to the Homeric apostrophe later, but for the moment, I want to focus on Aristeides' choice of *parakolouthein* to describe his awareness of his situation. The term arguably links his understanding of his condition with discussions in Galen about the patient's capacity 'to go along with' or 'to understand' what one experiences during illness.[18] At the same time, the reflexive *emautōi* speaks to a heightened sense of self-awareness of his own body, as does the use of first person form of *aisthanomai*; the stress on subjective awareness seems directly juxtaposed with the apologetic parenthesis; Aristeides suggests arguably that his level of perception is that of one who stands apart from his own body. Do his qualities of mind—his ability to remain mentally strong—allow him to view his

---

[18] Gal. *Loc. Aff.* viii.88–9K.

own body (and death) from the position of the other? Like Galen's ideal patient, Aristeides is able to understand his symptoms because of his detached mental acuity.

The interest in pain types—such as the 'numbing pain'—and in the process of perception suggests an anatomically-informed reading of the body and its pain. Importantly, however, for all his anatomical knowledge, it is worth noting that Aristeides' narratives embed the sensation and his perception of it in a much broader notion of physical discomfort and difficulty. Repeatedly throughout his *logoi*, Aristeides connects his sense of precise pain symptoms with more general metaphors and language for pain, hardship, and suffering. As critics have pointed out, in the opening lines of his first *Tale*, he refers to his experiences of the divine regimen as ἀγωνίσματα, 'contests' (47.1K); this metaphor links his experiences of the regimen with both rhetorical acts of performance and competitive striving through physical exertion that were undertaken by Aristeides' contemporaries throughout the Second Sophistic.[19] The slippage between physical hardship, exertions, and rhetorical competition helps to reify Aristeides' connection between his rhetorical performances and his endurance and performance of the god's recommendations. The painful and traumatic experience of illness and therapy (which were so heavily discussed in Galen and Aretaios) are rewritten in terms of competitive striving, physical regimen, and rhetorical training and performance. More significantly, he also recalls that his experiences were dominated by the 'tidal waves of the body' (ὑπὸ τῶν περὶ τὸ σῶμα τρικυμιῶν, 47.3K). There can be no doubt that the metaphor for overwhelming experience looks in a number of directions. It reiterates a connection with Odysseus and his experiences of the waves while escaping from Kalypso's island in book five of the *Odyssey*. At the same time, however, it is also a common metaphor for being overwhelmed by one's physical or psychological experiences.[20] It points to the way in which the body's *aisthēseis* and illness episodes are integrated into a sense of overwhelming and insurmountable experience.

---

[19] On the metaphors of rhetorical life and performance to conceptualize his illness and convalescence, see 48.70K and 49.44K for the description of his convalescence as a '*kathedra*'. On this issue: Israelowich (2012), 5. For the suggestion that the god was a rhetorical trainer: Bompaire (1989), 36–9.

[20] For the metaphor of being overwhelmed: E. *Hipp.* 1213 and Luc. *Dem. Enc.* 33. For its reference to psychological problems in the novel, see Ach. Tat. iii.2.5.1.

At other times, however, the sense of bodily hardship is figured in more precise terms. During his account of the plague, for instance, he refers to the fact that 'fevers attacked him and everything was difficult' (πυρετοὶ κατέλαβον καὶ πάντ' ἦν ἄπορα, 48.63K);[21] at other times, he recounts that because of his condition it was impossible to stand, his ears rang, and his body was 'troubled' or 'disturbed' (ἠνώχλει, 48.68K).[22] Taken together, such references continually emphasize a sense of bodily confusion and disarray, as well as mental and emotional disturbance and confusion. These terms do not always refer explicitly to pain symptoms, but they do help to locate them in a much broader context of physical destruction and disorder. Aristeides' very specific understanding of his pain is embedded in a more general theme of bodily difficulty and hardship.

2. NARRATING PAIN

In this section, I investigate how Aristeides continues to define his relationship with medical discourse by turning to the *Tales*' engagement with language and rhetoric. As I have discussed, Aristeides' vision of his pain is tied up with the ways in which he conceptualizes the relationship between his body and language: Aristeides tries out different modes of speaking and different types of voice to communicate his pain; some of these forms of language and narrative are drawn from medical contexts, while others have more in common with epic modes of narration or even the novel genre. This interest in different ways of speaking—their limitations and effectiveness for communicating pain—has a number of important consequences. As Aristeides moves away from a medical approach to language, he constructs different types of recognition, replacing medical forms of diagnosis with more nebulous forms of understanding. These different forms of recognition facilitate relationships with others around him and help to figure the body as both amazing and incredible.

---

[21] Cf. Aristid. 48.63K, 49.1K and 16K for the use of *aporia*.
[22] Aristid. 48.6K for another use of this term.

a. Rephrasing Case-History Contexts

Before I begin this discussion, I turn briefly to the ways in which the *Tales* intersect with medical case-histories in order to create a basis for thinking about the ways in which the *Tales* redefine medicalized modes of communication. Aristeides' opening lines in the first *Tale* develop a complex generic position which includes aretology,[23] medical case-histories, and epic. In a telling passage at 47.3K, he states that his aim was not simply to record his symptoms, but to narrate and reveal the forethought and power of the divine:[24] 'each of our [his and his fellow incubants'] days, just like our nights, has a story, if someone present either wished to record the symptoms or to narrate the forethought of the divine' (ἑκάστη γὰρ τῶν ἡμετέρων ἡμερῶν, ὡσαύτως δὲ νυκτῶν, ἔχει συγγραφήν, εἴ τις παρών, ἢ τὰ συμπίπτοντα ἀπογράφειν ἐβούλετο, ἢ τὴν τοῦ θεοῦ πρόνοιαν διηγεῖσθαι, 47.3K).[25] The implications of this line are far-reaching. Reference to the *pronoia* of the divine marks out Aristeides' aretological aims. The narratives are driven, then, by a twofold objective: to relate (and praise) the *pronoia* of the divine and to narrate the symptoms of the body. The aretological element of the texts constitutes an important aspect of their religious or mystical quality: these texts aim not only to communicate Aristeides' relationship with his god, but to convey a sense of the powerful, nebulous quality of the god. Aristeides' *logoi* use the communication of the body's experiences to allow readers to see or recognize the power and nature of the divine: producing a sophisticated, cagey, even crab-like narrative of his

---

[23] There does not seem to have been a rigid formula for such offerings. Nevertheless, they were often little more than carvings of particular body parts, such as the eyes (to signify blindness or some other ocular failing), inscribed with the name of the beneficiary: Petsalis-Diomidis (2005), 206–17. Although it is unclear whether aretology existed as a clearly defined genre, it is certain that there were literary works which provided extensive lists of, and praise for, the miracles (*aretai*) of divine figures. Such documents were often particularly associated with eastern cults. For a discussion of aretology, see Winkler (1985), 236–8. For the connection between the *Tales* and aretology, see Pearcy (1988), 378 and Petsalis-Diomidis (2006). For the *Tales* as case-histories, see Mattern (2008), 36–7.

[24] The division between a 'record' (ἀπογράφη) and a narrative (*diēgēsis*) of divine *pronoia* (τὴν τοῦ θεοῦ πρόνοιαν) is famous. For discussion, see Pearcy (1988). It is difficult to overestimate the importance of Pearcy's reading of this division. For further development of his position, see Whitmarsh (2004) and Tagliabue (2016).

[25] There is a textual problem here: Keil's edition reads τις παρ'ἔν. I follow Wilamowitz—and others, including Behr and Holmes (Holmes (2008), 81 n. 3)—in reading παρών, which can be defended on the basis of comparison with 48.56K and 50.20K. For discussion, see Behr (1968), 205.

experience of pain constitutes one of the strategies that help to communicate a truth about Asklepios. The *Tales*, for all their focus on the body, are narratives (*diēgēseis*) of and thank-offerings for divine favour. The religious aspect to the text provides a way of raising the stakes in the manner in which the body is transformed.

The connection between thank-offerings in general and the case-history narrative form has been documented by a number of scholars.[26] Aristeides' self-positioning at 47.2K also evokes the context of mortal case-histories: the phrase τις παρών recalls references throughout Galen, and other medical figures, to bystanders who observe the work of the doctor at the bedside, and who are responsible for the narration of a patient's symptoms to the physician; the reference to the 'record of symptoms' invites a reading alongside medical case-histories which provide lists of physiological conditions or experiences.[27] Throughout the *Tales*, Aristeides presents the reader with contexts in which he or she might ordinarily expect the type of case-history narrative familiar from Galen or other contemporary writers. In doing so, he develops expectations about the ways in which the internal body and its symptoms might be communicated, revealed, and understood.

The implications of this connection are strengthened by the final line of Aristeides' *proem*, where he informs his readers that, in light of the immensity of his various symptoms, he decided 'to submit, as truly as to a doctor, to the god to do in silence what he commanded' (παρέχειν ὡς ἀληθῶς ὥσπερ ἰατρῷ τῷ θεῷ σιγῇ ποιεῖν ὅ τι βούλεται, 47.4K). Thus, Aristeides constructs his relationship with the divine in terms of human medicine. While this line—for all the delicious irony of a phrase that emphasizes the silence of a most loquacious orator—figures the divine relationship, it also figures the human clinical encounter. The suggestion that he submitted 'in silence' speaks volumes about the power relationships inherent in human clinical encounters. For all its aretological ambition to reveal a divine relationship, this text also interrogates the politics of speaking in quotidian circumstances.

Aristeides' proem underscores the ways in which his text facilitates recognition and understanding of his symptoms. There are two

---

[26] See, esp., Mattern (2008), 31–7, with further references.
[27] For examples of bystanders at medical diagnoses: Gal. *Diff. Puls.* viii.572K and *Praen.* xiv.606K.

important implications to draw from the generic complexity of the *Tales*. The first concerns the mode of translation Aristeides adopts to transform his physical experiences into sophisticated discourse. Over the last decade, literary scholars have given increasing attention to the way narratives 'give witness' to or 'testify' to the experience of extreme trauma or pain.[28] Dominic LaCapra points out that narratives which recount the experience of extreme or prolonged trauma adopt a particularly poignant strategy for giving reference to that pain: rather than providing a structured, ordered narrative of experience, they testify to the intensity and immensity of their experiences by producing narratives which mirror their disorder and nebulous qualities. As Pearcy (among others) has acknowledged, the *Tales* attempt to provide a true account of the divine by breaking free from the constraints of genre and chronology.[29] In order to produce an effective narrative of his body, Aristeides translates his experience into a sophisticated story which communicates the nature of his experience by emphasizing, and displaying, the impact of his pain on language and narrative. Whereas Galen's reaction to the disordered narratives of sufferers was to exercise control over the editing and arrangement of material in order to produce precise understanding and diagnosis, Aristeides recasts that process in more difficult, cagey terms. Rather than translating his experiences into clear, structured discourse which explains the cause of pain, Aristeides' *logoi* reveal the nature of that experience by representing the way painful experience impacts on, confounds, and transcends the limits of clear, ordered narration.

The second implication raised by the testimonial nature of Aristeides' text concerns the type of recognition that *logoi* produce. If Galen aimed to produce a scientific understanding of the body's condition which was embodied in the process of diagnosis, then how might we approach recognition in Aristeides' *Tales*? Here I want to discuss two issues. Aristeides' primary aim is to produce a narrative which allows for an understanding of the power and nature of the divine by readers (primarily, but not always, doctors) both inside the text and outside the narrative. I suggest, briefly, that genuine understanding of

---

[28] LaCapra (2009), 60–2. I have been especially influenced here by Caruth's analysis of *Hiroshima mon amour* and the politics of understanding another's trauma: Caruth (1995), 25–56.

[29] Pearcy (1988), 388–90.

both Aristeides' experience and the nature of the divine is achieved by understanding the impossibility of pinning down Aristeides' body, the impossibility of producing an exact, scientific reading or understanding of Aristeides' experiences. As we shall discuss further, Aristeides' doctors continually fail to recognize or understand his painful symptoms. At 48.69K, he tells us that his doctors failed to 'recognize the complexity of his disease' (οὔτε ἐγνώριζον τὴν ποικιλίαν τῆς νόσου). The failure of doctors to diagnose Aristeides correctly is repeated throughout all of Aristeides' *Tales*. This failure to recognize the body's symptoms operates as a model for thinking about how the body is constructed as a form of text which can be understood or recognized by readers outside the narrative. Such internal misreadings emphasize the failure to pin down the body, to categorize its experiences in a single disease or cure within the terms of contemporary diagnostic culture.

If Aristeides' body resists straightforward reading, or diagnosis, so too his text undermines the process of understanding or recognizing completely the immensity of his experiences. Understanding Aristeides' past experiences is a slippery, difficult process. The type of problematic engagement with the process of recognition is dramatized in a subtle way in his second *Tale*: 'if', Aristeides claims, 'someone would take these things into account and look closely at how many and what sort of sufferings' (εἰ δὴ ταῦτά τις προσλογίσαιτο καὶ σκέψαιτο ἐφ' ὅσων καὶ οἵων τῶν παθημάτων) he endured throughout his illness, ' . . . he will say that everything is truly beyond wonders and he shall also see more clearly the power of the god and his forethought' (. . . φήσει πᾶν ὡς ἀληθῶς περαιτέρω θαυμάτων εἶναι καὶ τοῦ τε θεοῦ τὴν δύναμιν καὶ τὴν πρόνοιαν μειζόνως ὄψεται, 48.59K). Thus, Aristeides links understanding the god's power to the reader's understanding and ability to see his experiences. Aristeides' passage has been taken, by Perkins, as a straightforward statement of the author's facilitation of readerly understanding of his experiences, and through them, the divine.[30] Yet the passage is far from straightforward. The conditional nature of the clause appears to raise questions about the way that his narrative allows readers to 'see' the wonders of the divine; the conditional sentence (despite the future indicative in the *apodosis*) never quite confirms that the narrative will allow the reader to see his experiences. Furthermore, the reference to

---

[30] Perkins (1995), 182.

the ontological status of his experiences—his experiences are 'beyond wonders'—implies that the type of recognition his text creates lies outside the normal verification and scientific confirmation of the body's experiences. In order to create this type of recognition and understanding, Aristeides adopts a particular approach to the translation of his experiences into sophisticated discourse.

The combination of religious and corporeal concerns in Aristeides' *Tales* serves, then, to create a remarkable textual dynamic. The orator confronts contemporary medical practice by rephrasing the translation of bodily experience into sophisticated narrative. I adopt three themes from Aristeides' *Tales* in which the capacity to recognize or understand Aristeides' experiences are inflected by his engagement with the relationship between pain and language.

b. The Case-History and Voice

If it is true that Aristeides' *Tales* attempt to confront the politics of narrating the body which obtains in Galen's case-histories, then one of the primary strategies for that process involves refiguring the relationship between his narrative voice and pain. We have already seen that in Galen, especially, the authority of those who speak about pain and the ways in which such speech is affected by pain is a critical problem which needs to be overcome or managed to facilitate diagnostic recognition.[31] Aristeides' act of narration, however, is characterized by the ways in which he reclaims certain aspects of pain's damaging effect on voice and language.

Aristeides' *Tales* open with an emphasis on the limitations of his voice, his incapacity to narrate his experiences, and his consequent choice to remain silent. The claims of Aristeides' *prooimion* (47.1–3K), in which he stresses that he submitted to his doctor 'in silence', build on a lengthy quotation of the impossibility of describing his experiences; lines earlier, he claims that he refused the advice of his friends to speak or write about his experiences, fleeing what was for him an impossible task.[32] It is easy to see how his statement might be taken with a grain of interpretative salt: Aristeides claims to be silent and then immediately proceeds to narrate his experiences *ad nauseam*. Yet it is also susceptible to a more subtle, and supple, reading.

[31] Gal. *Loc. Aff.* viii.88–9K.   [32] Aristid. 47.2K.

Studies of trauma and the ways in which those exposed to extreme trauma recount their experience stress that the impact of the experience is often felt in terms of their consciousness of the incapacity to capture and convey the immensity of what has happened to them.[33] Testimonies of extreme trauma are often characterized by the vacillation between the compulsion to speak and the inability to capture all of their experiences. These references to silence and the impossibility of narrating his every experience are not just cues for an epic voice or a self-ironizing take on those who speak about their experiences. Aristeides' construction of his silence might well be seeded within the aretological and epic traditions of narration, but it also attests to the overwhelming power of pain to undermine the capacity for narrative description.

Aristeides' silence introduces a concern with aphasia which reverberates throughout the *Tales*. Early in the second *Tale*, he recounts how his early attempts to dictate his experiences were fundamentally limited by his bodily pain: 'the recording of these [events and experiences] was, from the beginning, impossible for me, because I believed I would not survive; and, in addition, the body was in such a condition that there was no leisure for such things' (ὧν τὸ μὲν ἐξ ἀρχῆς οὐδὲν ἡμῖν ἐπῄει γράφειν ἀπιστίᾳ τοῦ μὴ περιέσεσθαι, ἔπειτα καὶ τὸ σῶμα οὕτως ἔχον οὐκ εἴα σχολάζειν τούτοις, 48.1K). At other points throughout subsequent *logoi* this closeness between the effects of pain on the body and his incapacity to speak is linked to his inability to engage in oratory.[34] At other times, he tells readers that the symptoms of his pain reduced him to a state in which all he could do was scream: the effect of the pain was unspeakable (ἄρρητος) and 'would not allow [him] to be silent, but would force him to scream out more loudly' (οὔτε σιωπᾶν ἐῶσα καὶ πρὸς τὴν φωνὴν ἔτι μεῖζον ἀπαντῶσα, 49.17K). The silencing impact of pain seems reversed by the fact that Aristeides' pain forced him to overcome silence. Rather than inducing speech or other forms of communication, however, it results only in the non-linguistic register of the scream.

Such interest in silence is reiterated throughout this particular scene. He claims that the spasm which 'supervened on the fever'

---

[33] LaCapra (2009), 60-2.
[34] Cf. Aristid. 50.14K and 17K for reference to the 'matters of his body'.

was 'unspeakable' (οὔτε τις ῥητός) and that 'such a thing one could not even conceive' (οὔθ' οἷον ἄν τις καὶ διανοηθείη, 49.17K). The suggestion that certain experiences are *arrēta* is returned to on a number of occasions;[35] at other times, his symptoms are referred to as *amuthēta*.[36] The choice of *arrētos* to describe specific symptoms recalls Galen's discussion of the language of pain, in which experiences could be *arrēta* or that certain types of pain developed by Arkhigenes were *arrēta*.[37] In those instances, ineffability and the patient's inability to describe events were presented as critical fissures in the clear or indicative narratives which facilitated diagnostic recognition. They were, ultimately, problems to be overcome. In the *Tales*, ineffability and narrative failure are positively co-opted in order to emphasize the particular nature of Aristeides' condition as beyond the realms of language and understanding. In Aristeides' hands, the ineffability that undermined medical accounts of pain becomes a way of communicating the nature of his experiences.

Aristeides also figures a more general failure of *logos* or intelligible discourse. In the second *Tale*, for instance, Aristeides informs us that what he felt was 'not entirely easy to show in discourse' (ἐνδείξασθαι λόγῳ οὐ πάνυ ῥᾴδιον, 48.49K). At other times, he links this process with more explicit expressions of understanding on behalf of his readers: the condition was easy to understand for the god, but difficult to understand or to write about for mortals.[38] What commands my attention in these passages is the way in which they resist the cognitive reactions of certain kinds of medical readers. Narrative ineffability is linked to the capacity for recognition, but it seems to deny the possibility of a medical form of understanding on the basis of clear language and rational discourse.

c. Revealing the Anatomy of the Body

One of the primary strategies that Aristeides uses to confront a medical recognition and approach to the translation of bodily symptoms concerns the manipulation of the revelatory nature of the speeches, which are presented as an act of public revelation

---

[35] For *arrētos*, see, e.g., Aristid. 48.23K.
[36] See, e.g., Aristid. 48.6K, 62K, and 75K; also 49.46K.
[37] See Chapter 3 (text with nn. 33–4 and 37–8). [38] Aristid. 49.17K.

Sacred Pain in Ailios Aristeides

and display. At various points he claims 'to bring... into public' (ἄγειν ... εἰς μέσον) what he feels;[39] even their name—the *Hieroi Logoi*—emphasizes their public revelation of private religious material.[40] His continued claims 'to reveal' or 'to indicate' the internal conditions of the body through the use of the verb *dēloun* reiterates this desire. As we have seen, speaking in language that is clear is a central part of Galen's interest in patient narratives.[41] Aristeides continually recontextualizes the act of revealing the condition of his body and, in so doing, downplays the connection between the medical process of revelation and knowledge about the body, its internal states, and the diagnosis of the individual's conditions. This recontextualization forms a crucial part of the author's attempt to (de)construct the translation of the body's experiences into meaningful public discourse.

Aristeides begins the account of his conditions by telling his readers that he wishes 'to reveal to you the matter of my intestine' (τὸ τοῦ ἤτρου δηλῶσαι πρὸς ὑμᾶς, 47.4K). In the first example of physical description, Aristeides' language constructs the reader as a type of privileged viewer, looking in on the internal conditions of the narrator's body. This act of revelation is reminiscent of the process of revealing the body's internal physical structure in the public arena in contemporary medical discourse. Galen connected the knowledge of the body acquired through the public display of its internal structure and form by employing verbs such as *dēloun* and *sēmainein*. His *On Anatomical Procedures* is littered with claims that he has indicated, or will indicate, the nature of the body. At one point, for example, he claims that he revealed (ἐδήλωσα) the movement of the muscles about the thorax.[42] At other places, he claims that his works show or clearly reveal the inner structure and order of the body.[43] Aristeides' use of the verb *dēloun* immediately locates his revelation of the physical *minutiae* of his body within this medical

---

[39] Aristid. 48.2K. For the formula, see Hdt. 4.97; D.2.6, 18.139; and Isoc. 47.6; cf. D. H. *Antiq. Rom.* 1.78.3 for the connection with public revelation of secret business.

[40] See Heinrichs (2003) for a discussion of the notion of the *hieros biblos* (etc.) and its revelation and concealment of religious practice and knowledge. Although the title is modern, the suggestion that his works should be considered as *hieroi logoi* is figured at Aristid. 48.10K.

[41] Perkins (1995), 176-7.   [42] Gal. *AA.* ii.499K.

[43] Cf. the use of *sēmainein* at Gal. *Loc. Aff.* viii.111K and 381K. For the use of *dēloun* as part of the diagnostic and teaching process, see *Loc. Aff.* viii.231K, 311K, 313K, 314K, and 410K.

culture of public revelation and debates about the viewing of the internal body within medical dissection and vivisection.

However, as the process of revelation continues throughout the *Tales*, the reader's security about the way that the narrative allows for clear recognition of the body is gradually undermined. Perhaps the most important role of this term is to connect the act of bodily revelation with the way in which the god communicates with Aristeides: 'many other pronouncements...were revealed to both of us' (πολλὰ ἄλλα λόγια...ἀμφετέροις ἐδηλώθη, 48.36K).[44] On one reading, Aristeides' use of the term constructs the *Tales* as a form of translation. Just as Aristeides reveals to the reader the nature of the body, so too Asklepios reveals his prescriptions, treatments, and commands to Aristeides: the text replicates towards the external reader the internal narrative of dream revelation and bodily treatment which obtains in his personal relationship with the god.

If Aristeides assimilates revealing the body to the process of narrating his dreams, how does this influence the reader's capacity to understand the body? Divine revelation in Aristeides' narrative can be presented in language which suggests clarity. So, at 48.31K, we are told that the signs from the divine 'were revealed as vividly as possible' (ἐδηλώθη δὲ ὡς ἐναργέστατα), just as 'countless other vivid things from the god occurred for those who were present' (μυρία ἕτερα ἐναργῆ τὴν παρουσίαν εἶχε τοῦ θεοῦ, 48.31K). In this context, the god's revelations take on a clear quality. At this level, revealing both the commands of the divine and the internal conditions of the body seems unproblematic, providing a vivid path to understanding both the nature of Aristeides' conditions and experiences and the power of Asklepios. Having said this, at other points they are introduced in a manner which stresses the ineffable and mysterious nature of divine command. At one point, in describing a dream revelation, Aristeides tells us that '[he] suspected that fasting was indicated by these visions' (τούτων ὀφθέντων ὑπενόησα μὲν ἀσιτίαν δηλοῦσθαι, 47.55K). The uncertainty conveyed here is strengthened moments later when he

---

[44] Cf. Aristid. 47.75K (for others' communication with Aristeides), 49.48K, 50.21K. Other examples are discussed in the text; cf. also the usage at 50.76K, where it is used for his discussions with the emperors. See Israelowich (2012), 71–85 on the role of dream interpretation in Aristeides and the Asklepieion. On dream interpretation as a foil for Aristeides' interpretation of his body, see Holmes (2008).

Sacred Pain in Ailios Aristeides

asks Asklepios 'to indicate more clearly which of the two things he commanded' (σημῆναι σαφέστερον ὁπότερα λέγοι, 47.55K).

Aristeides' language implies problematic interpretation. Holmes' suggestion that this process presents Aristeides as something of a privileged interpreter of both dreams and his body is surely right.[45] For the present circumstances, I want to point out that the difficulty of interpretation in these uses of *dēloun* leaks into the ways in which readers react to the revelation of his body. Aristeides' treatment of the issue of revelation, figured through his use of *dēloun*, places the discussion and narration of the body's experiences within a highly medicalized narrative and revelatory context. Rather than affirming the audience's capacity to read and understand the body through this act of revelation, Aristeides undermines that process by assimilating his external act of revelation to the internal act of revelation from the god. This process dramatically undermines the security of both intra- and extra-diegetic readings of Aristeides' internal conditions. Aristeides' act of translation, here, seems to diverges from the goals of the Galenic process of narration that I discussed in Chapter 3. However, in this instance, it is the text's denial of clarity which testifies to the nature of painful experience.

By figuring his narrative's failure to provide precise knowledge, Aristeides refigures the engagement with vividness and clarity that we see in Galen's treatises. Galen's *On Anatomical Procedures*, for instance, is underpinned by claims that he will explain (*diēgeisthai*) the function of the human body.[46] Similarly, Galen's repeated use of verbs of seeing, visual wonder, and display throughout works such as *On Anatomical Procedures* or *How to Recognize the Best Physicians* constantly invites readers to see the body through his rhetorical narratives.[47] Yet Galen's interest in the display of different and unusual aspects of the body produces a remarkably different texture from that of Aristeides. Galen continually connects the sight and display of the body to clear and precise knowledge achieved through the process of narrative description. This connection is enforced by Galen's use of adverbs such as *akribōs*, *saphōs*, and *alēthōs*. At one point in his *On Anatomical Procedures*, for instance, he tells his readers that he will engage in dissection so that they will learn 'accurately' (ἀκριβῶς) about the heart.[48] Galen's narrative

---

[45] Holmes (2008), 131–3. [46] See, e.g., Gal. *AA*. ii.652K.
[47] See von Staden (1995a) and (1995b), 47–66, esp. 63–6.
[48] Gal. *AA*. ii.603K.

emphasizes the connection between narration, clear revelation, and readers' understanding of the anatomized body. Aristeides simultaneously points to that context and then downplays its usefulness for his own text. Throughout the *Tales*, that relationship is defined by the difficulty of reading the body, and the mysteriousness surrounding its linguistic, narrative, and oneiric revelation.

d. Belief and Certainty

The final issue that I wish to discuss in the context of Aristeides' capacity to shape the process of recognition concerns the *Tales*' cultivation and management of belief or *pistis*. Trust and faith in the reliability of Aristeides' account (and his body) are continually undermined by assertions that his experiences are incredible or amazing. Aristeides positions his narrative (and his experiences) alongside those of other novelistic and heroic figures like Apollonios of Tyana and Odysseus. Constructing belief thus operates as a strategy for not only figuring his own experiences as amazing, but also managing his readers' capacity to understand or recognize what he has undergone through the narrative that recounts them.

The *Tales* open with a Homeric allusion in which Aristeides claims that he will narrate like the poet's Helen. Aristeides presents himself as speaking in the mode of Helen because she narrates only part of the many deeds of 'long-enduring Odysseus' (47.1K).[49] What does it mean to speak like Helen? On one level, the passage refers (as much recent scholarship has pointed out) to Aristeides' inability to tell all of his immense experiences: Helen represents a primary model for Aristeides' summarization of his experiences.[50] At the same time, however, the reference to Helen's stories about Odysseus raises more difficult questions about the type of *logos* Aristeides will produce. Helen's story (*Od.* 4.235–64) appears to be a rhetorical performance which attempts to reshape her *kleos* by recounting an event in which she assisted one of the Greek heroes; it is a performance fraught with questions about her honesty. Although Helen herself tells us that her story is 'plausible' (ἐοικότα, *Od.* 4.239),[51] Menelaos

---

[49] Holmes (2008), 81–2, for discussion.
[50] Pearcy (1988), 380 and Whitmarsh (2004), 442–3.
[51] Her language here mirrors the treatment of Odysseus' act of disguise: NB the use of ἐοικώς at Hom. *Od.* 4.245. For a discussion of this: Gumpert (2001), 38. For Helen

tells us, only moments later, that she spoke 'according to her share of fate' (κατὰ μοῖραν) rather than accurately (*Od.* 4.266). Menelaos' response to Helen's speech suggests that her account might be less than factual.[52]

Aristeides' willingness to adopt Helen to emblematize his summarization of his experiences poses an interpretative challenge for his readers: will his account be the genuine and sincere account of a pained man and a devotee? Or does making a *logos* like Homer's Helen mean that he will produce something *like* the truth? The problems raised by the use of the *Odyssey* penetrate further. At a range of points throughout his *Tales*, Aristeides suggests that his stories need to be understood against Odysseus' *apologoi:* they are 'greater than the story told to Alkinoos (πέρα ἢ κατ' Ἀλκίνου ἀπόλογον, 48.60K). Aristeides is clearly playing on the proverbial meaning of the phrase Ἀλκίνου ἀπόλογον: the term's earliest recorded usage in Plato's *Republic* (at *R.* 614b) implies long-winded babbling. But the phrase also carries implications of mendacity. The phrase can recall Homer's placement of Odysseus' experiences in the outer ocean—a geographical and literary space characterized by incredible *thaumata* and lying tales of travellers.[53] Aristeides' self-conscious engagement with the *apologoi* raises questions about his truthfulness. Such questions are strengthened by Aristeides' willingness to refer to his *Tales* as a type of Odyssean journey,[54] and his reference to a dream in which Athena tells him that he is both Telemakhos and Odysseus and that the *Odyssey* was not a collection of 'fictional tales' (μῦθοι, 48.42K). Aristeides' denial of the *Odyssey*'s status as fictional is far from unproblematic. The suggestion that the *apologoi* should be read as more than fictional stories implies that their more modern analogues should themselves be seen as truthful. At a more fundamental level, however, Athena's denial of the *Odyssey*'s fictional status raises questions about where readers should situate both texts on the spectrum of narrative believability or facticity. Are we to approach the *Tales* as factual narratives in the same way that we approach the *apologoi*? By emphasizing its Odyssean nature, the

---

and rhetorical trickery in this passage: Zeitlin (1996), 410, who sees the passage as dominated by the figure of Proteus and the themes of deception and disguise. For Helen's story as a slippery act of public relations: Doherty (1995), 81–92, esp. 86–8.

[52] For Menelaos' story as proof that Helen is lying: Doherty (1995), 86–8.
[53] Tümpel (1893), 522–33.   [54] Aristid. 48.64–5K.

logoi allude to the problems that these narratives pose as true *logoi*, as opposed to *muthoi*.

The *Tales* are continually represented as a collection of stories which pose problems in terms of readerly belief or trust in them. Far from attempting to solve this interpretative problem, Aristeides attempts to augment uncertainty: at 49.40K, he exhorts readers who do not believe him to stop reading: 'regarding the event that took place after this, to the one who wants to trust, let him, to the one who doesn't, farewell!' (τὸ δὴ μετὰ τοῦτο ὅτῳ μὲν φίλον πιστεύειν, πιστευέτω, ὅτῳ δὲ μή, χαιρέτω).[55] This interest in the belief of the reader is, perhaps, reminiscent of another type of odyssey: that of the first-century-CE holy man, Apollonios, in Philostratos' *Life of Apollonios of Tyana*. During the account of Apollonios' travels to India, Philostratos tells the reader that it would be better neither to believe nor disbelieve anything written in his account.[56] How are we to read these authors' delicate flaunting of their texts' (un)believability? It is hard to accept that either Philostratos or Aristeides wants readers to treat them as either straightforwardly true or untrue. Rather, I suggest, it is more productive to see these authors as deliberately using the respective texts' problematic status to emphasize a type of truth about their subject matter: the truth about Aristeides' experience of Asklepios is that it—like the *apologoi* and Philostratos' Apollonios—strains at the boundaries of factual veracity and believability. It confounds attempts at factual or historical verification.

How others recognize his experiences depends on the ways in which they negotiate this and other aspects of Aristeides' representation of his own language and narrative. If we adopt a medical reading of the *Tales*, expecting the body's narration to provide diagnostic recognition and certainty, that process is explicitly and consciously undermined by the cagey nature of the narrative. If we approach it from other generic contexts, then it becomes easier to navigate the fissures and the crab-like nature of the account. In that context, the very points that resist certain knowledge and diagnostic reading represent his experiences as incredible, heroic, and wonderful. As

---

[55] Translation from Behr (1981).
[56] Phil. *VA*. 3.45 (61–2K): καὶ γὰρ κέρδος ἂν εἴη μήτε πιστεύειν, μήτε ἀπιστεῖν πᾶσιν ('for it would be a benefit neither to believe nor to disbelieve everything [in relation to the Indian stories about Apollonios]'). For discussion: Bowie (1978), esp. 1663–7 for the *VA*'s status as fiction, and Bowie (1994), 181–99.

he himself suggests: if one would consider his experiences, one would say that they are 'truly beyond wonders' (ἀληθῶς περαιτέρω θαυμάτων, 48.49K).

3. EMOTIONAL AND HEROIC SUFFERING

In this final section, I turn to some of the more affective aspects of Aristeides' representation of his pain and illness experience. I have tried to show, already, that Aristeides' act of speaking about pain and his body's experiences rewrites the doctor–patient relationship and the ways in which different groups of people understand or recognize his experiences through language or narrative. Here, I turn to the ways in which Aristeides attributes different emotional states—such as hope, despair, and joy—to his navigation of his illness and painful episodes. These help to shape affective relationships between Aristeides and his audiences.

Early in his fourth *Tale*, Aristeides describes travelling (at the instruction of the god) to Poimanenos for a cure to his long-endured disease. This scene is particularly telling because of its focus on the improving health of Aristeides and his return to his rhetorical career. At this time, he suggests that his 'indescribable catarrhs and the convulsions of his veins and nerves ceased' (ἀνώνυμενοι κατάρροι καὶ σφάκελοι περὶ τὰς φλέβας καὶ τὰ νεῦρα ἀπεπαύσαντο, 50.8K) and that he resumed his rhetorical career under the guidance of the god. What interests me about this scene is the way in which Aristeides describes the mental state that accompanied some of this process:

> ἦν οὖν οὐ μόνον τελετῇ τινι ἐοικὸς, οὕτω θείων τε καὶ παραδόξων τῶν δρωμένων ὄντων, ἀλλὰ καὶ συνέπιπτέ τι θαυμαστὸν ἀηθείᾳ· ἅμα μὲν γὰρ ἦν εὐθυμεῖσθαι, χαίρειν, ἐν εὐκόλοις εἶναι καὶ τῆς ψυχῆς καὶ τοῦ σώματος, ἅμα δ' οἷον ἀπιστεῖν εἴ ποτε ταύτην ἰδεῖν ἐξέσται τὴν ἡμέραν, ἐν ᾗ τις ἐλεύθερον αὑτὸν τῶν τοσούτων πραγμάτων ὄψεται, πρὸς δὲ καὶ δεδιέναι μή πού τι τῶν εἰωθότων αὖθις συμβὰν λυμήνηται ταῖς περὶ τῶν ὅλων ἐλπίσιν. κατεσκεύαστο μὲν οὕτω τὰ τῆς γνώμης καὶ μετὰ τοιαύτης ἡδονῆς ἅμα καὶ ἀγωνίας ἡ ἀναχώρησις ἐγίγνετο.

> It was all not only like an initiation into a mystery, since the rituals were so divine and strange, but also an amazing thing occurred in an unusual manner. For at the same time there was gladness, and joy, and a contentment of soul and body, and simultaneously, disbelief that it

will ever be possible to see the day when one will see oneself free from such great troubles, and in addition, a fear that some one of the usual things will again befall and harm one's hopes about the whole. Thus was my state of mind, and my return took place with such happiness and at the same time anguish.

Aristid. 50.7K[57]

Aristeides figures the movement from the state of illness into health in terms of a certain emotional ambivalence. The reference to delight, pleasure, and contentment on both physical and psychical levels points to the combined psychosomatic experience of illness and recovery that we have traced in other authors over the preceding investigations in Chapters 2 and 3. The transformation in experience is, at one level, marked by the emphasis of pleasure and *euthumia*. The choice of *eukolia* juxtaposes the continued use of *duskolia* throughout the *Tales* to emphasize physical discomfort.[58] What is particularly telling is the combination of those pleasant feelings with more problematic affective and psychological reactions to his situation. Disbelief, here, not only marks out the concerns of this moment, but returns readers to his continued references to his and others' disbelief in the possibility of his survival and recovery throughout the *Tales*.

There is a sense in which Aristeides plays out some of the emotional insecurities that Aretaios attributed to his patients in the *prooimion* of his *On the Causes and Signs of Chronic Diseases*.[59] In both situations, hope, confusion, and fear are part of the exposure to painful illness. In contrast to Aretaios' account, however, Aristeides connects that level of experience with the process of initiation. It is, perhaps, not surprising that Aristeides might represent his experiences in this way. Scholars have long stressed that his entire experience is figured as a type of mystical religious event, of which the *Tales* are a revelation.[60] What is telling is the way in which it continues to play into the exceptional nature of Aristeides' connection with the divine and his status as a sufferer. Reference to initiation seems to stress the exceptional nature of Aristeides'

---

[57] Translation adapted from Behr (1981).
[58] *Duskolia*: e.g. Aristid. 48.38K. For *euthumia*: 48.23, 73K, 49.13K, and 50.2K.
[59] Aret. *SD*. iii.1.1.2–2.7.
[60] Aristeides and the mystical: Downie (2013), 23–8. For a discussion of these and other 'sacred tales' (*hieroi logoi*) and mystery religion, see Heinrichs (2003).

recovery through its stress on the personal relationship that he is allowed to enter into with the divine.

The reference to hope in this context points to a consistent theme across the entire *Tales*. We have already encountered the suggestion that Aristeides' lack of effort in recording his experiences was due to his expected demise.[61] At other times, however, he is slightly more precise about exactly what emotions he, and others, feel during illness episodes. In one instance, Aristeides relates that after setting out for Rome he was afflicted by a number of conditions which caused excruciating pain. As a consequence, the doctors engaged in purges by prescribing the purgative *elatērion* until there were significant discharges of blood. At this point, 'fevers attacked him, and there was every kind of difficulty, and there was no such hope of safety' (καὶ πυρετοὶ κατέλαβον καὶ πάντ' ἦν ἄπορα ἤδη καὶ σωτηρίας οὐδ' ἡτισοῦν ἐλπίς, 48.63K). In the first instance, Aristeides' experiences seem to lead immediately to a hopelessness about his continued existence. This sense of hopelessness is, of course, familiar from other writings on illness: Aretaios' patients are often characterized by their sense of hopelessness.[62]

In one particularly telling scene in his second *Tale*, Aristeides describes the despair felt during an episode of the plague. We have already touched on this scene's interest in his own perception of his illness experiences. It is also relevant for thinking about Aristeides' sense of his heroic qualities. He begins by recounting how the plague upset the normal order of things: it affected members of his family and household, the livestock, and others who had come to the house to help the orator. Aristeides glosses these events with the remarkably blithe statement that it was no longer possible to sail easily through his current circumstances. As he continues, he elaborates on the emotional context in a great deal more detail:

πάντα δ' ἦν μεστὰ ἀθυμίας οἰμωγῆς στόνου δυσκολίας ἁπάσης· ἦσαν δὲ κἀν τῇ πόλει νόσοι δειναί. τέως μὲν οὖν ἀντεῖχον οὐδὲν ἧττον τῆς τῶν ἄλλων σωτηρίας ἢ τῆς ἐμαυτοῦ προνοούμενος, ἔπειτα ἐπέτεινέ τε ἡ νόσος καὶ κατελήφθην ὑπὸ δεινοῦ πυρὸς χολῆς παντοίας, ἣ συνεχῶς νύκτα καὶ ἡμέραν ἠνώχλει, καὶ τῆς τροφῆς ἀπεκεκλείμην καὶ ἡ δύναμις κατελέλυτο. καὶ οἱ ἰατροὶ ἀφίσταντο καὶ τελευτῶντες ἀπέγνωσαν παντάπασιν, καὶ

---

[61] E.g. Aristid. 47.1K.   [62] E.g. Aret. SA. ii.2.18.1–7.

διηγγέλθη ὡς οἰχησομένου αὐτίκα. τὸ μέντοι τοῦ Ὁμήρου κἂν τούτοις εἶπες ἂν τὸ 'νόος γε μὲν ἔμπεδος ἦεν'.

Everything was full of despair, groans, and wails from all kinds of difficulty, and there was terrible illness in the city. I persisted in my concern for the safety of others, no less than for my own. Then the disease increased and I was attacked by the terrible burning of every sort of humour, which troubled me continuously day and night, and I was prevented from taking nourishment and my strength failed. And the doctors gave up and finally despaired entirely and it was announced that I would die immediately. However, even in these circumstances, you would have said the Homeric phrase, 'his mind was steadfast.'

Aristid. 48.38–9K[63]

Aristeides' picture vividly recreates the emotional framework of this event. One point that is unclear is whether or not the emotions described are a reaction to Aristeides' particular condition or a more general reaction to the plague in the city. However this might be, what is clear is the way in which he figures the extreme—and highly tragic—emotional context of the situation: note the use of οἰμωγή to figure the cries of the people in the city. These emotional reactions of others to the 'terrible illness' are constructed as a foil against which Aristeides can distinguish his own *pathē* and those of others. When confronted with his worsening condition, those around him—specifically doctors—despair of saving him, and announce his imminent demise. In contrast to both emotional reactions—those who groan and those who despair—Aristeides claims that he remains mentally strong. Aristeides' emphasis on the Homeric phrase 'his mind was steadfast' stresses not only his emotional distance from those around him, but his heroic qualities in the face of his impending death.

There are two points that I wish to draw from this discussion of Aristeides' representation of his own psychological and emotional state. The emotional and psychological elements of his illness experience are familiar from other representations of medical experience. Aristeides' careful delineation of his different emotional states speaks to the ways in which pain-perceivers often felt about their experiences because he works within a framework which incorporates the emotional aspects of experience into a full understanding of what it means to be subject to pain. At the same time, however, rather than straightforwardly

[63] Translation adapted from Behr (1981).

reflecting that culture, Aristeides uses it to distinguish his difference and distance from some of those around him. Emotional states, here, serve to reify his relationship with his contemporary world and his superlative and special qualities. His affective navigation of his disease—in contrast to everyone else—is defined by that quality which underpins his connection with the Homeric heroes. Unlike the doctors who despair, and others who wail and lament, Aristeides', heroic qualities allow him to navigate his disease differently.

8

Pain and Language Recalibrated

Over the course of the last two chapters, I have tried to show how medical approaches to pain were reformulated in different literary contexts. The boundaries between medical culture and other areas of cultural activity were (and are) always fluid: medical texts and thinking always interacted with the language and ideas of tragedy or epic. What is particularly telling, however, in this context is the way in which the reformulation of pain is undertaken by these Imperial writers.

There are two particularly significant implications that I want to draw out at this point. The first concerns the ways in which these authors broaden the sense of pain developed in medical contexts. Aretaios and Galen, whom we encountered in Part 1, started from an understanding of physiological pain perception in which the symptom and specific pain types were given heightened significance. Here, those pain perceptions and symptoms are repackaged in broader terms. These texts look, increasingly, to the types of hardship and difficulty which are characteristic of some aspects of Imperial literature, such as the Greek romances.

The second common feature of these works is the way in which they redefine the relationship between pain and language or, more generally, the body and language. Lucian, for instance, not only combines the discussion of pain symptoms with avowedly tragic language and metaphors, but explores the ways in which pain (in the form of the goddess Gout) impacts on language: pain, in this context, literally teaches a new kind of linguistic register. Aristeides, too, takes up some of the assumptions about clear and informative language developed in clinical scenarios and recalibrates it. In so doing, he engages in a debate with medical writers about how one speaks about pain. Aristeides continually confronts questions about what language is indicative, communicative, or effective; what types of recognition it facilitates; and who speaks, and how, about their own experiences. Read against figures like Galen, this constitutes a powerful statement of authority concerning the body, language, and experience. At the same time, Aristeides also positions his readers in delicate ways. The expectations about belief and clarity readers bring to the text—the types of reader one wants to be—contribute greatly to how we navigate Aristeides' interest in the language and narratives of the body. Our engagement with Aristeides' experiences and the experiences of the gouty man in Lucian's paratragedy are ultimately conducted through their delicate positioning of the reader.

Part 3

Viewing Trauma, Seeing Pain

9

Ekphrasis, Trauma, and Viewing Pain

νοσώδη μὲν ἄνθρωπον καὶ ὕπουλον ὡς ἀτερπὲς θέαμα φεύγομεν, τὸν δ' Ἀριστοφῶντος Φιλοκτήτην καὶ τὴν Σιλανίωνος Ἰοκάστην ὁμοίους φθίνουσι καὶ ἀποθνῄσκουσι πεποιημένους ὁρῶντες χαίρομεν.

We flee the diseased man and the ulcerous one as an unpleasant sight, but when we see the Philoktetes of Aristophon and the Iokasta of Silanion, which are represented resembling those who are wasting away and dying, we are pleased.

Plut. *Quomodo Adulesc.* 18c

When Plutarch, in his treatise *How Young Men Should Listen to Poetry*, draws a comparison between viewing the body of the sick man and its representation, he speaks to a particular concern of Imperial society with how one views traumatic or distressing images of pain.[1] Plutarch's broader point is an educative one: we should train young children to view the mimetic representation of despicable subjects properly, teaching them to praise only the mimetic skill of the representation, not the subject matter, as good or appropriate.[2] Plutarch's point rephrases an assertion that is familiar within the literary tradition and can be traced back to Aristotle's *Poetics* at least.[3] Questions, nonetheless, abound about this comparison. How does

---

[1] For the broader point: Plut. *Quomodo Adulesc.* 18c–d. For the treatment of Philoktetes in art: *LIMC* VII. 1.376–85; for ancient references, see, e.g., *AP*. xvi.111 for the Philoktetes of Parahassios. Aristophon is mentioned at Plin. *HN*. 35.138. For the Iokasta of Silanion: *LIMC* V. 1.683–6.

[2] Plut. *Quomodo Adulesc.* 18d.

[3] Konstan (2005), 1–17 and Van der Stockt (1990), 27–31. For the connection of Plutarch's reading with that of Aristotle: A. *Po*. 1448b11–7, though note Aristotle's use of λυπηρῶς ὁρῶμεν.

one view the pained body? If the sick body is an important *comparandum* for the pleasures of viewing the representation of trauma or pain, what do such comparisons mean for the cultural positioning of pain and pain sufferers?

In this final investigation, I continue to probe the cultural positioning of pain by exploring its treatment in some aspects of ancient visual culture. I am particularly interested in how literary and rhetorical texts construct the pained body as an object of sight and theorize the ways in which audiences viewed this *sōma*. Certain visible aspects of physical deportment and condition—physical wounds and damage, the tightening of one's facial muscles, the grimace, the frown, or the contortions of physical posture—reveal much about the conditions or feelings of others; they are, very often, integral to a culture's understanding of, and interest in, the perception of pain.[4] I turn to these and other phenomena associated with the traumatized body in order to probe how others' pain is visualized in an Imperial context. By manipulating the visual aspects of the body and exploring the act of viewing itself, writers reflect on the nature of pain experience: they probe how those in pain feel and navigate their body's destruction, they explore how those who view them might understand and engage with the trauma and pain of others, and they construct and deconstruct the place of pain in this culture.

As has been acknowledged, Imperial society was casually violent; violence, physical abuse, and trauma saturated the social fabric; its representation is woven into most forms of literary, dramatic, and graphic media.[5] I approach the process of viewing trauma through the use of rhetorical *ekphrasis* and other tropes which were designed to construct the reader or listener as a viewer. I devote my attention to the *Imagines* of Philostratos, the *Leukippe and Kleitophon* by Akhilleus Tatios, and Plutarch's *On Flesh-Eating*. If this literary concentration circumscribes ancient society's interest in viewing trauma, then there are specific reasons for turning to this area of cultural production. In their formulations of viewing, they elaborate a careful relationship between pain and trauma (one in which trauma does not always involve pain), help to contextualize such experiences within broad cultural frameworks of understanding and meaning, and figure the visual, intellectual, and emotional engagement of

---

[4] Kleinman (2007), 17–18.
[5] Particularly influential for this study has been Barton (1992).

others. They create, in short, the body as both a culturally mediated sight and a site of pain. At the heart of that process lies their interest in pain as the centre of moral, quasi-emotional relationships between those who feel pain and the other.

The use of *ekphrasis* in this context raises two immediate issues. In the first instance, these three texts are drawn from very different literary genres, possess different rhetorical aims, and employ diverse narrative techniques. The *Imagines* is a collection of brief, self-contained rhetorical *ekphraseis* which seek to explore, in different ways, how one views art and how one writes about viewing art; *Leukippe and Kleitophon* is, at base, an extended continuous prose narrative about the trials and hardships of a young couple; while the treatise *On Flesh-Eating* is a rhetorical tract aimed at making a sustained argument for the humane consumption of animal meat. These differing contexts inflect their respective concerns with viewing culture (through the use of *ekphrasis* and other tropes) and their incorporation of pain and trauma into their works. The second issue that should be mentioned in this context concerns the centrality of pain to their respective texts. Unlike the medical treatises or the works of Lucian and Aristeides where pain takes centre stage, pain and trauma are not always the major issue of these works. Pain arises at specific points and is used strategically to facilitate certain rhetorical objectives or to explore particular issues of authorial concern. Despite these two points, it is valuable to talk about this variegated group of works in collective terms. The differences that these texts exhibit at the level of genre help to accentuate the significance of their common interest in pain: it underscores what is common across time, place, and context. Secondly, because pain is not the central or only concern of these narratives, they invite scholars to pay particular attention to the moments when it is treated in detail.

This group of texts speaks to different styles of viewing. I start with what might be seen as a type of prurient, desiring gaze in Philostratos' *Imagines*; here, trauma (and the pain that is potentially associated with it) is continually reformulated. If the wound raises questions about the presence of pain in the body, then Philostratos refigures both that connection and the ways in which viewers might engage with it, generally recasting experiences in terms of pleasure and viewerly desire. I then turn to a type of 'conflicted gaze' in Akhilleus Tatios and Plutarch. Here, I argue, the process of looking at the body continually oscillates between recognizing or downplaying the pain of others; consequently, it induces an array of quasi-emotional responses in the viewer, ranging from pleasure at others' pain to distress at, and pity for, it. These differing types of gaze incorporate the body into different styles of spectatorship and viewing, allowing us to probe the ways in which pain and trauma can be seen as part of a combined interpersonal experience which implicates both viewer and viewed individual.

1. VIEWING THE BODY AND THE POSSIBILITIES OF EMBODIED PAIN EXPERIENCE

The focus on the ways in which trauma and the pained body are viewed has a number of important implications which need to be discussed. In the last two investigations, I focused on people who felt themselves to be in pain and how they and their pain were treated by others. The experience of pain emerged from the dialogue between the perception of pain, the way that perception was represented, and how those processes contributed to relationships between the pained individual and the other (whether that be a lay person, doctor, or reader). There are significant reasons for my explicit focus in this section on the ways in which the external other looks at, and interprets, the pained body.

We have already learnt that anatomical approaches to the body were intimately connected with the ways in which the body was viewed. In turning explicitly to the issue of viewing, I draw out and elaborate upon a subject which has been left under the surface of the first two investigations. We saw, for instance, in the treatment of Aretaios, that the pained body—especially that distorted and contorted by tetanus—was conceptualized as a 'painful sight'.[6] In the rhetorical work of Aristeides, the suggestion that his pained body must be viewed is an almost constant theme: his *sōma* is repeatedly figured as a *thea* and a *thauma*; and his performance of miraculous feats of healing or physical endurance is continually presented as a theatrical spectacle which amazed and confused viewers.[7] The

---

[6] Aret. SA. i.6.8.6. For discussion, see Chapter 2 (text to nn. 39–40).
[7] See Chapter 7 (n. 30). Also relevant in this context is the connection with anatomy and revelation of the inner body: Aristid. 47.4K, with Chapter 7 (text to nn. 39–42) for further discussion.

intersections between the pained body, illness, and the process of viewing are also found in other areas of the cultural landscape. Galen's anatomical treatises are, of course, types of *ekphraseis* which offer up the opened body for readerly viewing; his own anatomical knowledge was developed through seeing—and then treating—the traumatized bodies of gladiators in the arena at Pergamon.[8] Qualities like the body's 'proportion' or 'symmetry' (*summetria*) cut across medical, aesthetic, and moral readings of the body: the healthy body was well-proportioned, just as those which are represented artistically, and those that are aesthetically pleasing.[9] These intersections between different engagements with how one views the pained body raise some important issues about the culture of the first three centuries CE: what is it about this society that facilitated the connections between these multiple ways of viewing the body?

There are, of course, other consequences of my turn to the dynamics of the gaze. One of the reasons the various theorizations of the gaze are important is that they treat two issues which impact on pain experience. Looking at the traumatized body—navigating what that body means for the viewer—involves imagining the close relationship between physical pain and what we can see has occurred to, or within, the *sōma*. These texts all ask one to imagine whether or not pain actually arises in the damaged body. Do audiences see it, and if they do not, why not? What physical and emotional qualities does the pain-perceiver display or what are the contextual factors which allow the viewer to disassociate trauma and the perception of pain? In elucidating how the audience might (or might not) imagine pain in the viewed body, these authors also speak to the broader cultural values which underpin Imperial society's understanding of the sensation. Plutarch's words (which I quoted at the start of the chapter) place the experience of pain on an aesthetic spectrum which maps how audiences feel about viewing the pain of the individual and how their culture makes judgements about those in pain. These discussions of how viewers 'feel' and what their reactions to it are— is it viewed pleasurably, erotically, piteously, or in a distressing

---

[8] See, e.g Gal. *Comp. Med. Gen.* xiii.599–601K. For further discussion, see Introduction (text with nn. 35–8, esp. n. 38), for further references to Galen's anatomical practices and viewing.

[9] See Gal. *Temp.* i.565–6K for his praise of the *Kanon* of Polykleitos for its healthful qualities. For further discussion of medicine and aesthetics in a Classical context, see Leftwich (1995), along with the Introduction (text with nn. 41–4).

manner?—help to construct and reify the cultural, aesthetic, and emotional status of those who perceive pain. In short, they construct what it means to be in pain in this society.

2. THE WOUND, GESTURE, AND 'SEEING' PAIN

The way in which physical trauma or violence—especially torture—is presented as a spectacle to be viewed or witnessed has been subjected to extensive critical analysis over the last three decades. In his groundbreaking work *Discipline and Punish*, Foucault argues that pain, when created through public displays of torture, speaks metaphorically of the power of political and juridical regimes.[10] For Foucault, the body acts as a script, its physical abuse is (re)written as power and justice and 'read' or 'seen' by a viewing public as such. Foucault's discussion has been pivotal to classical and early-modern scholarship on torture and the spectacle of violence. Page duBois's seminal study *Torture and Truth* employs this model to analyse the importance of torture within Athenian society and Archaic and Classical Greek literature.[11] Perhaps Foucault's influence has been most strongly felt in the context of the critical work on the Roman Imperial arena and Christian martyrdom. As Shaw and many others have noted, Christian texts rewrite the power discourses of the Roman world by reconceptualizing the relationship between torture, pain, and endurance.[12]

Some of the assumptions of Foucault's work have been taken up by Jennifer Ballengee in her fascinating and deeply Foucauldian discussion, *The Wound and the Witness*. Following Foucault, she argues that the 'ideological truth' of pain is linked with the ways in which literary representation structures readers as 'witnesses' of physical violation. Ballengee is primarily concerned with situations in which 'bodily injury' and 'suffering' are 'presented as torture...before a witnessing audience':[13]

---

[10] Foucault (1991). For torture as a public spectacle, 3–14 and 41–7, and for pain as the objective of juridical mechanisms, 30–69.

[11] duBois (1991) and Ballengee (2009).

[12] Shaw (1996), 300–1. See Potter (1993) and Frilingos (2009) for further formulations of the power–torture relationship.

[13] Ballengee (2009), 5.

The association of bodily pain with understanding resonates... within the idea of being a witness. The texts addressed in this study all demonstrate a consistent association between bodily pain and an essential, ideological 'truth' that is conveyed by means of the representation of torture.[14]

Ballengee's broad point is that the meaning of torture is constructed through the process of viewing; the viewer is complicit in the act of understanding the tortured body's 'meaning'. For all that is valuable in this work, Ballengee does not give enough attention to the distinction between torture, physical injury, 'suffering', and pain. Different types or levels of experience are elided here: does bodily injury entail 'suffering' or pain, and are they necessarily equatable to torture? It is a truism that the metaphors of 'torture' and 'suffering' mean vastly different things in Christian and pagan contexts, such as tragedy or the Athenian law courts. While Ballengee's reading is (often very) sensitive to nuances of meaning over time and cultural context, it is less sensitive to the (potential and real) distinctions between the different categories of experience. Martyrs, it seems to my mind, experience pain in very different ways from the subject of an anatomical dissection by the doctor Galen or a sacrificial victim. While it is hard to disagree with the general assertion that the viewer is complicit in the construction of meaning of spectacular scenes of torture, it is also true that there are different types of witnessing across ancient scientific, literary, and religious culture which allow for different pain perceptions to be seen or not seen, understood, verified, and engaged with.

I start, like Ballengee, from a focus on physical injury—what was commonly designated in ancient texts as *trauma* or *helkos*. The wound is at once both a broader and more specific category of discussion than torture. There are, of course, plenty of wounds that occur on the body that do not arise as part of torture. It is more specific because of the way in which it returns the viewer to the physical body. There are times when the term 'wound' (*trauma*) holds a certain amount of metaphorical significance—'the wound of love' is a common theme in erotic poetry and prose[15]—but, unlike the categories of torture or suffering, it is visible on (or in) the *sōma*. Secondly, the wound is connected with the ways in which that body is

---

[14] Ballengee (2009), 5–6.
[15] See, e.g., Chariton i.1.7 and Ach. Tat. i.4.4.

presented to the reader: it has the potential to expose the viewer to aspects of the body not normally encountered, such as blood and gore and the internal organs. Like anatomical demonstrations and descriptions, the wound takes the viewer inside the body, transforming that which is (under normal circumstances) hidden and closed off into that which is apparent. As well as discussing wounds, I will branch out into a number of other areas of corporeal presentation. I am particularly interested in some of the broader aspects of physical deportment that are often connected with wounds, including scars (the visible traces of some form of physical destruction), a range of physical contortions such as the contraction of the body or hands, facial expressions, and screams. Like the wound, they have the advantage of returning the discussion to the visual qualities of the body.

One of the reasons why I want to start with the basic physical (and visual) aspects of the body is because, I argue, ancient texts continually explore the ways in which these visible phenomena act as signs of, or are imagined to be part of, the perception of pain. Paradoxically, pain is a fascinating subject precisely because the *aisthēsis* itself has little or no visual content: wounds, physical damage, and contortions—body language—operate as visible *sēmata* of the invisible perception. The recognition of pain on the visual body requires a specific act of reading or imagination by others; an act of reading into the body, its conditions and superficial signs, what one imagines to stand behind them. In making (or denying) the connections between external signs and pain, these authors allow scholars access to their thinking and (sometimes unspoken) assumptions about the perception of pain in the violated body.

There are two implications which emerge from this point. The first is that the act of reading the signs of the body requires a particular engagement with one's cultural assumptions and ideas about pain and its visible evidence. Certain physical phenomena operate as metaphors for pain because they might be habitually associated with the perception. In a medical context, for example, we have seen that the wound is part of the definition of pain among rational medical writers: the destruction of the body's continuity through cutting, burning, or other violent activities leads to the perception of pain.[16] In this context, trauma and pain are closely

---

[16] See, e.g., Gal. *MM*. x.232K: 'the destruction of continuity' (ἡ τῆς συνεχείας λύσις) is called 'a wound' (ἕλκος) when it occurs 'in the fleshy part of the body' (ἐν σαρκώδει

associated—one almost stands in for the other. In other contexts, the tearing of one's neck and hair in mourning might operate as a metaphor for the emotional distress associated with bereavement precisely because it is habitually associated with mourning and its associated *pathē*.[17] Douglas Cairns has suggested that 'shivers' (φρῖκαι) operate almost as metonyms for the emotions of fear and terror precisely because of their habitual association throughout Greek culture.[18] With this in mind, seeing pain in the wound involves reading into, imagining into the body's visible qualities, something one assumes to be present in the *sōma*.[19]

The second implication concerns how these authors (re)write some of their shared cultural assumptions. It might be a natural assumption to imagine pain as a central aspect of trauma. These writers, however, suggest that it is often not the case. They often downplay the presence of pain in favour of other internal feelings of the wounded or traumatized. At other times, they redirect the viewer's gaze away from pain, denying its presence or simply eschewing the perception. In so doing, they not only recalibrate or nuance the connection between pain and trauma, but also begin to explore where, in what contexts, and under what conditions one might imagine another as feeling pain and the extent to which the wound might be associated with other, less distressing perceptions or emotions. The pain that Ballengee and others assume to exist in acts such as torture is often denied and rewritten in different viewing contexts. On one reading, that process adds to the understanding of the complexity of the ancient landscape, contextualizing the medical connection between bodily destruction and pain. It also attests to the variety of viewing practices which facilitated differing approaches to the presence of pain in the body.

μορίῳ). For further connections: Aret. *SD.* iv.12 with further discussion, Chapter 2 (text to nn. 11–12) and Chapter 3 (text to nn. 16–18).

[17] For other physical symptoms, see Dio of Prusa on the 'external practices' devised by those in grief: D. Chr. 16.2. For fuller discussion of the ways in which bodily deportment acts as a metaphor for pain or other invisible phenomena, see Kirmayer (2007) and Kleinman (2007).

[18] Cairns (2013), esp. 87–9.

[19] I have been very much influenced in my thinking about 'seeing in' vs 'seeing as' by Squire (2013), 104–7, with further references.

170 Ekphrasis, *Trauma*, and Viewing Pain

3. FRAMING EMOTIONAL RESPONSES
TO TRAUMA

Just as these texts investigate the connection between pain and trauma, they also develop affective and intellectual responses to these experiences. Philostratos, Akhilleus Tatios, and Plutarch all employ the rhetorical trope of *ekphrasis* (and the related quality of rhetorical vividness) to bring the traumatized body before the eyes of the reader. The act of viewing underpins a range of quasi-emotional responses to pain and trauma. These responses shape the individual's navigation of their own pain and the viewer's reaction to the pain of others.

In discussing the affective consequences of viewing, I turn to a subject which has received considerable critical discussion.[20] Central to scholarly treatments of the way in which *ekphrasis* shapes the viewing experience has been a process in which the viewer is thought to exercise control over the image and its powerful emotional effects. As Kathryn Gutzwiller notes in relation to Hellenistic epigram, *ekphrasis* presents a viewer negotiating the 'powerful emotive impact of an image in order to tame it in the articulation of thought'.[21] Gutzwiller's suggestion chimes with a range of other scholarly readings of *ekphrasis* from the Hellenistic and Imperial worlds. For Simon Goldhill, *ekphrasis* constructs a *sophos theatēs*, who, rather than being overawed or emotionally stunned by art, responds in sophisticated and educated acts of speech and praise.[22] This reaction to art is explicitly dramatized at a number of critical points in Imperial literature. Lucian's *On the Hall*, for instance, stresses that the emotional responses of wonder and stupefaction are characteristic of the uneducated, while those who have been educated—the *pepaideumenoi*—are able to speak about what they see.[23] On this reading, forming oneself as an educated (and elite) viewer involves navigating the emotional impact of visual objects and then responding in appropriate, sophisticated

---

[20] Goldhill (1994), 197–223 for the culture of viewing in Hellenistic poetry and, for critical engagement with his argument, Zanker (2004). For Imperial culture: Goldhill (2001b), (2002), and (2007). For *ekphrasis* in general: Elsner (2002b) and the individual contributions to that volume, Bartsch and Elsner (2007), Webb (2009), and Squire (2013).

[21] Gutzwiller (2002), 110. See also Squire (2013), 128 for the application of this to Philostratos.

[22] Goldhill (2001b), 154–94.

[23] Luc. *Dom.* 1–2; cf. the discussion of self-control at Longus *D&C. praef.*

ways. The promotion of such a sophisticated response plays down, at one level, the ways in which such descriptions explore the affective reactions of the viewer. I argue that traumatic scenes emphasize a type of conflicted quasi-emotional (or emotion-like[24]) reaction to trauma and pain. In so doing, they shape the connections between the viewer and those who feel pain.

There are three areas of emotional responses to traumatic images that I am particularly concerned with: shock, pity, and desire. 'Shock' or 'amazement', often designated with the term *ekplēxis* or forms of *thaumazein*, is famous from discussions of the impact of vivid rhetorical language on the reader. It is commonly associated with powerful images, language, and rhetorical works and their capacity for *phantasia*. Pseudo-Longinos, in the treatise *Concerning the Sublime*, argues that poetry and rhetoric both aim at creating pathetic responses in their listeners. Although their techniques are different, since poetry aims at *ekplēxis* and rhetoric aims at *enargeia*, it is true that 'both...equally seek out the pathetic and the sympathetic emotions' (ἀμφότεραι...ὅμως τό τε παθητικὸν ἐπιζητοῦσι καὶ τὸ συγκεκινημένον, 15.2). Powerful rhetorical or poetic imagery, Pseudo-Longinos suggests, has the capacity to transcend rational aspects of readerly experience. Powerful astounding imagery overpowers the reader's rational engagement with both the medium and the material: 'in every way, that which is amazing always dominates that which is convincing and that which is pleasing through its ability for shock' (πάντη δέ γε σὺν ἐκπλήξει τοῦ πιθανοῦ καὶ τοῦ πρὸς χάριν ἀεὶ κρατεῖ τὸ θαυμάσιον, 1.4). Conviction is 'up to us' (τὸ μὲν πιθανὸν ... ἐφ' ἡμῖν), but things that are amazing and produce *ekplēxis* carry with them an 'irresistible power and force' (δυναστείαν καὶ βίαν ἄμαχον προσφέροντα) 'which dominates every reader' (παντὸς ἐπάνω τοῦ ἀκροωμένου καθίσταται, 1.4).[25] What commands my attention (as it has other commentators) is the interplay between conviction—with all its rational assumptions—and amazement and shock. The suggestion that 'conviction' is 'up to us' will, of course, remind readers of Epiktetos' suggestion that Stoic decision-making (and their concept of the self's

---

[24] I use the cumbersome phrases 'emotion-like' and 'quasi-emotional' because I want to stress that some aspects of the responses to traumatic art fit properly within the history of emotions—desire, pity, and fear all sit within ancient definitions of the *pathē*. Others, however, have a status that is difficult to classify, such as 'shock' or 'awe'.

[25] For the discussion of slavery, see Goldhill (2007), at 4–5.

relationship to the external world) is defined by the differences between what is 'up to us' and what is not.[26] Pseudo-Longinos conceptualizes rhetoric as transcending the boundaries of rational and aesthetic judgements about the world or subject matter through its capacity to stir emotion. In figuring the power of language thus, Pseudo-Longinos paves the way for a range of emotional responses to the images created by vivid, powerful rhetoric.

Ekplēxis, then, speaks to the emotive power of images and vivid language. Determining how we are to map this type of experience onto Imperial culture's emotional landscape is slightly more difficult. A number of authors connect the experience of 'shock' and 'amazement' with pleasure.[27] At other times, it seems to occupy a more problematic position. Throughout the treatise *How Young Men Should Listen to Poetry*, Plutarch continually stresses that mythical narratives which combine truth and falsehood facilitate 'pleasure or shock' (πρὸς ἡδονὴν ἢ ἔκπληξιν, 17a).[28] It is, of course, difficult to determine precisely what is intended by the use of the conjunction in this (and other) instances. Plutarch locates the experience of 'shock' at mythic narratives alongside their pleasure: *ekplēxis*, in this context, seems to sit alongside but not map exactly onto feelings of *hēdonē*. Further nuance to this type of emotional experience seems to be added by Plutarch's more general concern, at this point, with theatrical passages in poetry which are emotionally distressing for the reader and induce emotional disturbance (*taraxia*) and fear (*phobos*). Indeed, part of Plutarch's message is that poets who are able to render visions and images of flaming rivers, terrible places, and harsh punishments combine falsehood and mythical material that produces this concatenation of emotions in readers.[29] Plutarch's complex positioning of *ekplēxis* between pleasure and more distressing emotions is, I suggest, reiterated at other points in the cultural landscape. The quality is, for example, repeatedly connected with the overwhelming and (distressing?) viewing of anatomical procedures in Galen's *On Anatomical Procedures*.[30] In *On Hygiene,* Galen links the

[26] Epict. *Ench.* 1.1.
[27] Plut. *Quomodo Adulesc.* 17a and 25b; Plb. 34.4.3; and Strb. 1.2.17.
[28] For further references, see Plut. *Quomodo Adulesc.* 25d.
[29] Plut. *Quomodo Adulesc.* 16e for that which produces *taraxia*, and 17b for the working of 'fearful words and images and visions' of flaming rivers, wild places, and harsh punishments in the underworld.
[30] Gal. *AA.* ii.669K and 693K.

experience of shivers and shudders with shock (*ekplēxis*) and fear (*phobos*) at certain sights or sounds.[31] The condition of shock or amazement, at one level, operates as a type of shorthand for expressing the overwhelming qualities of particular events. As we shall see, it also helps to communicate the immensity of one's viewing experience, the capacity of certain sights and events to overwhelm the individual.

The second major emotional response that I am concerned with is pity. We learnt in the Introduction that an important aspect of this emotional experience focused on the way in which sufferer and other were connected. We have already discussed Aristotle's definition of pity in the *Rhetoric*. Importantly, this view of pity links viewer and viewed in a number of ways. In the first instance, it involves assumptions that must be made on the part of the viewer about whether or not the pitied deserves that which has befallen them: it involves intellectual judgements about what has happened and the character of those who are exposed to certain events. Secondly, it emphasizes the way in which the pitier understands their common ground with those who are exposed to pitiable events. David Konstan has famously suggested that, on Aristotle's reading, Greeks felt pity for those who were distant from themselves. Pity is felt towards those who are one step removed from the viewer.[32] Pity, on Aristotle's reading, involves a view of what might happen to one or one's loved ones which is created by viewing the experiences of others.[33] Aristotle's view of pity is culturally specific to Classical Athens. Aristotle's model (if it was ever the definitive model of the emotion for the ancient world)— while not consciously rewritten by these authors—is presented in ways that expand upon different nuances of the emotion. My objective in starting from the Aristotelian model is to explore the ways in which it figures the relationship between viewer and viewed: pity is, ultimately, one way in which these authors figure how audiences react to pain.

The last area of quasi-emotional response to which I turn is desire (erotic or otherwise). Desire, especially in its relationship with beauty, is a common trope in the way these texts figure the viewing process. Philostratos, Akhilleus Tatios, and Plutarch all explore the

---

[31] Gal. *San. Tu.* vi.278K. For the continued association of *ekplēxis* with fear and confusion: Plut. *Consol. ad Apoll.* 108b7–8 and D.Chr. 1.25.
[32] Konstan (2001), 128–36. For the discussion of pity, see the Introduction.
[33] Pelling (2005).

connections between trauma, physical beauty, and viewerly desire, repeatedly interrogating how trauma, pain, and beauty are related: how does one physiological experience influence the other and how do both change the way in which the viewer reacts to the body? At the same time, however, desire and beauty are linked with the process of looking at the wound itself. Trauma holds an almost irresistible attraction—it forces the reader to look; the viewer (is often conceptualized as one who) desires to see it—to consume it— and struggles to look away. In both of these aspects, these texts elaborate on the dynamics of how viewers engage with pain and trauma—how it is consumed visually or otherwise by the other. Pain and trauma are mapped onto an aesthetic order defined, in a large part, by beauty, pleasure, and viewerly desire.

All of these quasi-emotional reactions speak, then, to the intricacies of the pain experience and to the ways in which pain is incorporated into cultural discourse. One final point needs to be raised here. Of course, the ways in which one views these images are shaped by the types of context which are created for particular images or scenes. The *ekphraseis* discussed in Chapters 10, 11, and 12 go to significant lengths to contextualize the scenes they present. They do so by situating certain events or images against literary and mythical traditions and embedding them within cultural (often literary) contexts. By likening different images or scenes to ritual sacrifice and others to scenes of tragic recognition, writers shape not only how readers understand these scenes, but how they navigate their emotional reactions. There is an important connection between the literary and cultural intertextuality of various images and their capacity to shape viewers' cognitive and affective reactions.

10

Philostratos' Prurient Gaze

There are few figures whose shadows loom larger over Imperial Greek literature than Philostratos the Elder.[1] In this chapter, my focus is primarily on one of Philostratos' works of art criticism, the *Imagines*. Philostratos' masterful collection of sixty-five *ekphraseis* of paintings reputedly collected in a Neapolitan art gallery has been less well studied than some of his more famous works, such as the *Lives of the Sophists* or the *Life of Apollonios of Tyana*.[2] It is, nonetheless, critical to the understanding of Imperial society: it offers one of the most sustained reflections on both viewing art and writing about viewing to emerge from the first three centuries of Imperial Greek literature. Written in the early third century CE, this work is seminal to my investigation of the ways in which authors reflect on how audiences view, understand, and react to trauma and pain. Philostratos' approach to these issues is inflected by a specific and sustained focus on the nature of ekphrastic practice, the process of 'seeing' through rhetorical or literary description. That general interest shapes a more specific treatment of the violent destruction of the human body in which pain is often renegotiated, glossed over, or occluded. Paradoxically, it is this relationship between trauma and physical pain

---

[1] For general introductions to Philostratos the Elder and his corpus, see Anderson (1986), and Bowie and Elsner (2009), especially Elsner's chapter in the same volume (3–18). On Philostratos' biography and his relationship with the family of Philostratoi, see Bowie (2009), 19–20, with further bibliography. See also Flinterman (1995) for his representation of the political and philosophical import of sophistry in this period. For the difficulty of connecting specific members of the family with the surviving works attributed to 'Philostratos', see Bowie (2009), 19–20.

[2] On the authorship of these texts, see Men. Rh. ii.390.2–3 and Anderson (1986), 291–6, esp. 295. The question of whether or not the *ekphraseis* reflect real paintings is now obsolete. For discussion with further bibliography, see Squire (2013), 105 and, for an example of the previous orthodoxy, Lehmann-Hartleben (1941).

which is telling for how and why both experiences might be understood as part of the viewing ideology and visual culture of this period. By shaping how and what audiences visualize, Philostratos investigates what meanings audiences might attribute to trauma, what counts as painful, and how audiences might react affectively to it.

One of the reasons for turning to Philostratos is his determination to acculturate young men to the proper way to view art. In elaborating a description of the portico in which he claims the paintings are held, Philostratos stresses the connection that the Neapolitans have with Greek sophistication. Neapolis, he claims, was founded by a 'race of Greeks' (γένος Ἕλληνες) who are 'urbane' (ἀστικοί) and, therefore, 'Greek with respect to their eagerness for discourse' (τὰς σπουδὰς τῶν λόγων Ἑλληνικοί εἰσι, Phil. *Im.* 295.15–16K). The ascription simultaneously marks out the inhabitants of the city as both cultured and worthy of Greek *paideia* and emphasizes the important issue of cultural taste among the internal audience of his epideictic oration: his listeners might come from a cultured race, but they have much to live up to! Philostratos' discourse is an exercise in the inculcation of cultural values: 'we relate the forms of the paintings themselves in lectures we have put together for the young, from which they will interpret and also will care for what is esteemed' (ἀλλ' εἴδη ζωγραφίας ἀπαγγέλλομεν ὁμιλίας αὐτὰ τοῖς νέοις ξυντιθέντες, ἀφ' ὧν ἑρμηνεύσουσί τε καὶ τοῦ δοκίμου ἐπιμελήσονται, 295.10–12K).[3] Philostratos' epideictic work is an act of cultural training which aims at producing the very *paideia* that underpins his own (authoritative) readings or viewing in his listeners.[4] Particular emphasis must be given, I think, to the phrase 'they will care for what is esteemed' (τοῦ δοκίμου ἐπιμελήσονται). This act of paedeutic instruction reiterates cultural values by enforcing what is interesting in these paintings, what is worthy of one's cultured attention. From the opening lines of his *prooimion*, then, Philostratos' interest in education colours his desire to direct the gaze; what is emphasized and occluded is figured in terms of cultural significance. As we shall see, this has important implications for thinking about the representation of pain.

The *Imagines* develops a particularly nuanced relationship with painful or traumatic experience. In elaborating the value of painting, Philostratos tells readers that the craft partakes of wisdom (*sophia*)

---

[3] For the importance of interpretation in this context, see Newby (2009), 323 n. 8.
[4] For the text as educative: Newby (2009), 323–4.

and truth (*alētheia*); he then accentuates its value by comparing it to a number of other mimetic arts. *Mimēsis* in painting, he claims, is an ancient discovery and one that is 'most closely related to nature'.[5] In comparison to the other plastic arts, such as sculpture or gem cutting, painting gives especial access to the emotions and deeds of heroes because it 'displays shade' (σκιάν τε γὰρ ἀποφαίνει, 294.18–19K) and, thus, 'one recognizes the face of one who rages, another who is in pain,[6] another who rejoices' (βλέμμα γινωσκει ἄλλο μὲν τοῦ μεμηνότος, ἄλλο δὲ τοῦ ἀλγοῦντος ἢ χαίροντος, Phil. *Im*. 294.19–20K). The depiction of painful and pleasurable experiences appears intimately connected with the very nature of painting, and this connection is facilitated precisely because of painting's unique capacity for colour. The choice of *gignōskein* implies more than just seeing the presence of such emotional or physical states in paintings, but also facilitating the understanding or recognition of the look and form of one who is either feeling pain or pleasure. If painting should be valorized for its relationship with *alētheia* and *sophia*, the use of *gignōskein* suggests that this should be done on the basis of its capacity to facilitate a truth about those in anger, pain, and pleasure.

This programmatic reference to *algō* is telling, given the regular treatment of traumatic scenes or physical destruction throughout the work. If the *Imagines* repeatedly returns readers to scenes of violence and bodily destruction, it does so in a manner which often occludes explicit reference to pain or focuses on different aspects of the traumatic experience. While the description of *ta traumata* often implies pain, and it is certainly possible to imagine that pain is present in the scenes of physical trauma that Philostratos describes, it should be understood that pain is only rarely explicitly flagged by the author's language.[7] This raises the immediate question about how

---

[5] Phil. *Im*. 294.9–10K: ξυγγενέστατον τῇ φύσει.

[6] The translation of ἀλγοῦντος is problematic. It is rendered 'grieving' at Newby (2009), 325 and in Fairbank's Loeb translation (Fairbanks (1931)). While this translation might accord with the other emotional states (rage? and pleasure?) mentioned in this context, it misses some of the complexity of the term throughout Philostratos. Given that the subject matter of so many of Philostratos' paintings is physical trauma and its emotional consequences, it seems that ἀλγοῦντος might be better translated here as 'in agony' or 'in distress'. This is supported by the continued use of *ania* and *penthos* to describe states which are more clearly 'emotional'. For πένθος: 305.10K, 349.30K, 350.15K, and 379.29–30K.

[7] There are few references to physical pain throughout the entire text. For one example, see *Im*. 296.22K (Skamander). It must be telling that it is the first *ekphrasis* of

to reconcile the *ekphraseis* with Philostratos' programmatic comments. Thinking about the paintings and their description through this lens heightens the significance of Philostratos' authorial decisions: what he chooses to 'see' in terms of painful experience is marked as telling precisely because he flags the issue as something fundamental to painting; do his paintings offer access to the experience of pain by, paradoxically, refiguring and occluding the perception? If we are supposed to recognize the look of one who is 'in pain', what does it say when this process is commonly presented in language that does not explicitly emphasize physical pain?

The third point that I wish to raise in this context concerns the ways in which Philostratos manages the symbiotic relationship between the image, viewing, and textual representation. Scholars have been particularly awake to the games that Philostratos plays in constructing and regulating the viewing subject. There are two points that are particularly important for my interpretation of the *Imagines*. Firstly, Philostratos' engagement with earlier literature constantly shifts readers'/viewers' attentions between different media. As Jaś Elsner argues in *Art and the Roman Viewer*, one of the important consequences of the intertextuality of Philostratos' *ekphraseis* is contextualization: it is through reference to various literary works that the viewer is able to negotiate the 'other' of the painting and make sense of it; to tame it for the purposes of interpretation, to incorporate the painting into the social reality of the viewer.[8] As one prominent commentator put it, the purpose of the literary glosses is to help 'control' the overpowering wonder created in some contexts in the *Imagines:* for Zahra Newby, literary erudition helps to manage the overpowering effects of amazing scenes.[9] It is hard to disagree that literary references facilitate the incorporation of the painting and the subject matter into the common experience and understanding

---

the entire collection. For another provocative example, see the description of Antilokhos at *Im.* 351.6–8K: ἡ ψυχὴ κατέλιπεν οὐχ ὡς ἤλγησεν, ἀλλ' ὡς ἐπεκράτησε τὸ εὐφραῖνον ('the soul left him not when he felt pain, but when happiness dominated').

[8] Elsner (1995), 30–1 for 'contextualization'.

[9] Newby (2009), 323: 'a continual movement between absorption in the world of the image and a detached intellectual viewing which seeks to constrain the power of the visual through subjection to textual or verbal explanations'. See also Squire (2013), 128 n. 6, quoting Gutzwiller (2002), 110: 'like epigram, Philostratos represents "a viewer working through the powerful emotive impact of art so as to tame it in articulation of thought"'.

of the viewer. As we shall see (and as Elsner is at pains to point out), that process is far from straightforward. Rather, it offers simultaneously a multilayered process of literary, artistic, and scopic reception of earlier Greek culture. This interplay between emotional and interpretive reactions among viewers is particularly telling. While it is true that, in many instances, the emotional elements of these descriptions are controlled through the process of interpretation and articulation, it is also true that the process of interpretation and literary contextualization facilitates a more nuanced emotional engagement with what is being depicted and the picture itself.

In what follows, I look to several examples of trauma: the death of Menoikeus, the related scene of Antilokhos, and the suicide of Pantheia. There are many other examples of physical destruction narrated throughout the *Imagines*. What interests me in these contexts is not only their prolonged focus on the body's wounds, blood, and physical deportment, but also their willingness to develop and explore different kinds of emotional reactions to these phenomena. They all connect the wound with a discussion of what it means 'to see' or 'to look at' trauma. That process of looking—what one sees or fails to notice, or how one sees—is allied to the ways in which Philostratos explores the emotional impact of these scenes. As I shall show, Philostratos emphasizes not only the theme of desire and pleasure in viewing such images, but also other emotional reactions such as pity and distress.

1. MENOIKEUS AND OTHER DYING HEROES

Let us begin with an early description of a painting of the young dying hero Menoikeus, analysed in detail at *Imagines* 299.16–300.22K. Philostratos' account homes in on the body of the young man as he dies before Thebes. This focus explores the ways in which viewers engage with the trauma Menoikeus endures and his destroyed body. It does so, however, by stressing pleasure, understanding, and recognition, rather than some more distressing or ambivalent emotive responses. Philostratos' *ekphrasis* rephrases Menoikeus' death in terms of the beauty of his body and viewerly desire or pleasure.

In the first instance, the entire scene is geared towards viewerly pleasure and eroticism which combines the interpretation and praise of the artist's skill with the aesthetic appreciation of Menoikeus' body. In the initial description of the scene around the city of Thebes, Philostratos pays particular attention to 'the artifice of the artist, which is pleasing' (ἡδὺ τὸ σόφισμα τοῦ ζωγράφου, *Im.* 299.24–5K). Praise of the artist at this point is reiterated moments later when he turns to the description of Menoikeus' body. He tells his readers 'to look at the effects of the painter' (ὅρα γὰρ τὰ τοῦ ζωγράφου, 300.7K) because he paints the youth not white or luxurious, but as breathing from the *palaistra*; his body is 'like a flower which is honey-coloured, the sort which Ariston's son praises' (οἷον τὸ τῶν μελιχρόων ἄνθος, οὓς ἐπαινεῖ ὁ τοῦ Ἀρίστωνος, 300.9–10K); he has been equipped with a deep chest, 'well-proportioned' (συμμέτρῳ) thighs and hips, and there is strength in his shoulders. The lingering focus on the body is deeply erotic and reflects a tendency throughout the *Imagines* to view the youthful male body as desirous and its corpse erotically. Philostratos' allusion to the praise of Ariston's son perhaps points the reader to Plato (Ariston's son) and the praise of the youthful male body in Plato's *Republic*. Indeed, it recalls a passage in which the philosopher describes the beautiful bodies of youths and the erotic fantasy of attachment felt by their lovers at *Republic* 474d–e. In turning to Plato's text, Philostratos connects the praise of the boy's body, praise of the painter's ability, and the literary erudition of the reader or viewer. The allusion adds an intellectual gloss to the ways in which the body and the painting are read simultaneously in terms of pleasure and desire; both are elaborated through a veneer of erudition and allusion which facilitates interpretation, intellectual and stylistic criticism of the painting's skills, and the aesthetic appreciation of Menoikeus' beauty.

The stress on erotic desire and beauty created through the reference to the *Republic* is reiterated when Philostratos returns to the moment of the hero's death:

ἕλκον τὸ ξίφος ἐνδεδυκὸς ἤδη τῇ πλευρᾷ, καὶ δεξώμεθα, ὦ παῖ, τὸ αἷμα κόλπον αὐτῷ ὑποσχόντες, ἐκχεῖται γάρ, καὶ ἡ ψυχὴ ἤδη ἄπεισι, μικρὸν δὲ ὕστερον καὶ τετριγυίας αὐτῆς ἀκούσῃ. ἔρωτα γὰρ τῶν καλῶν σωμάτων καὶ αἱ ψυχαὶ ἴσχουσιν, ὅθεν ἄκουσαι αὐτῶν ἀπαλλάττονται. ὑπεξιόντος δὲ αὐτῷ τοῦ αἵματος ὀκλάζει καὶ ἀσπάζεται τὸν θάνατον καλῷ καὶ ἡδεῖ τῷ ὄμματι καὶ οἷον ὕπνον ἕλκοντι.

He draws the sword which has already been plunged into his flank. And let us receive the blood, child, holding under it a fold of our clothes. For it pours out, and the soul is already leaving, and a little later you should hear its gibbering cry. For desire for beautiful bodies souls have too, and because of this they leave the body unwillingly. As the blood leaks out of him, he sinks to his knees and receives death with beauty and pleasure in his eye, even as one receives sleep.

Phil. *Im.* 300.14–22K

As has been acknowledged, the description of Menoikeus' wounds and his death in the final sections of the *ekphrasis* plays on a fantasy of incorporation in which viewers are invited to (almost) participate in the reality of the painting.[10] The close engagement with his blood also shapes the affective (and interpretive) responses to the wound. The suggestion that the soul has left Menoikeus, and that readers will hear 'its gibbering cry', creates a multisensory viewing of the painting: audiences 'hear' the action of the painting. The gibbering cry, however, seems not only to render the reader particularly close to the action, but to shape emotional responses in a particular way. The choice of τρίζω looks to its use in *Iliad* 23 to describe the death of Hektor and *Odyssey* 24 to describe the wailing of the souls of the suitors in the underworld.[11] There is a complex layering to the intertextual texture of these references. The references recall not only the epic context of such screams, but arguably the cultural significance of them for later writers. Importantly, the passages from both epics are listed by Plato as passages which should be excised from the educative agenda of youths, as they induce 'terror' and 'fear' towards the underworld and encourage less than praiseworthy values in young men.[12] Philostratos incorporates into his own paedeutic text that which Plato had explicitly eschewed from his own (culturally authorative?) discussion of education. The potential for a problematic reaction among viewers to such shrieks is rewritten, however, by the following lines, where the soul's gibbering cry is rephrased in terms of the desire which souls hold for beautiful bodies and their unwillingness to be separated from them (a point which my clunky translation tries to underline). Philostratos' explanation, with all its allusions and intimations of erudition, takes readers on a type of emotional roller coaster: emphasizing, firstly, the more distressing elements of viewing

---

[10] Newby (2009), 335–6.
[11] Hom. *Il.* 23.101, for the use of τετριγυῖα in the death of Hektor. Cf. τετριγυῖαι at *Od.* 24.9.
[12] Pl. *R.* 387a-e for the discussion of terror and fear.

Menoikeus' death and then dramatically turning the tables by refiguring this through the theme of desire. Philostratos takes a potentially distressing aspect of the painting and reframes it in terms of his own educative agenda.

If we 'hear' the moment when the soul leaves the body, then so too do we see, through Menoikeus' own facial expressions, the moment at which death arrives. The suggestion that he 'receives death' with 'beauty and pleasure in his eye' continues the focus on the erotics of beauty and viewing pleasure. Importantly, it is reminiscent of Philostratos' opening programmatic lines about how painting—through its depiction of the eyes—is able to communicate deeper truths about those who feel anger, *algos*, and pleasure. The reference to *kalos* in the final description of Menoikeus' gazing at his wound is particularly problematic—does it refer to Philostratos' interpretation of the boy's expression or the objective qualities of his eyes as they look upon death and sleep? Is their beauty in his eyes? Or, does he (Menoikeus) look at something beautiful and pleasing? Or both? If Menoikeus' act of looking guides the act of viewing outside the text, then it becomes increasingly difficult to separate the process of viewing desire in the pained, traumatized body, the desirous viewing of it, and the assumption that the wounded body is beautiful.

There are a number of important connections between the treatment of Menoikeus' death and Philostratos' bigger project. The beauty and pleasure that characterize this hero's reaction to death speak to an enduring interest in the moment that death occurs and the types of facial expression or countenance of those who encounter violent deaths. Indeed, a number of Philostratos' descriptions focus on the transformations between life and death; he explores the ways in which people look at the moment of death, the relationship between the violence and trauma that led to that eventuality, the possibilities of painful feelings, and the apparent serenity that often characterizes the body and the face at the point of death and just after it.

2. ANTILOKHOS

One *tableau* which goes to some length to dramatize that dynamic is the treatment of Antilokhos. This description explores not only pain and other feelings at the moment of death, but their relationship with the emotional reactions of those around them. Philostratos begins by discussing Antilokhos' role in relaying the message of Patroklos' death to Akhilleus in *Iliad* 18. Philostratos' reading of the *Iliad* stresses that Akhilleus loved Antilokhos and that this desire helped to assuage the grief that Akhilleus felt at Patroklos' death. Indeed, Philostratos' reading plays up the intersection of grief and pleasure: Akhilleus 'wails for his beloved in grief' (καὶ θρηνεῖ ἐρωμένου ἐπὶ τῷ πένθει, Im. 349.29–30K) but 'he is, I think, pleased at the touch [of the hand of Antilokhos], who weeps too' (ὁ δ', οἶμαι, καὶ ἁπτομένῳ χαίρει καὶ δακρύοντι, Im. 350.1–2K). Philostratos' reading of the scene seems slightly misdirected, particularly in its focus on the desire felt by Akhilleus for the messenger. The contingency of this reading (which is perhaps flagged by the use of *oida*?) suggests, however, that Philostratos is using the epic to frame a concern of the painting and the affective reactions of the bereaved to trauma and death.

As the *ekphrasis* continues, there is an increasing focus on the intersection of multiple affective responses to Antilokhos' death. Antilokhos' slaying at the hands of Memnon causes great grief to the Akhaians: the Greek heroes 'lament' (ὀδύρονται, 350.7K) Antilokhos, 'the army grieves... for him with a dirge' (ἡ στρατια πενθεῖ... αὐτὸ θρήνῳ, 350.14–15K), and 'in grief' (ἄχει, 350.19K), Akhilleus throws himself on the chest of the hero 'in lament' (θρηνεῖ, 350.22K). This focus on grief for Antilokhos, of course, mirrors the treatment of grief in Philostratos' reading of Homer and the passage from the *Iliad* on which it is based. It directly juxtaposes the erotic connotations of Antilokhos' body and sets up the viewing context for that body. Philostratos, having recounted these feelings of grief, immediately asks readers to turn to the 'well-proportioned body' (τὸ σῶμα σύμμετρον, 350.31–2K) of the hero. The body and its wound are described in terms reminiscent of the description of Menelaos' bloodstained thigh at *Iliad* 4.141–2. As in the description of Menelaos' wound, Antilokhos' blood—which emerges from the point where the spear was driven through his chest—takes on the colour of ivory as it stains his body. Reading the scene through the erotic lens of Homer's presentation of Menelaos' thigh returns the viewer to the precise point of trauma and the wound and does so in a manner that emphasizes not only its erotic connotations, but also frames this against the more distressing emotional reactions of those who viewed the corpse.

This ambivalence between erotics and distressing emotions is mirrored in the treatment of the youth's own feelings:

κεῖται δὲ οὐ κατηφὲς τὸ μειράκιον, οὐδὲ νεκρῷ εἰκάσαι, φαιδρὸν δὲ καὶ μειδιῶν, τὴν γάρ, οἶμαι, χαρὰν τὴν ἐπὶ τῷ τὸν πατέρα σῶσαι φέρων ἐν τῷ εἴδει ὁ Ἀντίλοχος ἀπώλετο ὑπὸ τῆς αἰχμῆς, καὶ τὸ πρόσωπον ἡ ψυχὴ κατέλιπεν οὐχ ὡς ἤλγησεν, ἀλλ' ὡς ἐπεκράτησε τὸ εὐφραῖνον.

And the youth lies there, not downcast, not even like a corpse, but bright and smiling, for, I think, Antilokhos, having pleasure in his form since he saved his father, died by the spear, and with regard to the face, the soul left him not when he felt pain, but when happiness dominated.

Phil. *Im.* 351.2–8K

There is much that is arresting in this description. The continued stress on pleasure is telling for how we understand Antilokhos' experience of trauma. Despite the wounds and death caused by the spear, there is pleasure in his form. Pleasure in the face of trauma is reminiscent, of course, of Menoikeus' description (not to mention the programmatic lines of the entire *Imagines*); Menoikeus' feelings are underpinned by his sense of his own beauty and his understanding of his own actions. The context (which Philostratos reads into the painting) changes how and what the pained and traumatized individual is assumed to feel. That reading of Antilokhos' experience is reiterated in the final emphasis on his facial expression, which stresses the transformation of pain into pleasure. The moment of death—in both this scene and the description of Menoikeus—is presented as one in which pain is overridden by more pleasant feelings, transformed into feelings of cheer by the emotional context of trauma. Philostratos seems particularly interested in this critical juncture when the soul leaves the body and how individuals confront that moment. It induces reflections on the beauty of the body, the emotional contexts in which the traumatized and those around them place the destruction of the body, and the individual's and audience's respective feelings of pain, pleasure, and distress.

3. PANTHEIA

The rewriting of the wound and pain is clear, too, in the description of the death of Pantheia. The description of her suicide is set against the earlier death of her husband Abradates. His death provides a contrasting scene which highlights some aspects of the depiction of Pantheia and Philostratos' engagement with pain. As with Menoikeus' depiction, the literary erudition of both deaths helps to phrase a number of important emotional responses: allusions to Homer and the explicit framing against Xenophon's account of their demise stress the ways in which bodily experience is read in terms of the emotional qualities of the actors and shape the ways in which external viewers see and react to both.

Philostratos' *tableau* begins by drawing immediate links with Xenophon's account of Pantheia. The relationship with this urtext is characterized by the author's and the painter's different depictions of her beauty and character. According to Philostratos, Xenophon wrote 'her beauty' (ἡ καλή) 'from her character' (ἀπὸ τοῦ ἤθους, *Im.* 353.1–2), whereas the painter (although not unfamiliar with Xenophon's account, according to Philostratos), depicted her 'in such as a way as he divined from her soul' (ὁποίαν τῇ ψυχῇ ἐτεκμήρατο, Phil. *Im.* 353.17–18).[13] The comparison initiates a situation in which both depictions attempt to read inner qualities and outward form against and through each other—the Xenophontic account depicts her character and thus displays her beauty from it, whereas the external qualities of the painting are predicated on an understanding of her soul. This interplay paves the way for Philostratos' own reading of the body, in which outer form reveals inner qualities and experiences. What we can see on her body appears to speak of her inner condition, her experiences of pain and pleasure, and her virtues. Philostratos' account is continually energized by this toing and froing between the moral and experiential elements which are not visible and the external visible signs of her body.

The description proper begins with an account of the death of Pantheia's husband Abradates. Philostratos describes him as a 'young man still with down on his chin' (νέος ἔτι ἐν ἁπαλῇ τῇ ὑπήνῃ), who has been removed from life too soon. Indeed, he is cut down at the very moment:

ὁπότε καὶ οἱ ποιηταὶ τὰ δένδρα τὰ νέα ἐλεεινὰ ἡγοῦνται τῆς γῆς ἐκπεσόντα. τὰ μὲν δὴ τραύματα, ὦ παῖ, οἷα ἐκ μαχαιροφόρων, τὸ γὰρ κατακόπτειν πρὸς τρόπου τῇ τοιαύτῃ μάχῃ, τοῦ δὲ αἵματος ἀκραιφνοῦς

---

[13] For reading the soul and body through each other, see Gleason (1995), 21–54.

ὄντος τὸ μὲν τὰ ὅπλα χραίνει, τὸ δ' αὐτόν, ἔστι δ' ὃ καὶ διέρρανται κατὰ τοῦ λόφου, ὁ δὲ ἄρα χρυσοῦ τοῦ κράνους ἀνέστηκεν ὑακίνθινός αὐτῷ τῷ χρυσῷ ἐπαστράπτων.

When even the poets hold that the trees, the young ones, are pitiable when they have been torn out of the ground. As for the wounds, child, they are the kind that come from sword fighting—for the cutting down [of the foe] occurs in this way in this kind of fighting—some of his pure blood stains his armour, some him, and there is also some spread across the crest which stands up hyacinthine-like from the golden helmet and shines on the gold itself.

Phil. *Im.* 353.29–354.6K

At one level, the passage appears to be fascinated with the violent destruction of the body. The emphatic focus on 'the wounds' (τά τραύματα), 'the cutting down' (τό κατακόπτειν), and 'the blood' (τοῦ αἵματος), all of which begin new clauses, invites both the internal audience and the external reader to focus on the *minutiae* of the violent destruction of the body. That focus is further developed by the elaboration of the details of the wounds. We might see the intellectual gloss concerning the nature of the weapon and the sword fighting as a way of shifting focus from the wounds themselves. Yet by asking one to consider the specific weapon that was used (a *makhaira* is a short Persian sword) and the method of fighting which has produced the wounds, the narrative asks both internal and external audiences to contemplate the violent and traumatic history or *praxis* that lies behind the visible *tableau*. For all its intellectual detachment, the comment on sword fighting returns viewers to the trauma at hand. This interest in the wounds is compounded by the ways in which the audience is asked to trace the splattering of blood across the body. At one level, such a focus on the spreading of blood might recall the treatment of figures such as Menelaos in *Iliad* 4.[14] As the passage continues, the lingering description of the ways in which the blood 'stains' his armour, him, and the crest of his helmet returns us again to the violence enacted on Abradates' body.

Philostratos' description taps into the trope of the eroticized body of dying or dead boys, but it is also true that this process of depicting the erotic connotations of the youth's body explores other affective and intellectual reactions to the death. In the first instance, for all its conspicuous focus on the damage to the body, there is little explicit

[14] Hom. *Il.* 4.141–7.

reference to the pain Abradates might have felt during this event. This is, perhaps, not surprising, given the fact that in the narrative arc of the painting and the *ekphrasis* Abradates is already dead. The erotic depiction of the youthful hero seems to overshadow any interest in his feelings of pain. At the same time, the passage is also defined by a consistent focus on the *pathos* of pity. The passage begins with a reference to the poets who consider young trees pitiable when they are ripped from the ground too soon. The reference to poets in this context emphasizes the connections with Homer and the description of heroes who died young in the *Iliad*, especially during books 16 and 17 and Akhilleus' rampage in 20 and 21.[15] Philostratos rereads and adjusts the links that he creates in order to redefine how we view the youthful figure in the picture before us. Here it seems to be the temporality that excites the sense of pity in both the Homeric and the Philostratean context rather than any sense of pity for Abradates' exposure to painful and traumatic experiences. The final reference to the hyacinth-red plume on Abradates' helmet (an allusion to the Xenophon account)[16] seems to stress a similar point. In the context of youths who die young, the hyacinth is particularly evocative. The colour of the flower perhaps recalls the splattering of blood in the previous lines; the reference to the flower itself evokes the figure of Hyakinthos, the youth who was the erotic object of Apollo. For all its connection to the regalia and the arms of the Xenophontic Abradates, the death scene is linked with the heroic and mythic world in which beautiful, desirable youths are taken before their time.

One of the reasons for spending considerable time discussing the death of Pantheia's husband is that the absence of pain in that scene serves to heighten certain aspects of the depiction of Pantheia in which pain is given more explicit discussion. Her description is infused with erotic readings which combine a fascination with the act of trauma upon the body, explicit reference to her pain, her moral qualities, and her beauty. The description begins by lingering over Pantheia stabbing herself in the breast:

τὸν μὲν δὴ ἀκινάκην διελήλακεν ἤδη τοῦ στέρνου, ἀλλ οὕτω τι δὴ ἐρρωμένως, ὡς μηδὲ οἰμωγὴν ἐπ᾽ αὐτῷ ῥῆξαι. κεῖται γοῦν, τὸ στόμα ξυμμετρίαν τὴν ἑαυτοῦ φυλάττον, καὶ, νὴ Δί᾽, ὥραν, ἧς τὸ ἄνθος οὕτω τι ἐπὶ χείλεσιν, ὡς καὶ σιωπώσης ἐκφαίνεσθαι. ἀπήρτηται δὲ οὔπω τὸν ἀκινάκην.

---

[15] See, e.g., Hom. *Il.* 17.53.   [16] X. *Cyr.* 6.4.2.

Clearly, she has already driven the dagger through her chest, but in some way so forcefully that she does not let out a groan at it. So she lies, and maintains the orderliness of her mouth and, by Zeus, the flower, the bloom of which is such on her lips that it even shines out from her silence. She has not yet drawn out the dagger.

Phil. *Im.* 354.13-19K

This initial description of the body of Pantheia plays heavily on her inner qualities, their consequences for her outer form, and their role in shaping her experiences. The initial description of driving the dagger in is particularly telling. The adverb ἐρρωμένως, which I translated as 'forcefully', could refer to the physical strength that she has used to drive the dagger into her chest. On this reading, the force of the damage to the body undermines her capacity for speech. At the same time, it can also refer (especially in its middle form) to qualities of good health and mental strength: 'she has driven the dagger through her chest, but with such strength that she does not let out a groan' suitably captures the ambiguity of the reference to either the physical strength or the mental fortitude she displays.[17] The use of ἐπ' αὐτῷ, could also refer either to her husband, over whose funeral pyre she offers herself as a final funeral gift, or to the knife itself. The first, stressing the potential for grieving and emotional trauma felt over the death of her husband Abradates, is supported by the emotionality of the reference to her 'groan' or 'wail' (οἰμωγή) and its connotations of lamentation.[18] It is arguable, however, that ἐπ' αὐτῷ could additionally refer to the knife which has just been pushed into her body—she does not groan at 'it'. The ambiguity of this depiction is never quite worked out and this indeterminacy suggests two points. The ambiguity of what she feels speaks, in the first instance, to the indeterminacy that lies behind the programmatic references to *algeō* in the first lines of the *Imagines*. Pantheia is a type of test case for the emotional and physical effects and affects of war, trauma, and death. Her ambiguity speaks to the inherent combination of physical pain associated with the wound

---

[17] For implications of physical strength: Phil. *Im.* 371.26K, 376.13-14K, and 384.11K. For the connection with a mental condition: *Im.* 378.29K, where it is connected with Herakles' *dianoia*. Cf. also Plut. *Cons. ad Apoll.* 118f, where Perikles is seen 'bearing his griefs manfully' (τὰ ἑωυτοῦ πένθεα ἐρρωμένως φέροντα). For the implication of 'good health': D. 2.21.

[18] Hdt. 3.66: ταῦτα κατηρείκοντο καὶ οἰμωγῇ ἀφθόνῳ διεχρέωντο ('at these things they rent their garments and employ plentiful wailing'); for a reaction to physical (and?) emotional anguish, see πικραῖς οἰμωγαῖς ('bitter wails') at S. *Ph.* 189-90.

and its broader emotional ramifications. The second point to make concerns the ways in which Pantheia confounds one's expectations. By raising the possibility of her distress only to deny its presence, Philostratos points to Pantheia's exceptional mental qualities. This interest in her apparent serenity is emphasized in Philostratos' focus on the 'orderliness' (which translates ξυμμετρίαν) of her mouth, which stresses inner calmness and emotional self-control and moderation. The noun *summetria* often refers to either physical or psychical moderation and mental fortitude in the face of extreme emotional situations.[19] Silence and order speak volumes for her qualities and her experiences. By juxtaposing these with the audience's expectations for her scream, Philostratos accentuates the exceptional inner strength of the woman and, in the process, recasts her reaction to, and navigation of, her physical trauma and emotional distress.

The reversal of expectations about pain and the wound permeate the following lines and their focus on erotics and pleasure. Indeed, Philostratos demonstrates a prurient interest in her pained body, subjecting Pantheia to a type of erotic, fetishizing gaze:

ἀνήρτηται δὲ οὔπω τὸν ἀκινάκην, ἀλλ' ἐνερείδει ἔτι ξυνέχουσα τῆς κώπης αὐτόν—ἡ δὲ κώπη ῥοπάλῳ χρυσῷ εἴκασται σμαραγδίνῳ τοὺς ὄζους. ἀλλ' ἡδίους οἱ δάκτυλοι—μεταβέβληκέ τε οὐδὲν τοῦ εἴδους ὑπὸ τοῦ ἀλγεῖν, ἤ γε μηδὲ ἀλγεῖν ἔοικεν, ἀλλ' ἀπιέναι χαίρουσα, ὅτι αὐτὴν πέμπει...

She has not yet drawn out the dagger but still pushes it in, holding it by the hilt—the hilt like a golden stalk with emeralds for its branches—but the fingers are more charming; nothing of her form has been altered by her pain, and indeed she does not seem to feel pain, but rather she appears to depart feeling pleasure because she sends herself...

Phil. *Im.* 354.18–24K[20]

The focus on the wound fetishizes the body as an object of viewing pleasure where the aesthetic qualities of her image are allied to what she is assumed to feel. Philostratos creates a sense of temporal delay throughout this passage: οὔπω ('not yet') picks up the use of the perfect διελήλακεν ἤδη ('already she has driven') earlier in the description and invites the reader to contemplate the length of time that

---

[19] LSJ s.v. συμμετρία. For further discussion of this term as depicting aesthetic beauty and physical proportion, see Introduction (nn. 42–5).
[20] Text (here and at 354.28-30) follows, and the translation is modified from, the Loeb of Fairbanks (1931).

the blade has remained in Pantheia's chest. The emphasis on the continuing activity of holding the dagger in her body forces the reader to linger over her wound and the insertion of the weapon. Looking at the wound and its cause asks the reader not to consider her pain, but to reflect on the comparison between the weapon's refinement and the beauty of her fingers. In contrast to Abradates' description, the treatment of Pantheia goes further in examining the relationship between these different qualities. Philostratos' narrative constantly oscillates between the beauty of her form and the consideration of her pain. The suggestion that 'nothing of her form has been altered' (the term can also mean 'damaged') 'by pain' is particularly telling: her pain is not visible on her form, it has not undermined the possibilities of viewing her body pleasurably. It posits, arguably, the possibility of a mutually exclusive relationship between pain and beauty: does pain transform beauty? Does the maintenance of beauty require overcoming the potentially displeasing visual aspects of pain? In this scene, rather than occluding or ignoring pain (as he had in the description of Abradates), Philostratos explicitly navigates the relationship between aesthetics and *aisthēsis*.

Philostratos' final clause is also stressed as an act of readerly interpretation. Note the weight given to the language of appearance: 'she seems' not to be in pain precisely because of her decision to dispatch herself; the use of ἔοικεν underscores the contingency of his surface-level reading. Philostratos' appraisal of her actions—the fact that she dispatches herself—and her body's lack of damage or change underpins the assumed absence of her pain. The moral reading of her actions inflects the interpretation of her perception and the construction of her experience. This juxtaposition between the feelings of pain and pleasure (note the use of ἀλγεῖν and χαίρουσα) recalls his earlier programmatic statements about pain and pleasure in painting. Philostratos' treatment of Pantheia's body—his reading of her inner qualities and experiences—speaks to his conception of painting's capacity to communicate truths about the body, its status as a mimetic art which partakes of both *sophia* and *alētheia*.

The fascination with her dead or dying body and its damage remains constant throughout the *tableau*. Moments later, he tells his readers that, unlike other mythical examples of wives who have killed themselves, she keeps 'her beauty unadorned'; she pours her abundant black hair over her shoulders and neck (χαίτην μὲν οὕτω μέλαινάν τε καὶ ἀμφιλαφῆ περιχέασα τοῖς ὤμοις καὶ τῷ αὐχένι, *Im.* 354.29–30K) and reveals her white skin, which she has torn (δέρην δὲ λευκὴν ὑπεκφαίνουσα, ἣν ἐδρύψατο, 354.30–31K); her white throat, though she had torn it in her grief, is, however, not shamed by the marks, since they become 'signs more sweet than a painting' (τὰ σημεῖα τῶν ὀνύχων ἡδίω γραφῆς, 354.31–2K). The reference to tearing the white neck combines not only the erotic overtones of the white female body suddenly revealed to prurient eyes, but also the intensity of Pantheia's situation. The allusion to the process of mourning reveals the nature of Pantheia's emotions, which underscore her willingness to engage in acts of physical violation; at the same time, they emphasize the dissonance between the reader's interpretation of their meaning—in Philostratos' hermeneutic text they become signs of pleasure and a testament to her enduring beauty—and Pantheia's experience. In a similar fashion, the redness of her cheeks has not left her as she dies, but they are made beautiful by her moral qualities, by her *partheneia* and modesty. The concatenation of different body parts sketched and lingered upon allows the reader/viewer to trace Pantheia's pained and traumatized body with prurient eyes.

This process is commonly seen as one in which the female body is fetishized. In other words, Pantheia's body is broken up by the act of description into a series of parts which can be viewed erotically by the principally male audience. On one reading, this treatment of the female body is familiar from a range of rhetorical depictions of women across the ancient world.[21] Indeed, the phrase returns us directly to the opening lines of Philostratos' *Imagines*, in which he told his readers that painting was an effective artistic medium because it revealed the looks of those who were in distress and those who were rejoicing. If Pantheia's death is laboured, it is with good reason: it speaks directly to the way in which Philostratos wants his readers to think about the nature of painting and to structure our reading of it. In so doing, he explicitly navigates a complex relationship between pain and beauty and viewing pleasure.

Philostratos, then, is particularly interested in the ways in which the destroyed body might be seen and understood by those who experience trauma and those who view it. Philostratos' monumental work repeatedly returns to scenes in which the body is violently destroyed. These scenes are characterized by, among other things,

[21] Morales (2004), 20–9.

the way in which the individual looks—and feels—at the moment trauma is enacted and the poignant moments between that event and the death of the individual. As we have seen, that discussion is further defined by the ways in which pain experience is thought about and presented in these situations. In many instances, the act of wounding or the soul leaving the body is presented in terms that lead the audience to expect pain to accompany the event. That experience is, however, recast: the context in which the individual was traumatized, and their internal feelings about the event, are consistently used to rewrite the assumed presence of pain and its relationship to aesthetic pleasure (and desire) or other affective reactions like pity.

It is, perhaps, well known that Philostratos' text is not entirely concerned with pain. Nonetheless, the pleasant feelings of those who are violently traumatized are consciously and actively rewritten through a creative act of reading the body and the context of death. In many of the situations that we have discussed, the process of reading the body and the signs of the wound allows for a greater understanding of the 'inner feelings' of Philostratos' subjects. What is so telling about that process is that Philostratos engages in an act of interpretive ping-pong: reading the internal and psychological characteristics of pain through their visual representation, before returning to (re)read and explain the external signs of the body in terms of inner feelings. From the perspective of this discussion, that process is not only significant for the interpretive leaps it makes (and which are often left unspoken), but also for the ways in which that process shapes both the relationship between pain and trauma and the broader understanding of the pain experience. Philostratos explores the ways in which pain, trauma, and the inner feelings of individuals who experience them are connected. The experience of pain lies at the intersection between pleasure, internal feelings of joy, and trauma.

11

Viewing and Emotional Conflict in Akhilleus Tatios

Akhilleus Tatios' *Leukippe and Kleitophon*, commonly seen as the raciest of the five 'ideal' Greek romances, provides a fascinating and provocative example of ancient viewing culture. Ancient testimonies of the author, and the *Souda*, suggest that he was a resident of Egypt, but are unreliable in other details, especially his name and date.[1] A number of papyrus fragments suggest that the text was composed before the middle of the second century CE, but more certain dating is difficult to ascertain.[2] The text is generally seen as subversive[3] of a basic narrative type in which a young couple meet, are separated on various journeys throughout the Mediterranean, and then are reunited and (re)integrated into the community, often through the institution of marriage. Akhilleus Tatios' narrative manipulates this basic structure (the couple do not seem to live happily ever after), and offers his readers a guide to sexual and gender relations, describes the torture and (*faux*) murders of Leukippe, and finally ends with the

---

[1] For ancient testimonies of the author: Vilborg (1955), 163–8. For the entry in the *Souda*, see *Souda* s.v. Ἀχιλλεὺς Στάτιος. The suggestion, at this location, that he became a Christian priest seems wrong. The *Souda* is also the only text to refer to him as Statios and lists a number of other works by him.

[2] Vogliano (1938). See also Laplace (1983).

[3] The bibliography on Akhilleus Tatios' subversive qualities is extensive: Morgan (1996), 188. On its odd standing within the genre: Reardon (1994), 80–5 and Chew (2000). See Durham (1938) for the now outdated view of the *Leukippe* as a parody of Heliodoros. For parody throughout the novel: Fusillo (1991). The precise nature of its relationship with *Daphnis and Khloe* remains disputed; see Alvares (2006) for their combined interest in Second Sophistic issues and Whitmarsh (2011), 93 for the commonplace that one read the other.

specious and deceitful manipulation of virginity tests.[4] Within this frame, Akhilleus Tatios presents a sustained engagement with the possibilities of viewing, reading, and negotiating spectacular violence and trauma. He continually manipulates rhetorical *enargeia*, and other tropes, to explore the ways in which the other—internal and external readers and viewers—understand and react to violence and pain.

My use of 'ideal' to designate the Greek romances points to an erstwhile belief in the ways in which the five major extant Greek romances consistently conformed to, and confirmed, an elite ideology (which is most evident in their promotion of a socially validated relationship between two elite protagonists).[5] Scholarship over the last decade has done much to dispel this ideal on a number of different levels.[6] Nonetheless, while these texts are not simple univocal manifestations of elite ideology, they do offer clues to the ways in which Imperial society negotiated the relationship between the individual, their experiences, and their community. The treatment of the body, in particular the female body, is fundamental to this. Across the novels, the beauty of the protagonists often lies at the heart of social hierarchies, suggesting that viewing the body is imbued with political (and even martial) implications.[7] As Brent Shaw argues, Akhilleus Tatios' interest in the physical endurance of Leukippe is part of a growing Imperial sense of the moral and social worth of patient or passive endurance;[8] the theme of *partheneia* is also one which reflects the import of virginity for social, cultural, and gender

---

[4] For murder: e.g. Ach. Tat. iii.14–15, v.7. Torture: vi.21–2. How to court young girls: i.9–10. Sex is best with boys or women: ii.35–8. Virginity tests: viii.6 (Leukippe) and viii.11 (Melite). For the failure to return to the original narrative frame: Repath (2005).

[5] Foucault (1986), 228–32, Konstan (1994), Perkins (1995), 41–76, esp. 44–5, and Swain (1996), 101–9.

[6] On Foucault's misrecognition of the novels' complexity, see Goldhill (1995), x–xi. On genre: Whitmarsh (2008), 6–7 and (2011) for the novels' complex and varied framing of identity in the Imperial period.

[7] For Kallirhoe: X. Eph. v.3.2, with discussion in Elsom (1992) and Egger (1994). Daphnis' and Khloe's beauty marks them out as socially superior: Longus *D&C.* i.7. For the politics of looking at Leukippe: Morales (2004), 156–226. On the power of Leukippe's beauty, see, e.g., Ach. Tat. i.4.

[8] Shaw (1996), 269–71 and 275 for the notion of the body as a 'silent script'. King (2012) on the importance of resistance, bodily narratives of display, and Leukippe's authority in this text. For my views on Shaw's contextualization of the novel, see Introduction (text to nn. 72–5). For further discussion of the viewing of violence, see Frilingos (2009) and Chew (2003), who both argue for a Christian context for viewing the traumatized or violated female body.

identities in Imperial communities (especially in Christian ones).[9] Viewing the violated, traumatized body is part of a much broader interest in the ways in which the *sōma*, along with its experiences and form, helps to phrase, solidify, or problematize social values.

Akhilleus Tatios' novel is, as one astute commentator put it, 'profoundly ocularcentric; it is a scopophiliac's paradise'.[10] This visuality encompasses the use of *ekphrasis* to describe specific (fictional) works of art,[11] and a range of other visual *tableaux: Leukippe and Kleitophon* revels in descriptions of natural wonders, flora and fauna, great physical beauty (especially, but not limited to, Leukippe), the human body, and man-made spectacles. Two themes dominate the treatment of this visual aspect of the novel. Shadi Bartsch, famously, argues that the set-piece descriptions of the novel provide a series of hermeneutic clues which allow later events in the novel to be decoded.[12] While Bartsch's interpretation is important for stressing the ways in which ekphrastic 'digressions' are closely connected to the broader narrative, it ensures that pictures are treated primarily as texts to be deciphered in such a way as to unlock the meaning of the narrative; not enough space, to my mind, is given to treating specific descriptions as images which are designed to be viewed. Bartsch leaves unanswered some important questions about how the viewing process works, how the subject matter of the image might impact on the viewer, and how one is asked to engage—emotionally or otherwise—with what is seen. These questions have, in part, been taken up by Helen Morales (and, more recently, by others such as Ballengee).[13] Morales points out that the way readers view the female body helps to construct Leukippe as

---

[9] For the continued emphasis on virginity in Akhilleus Tatios, see, e.g., the use of *parthenos* and related forms throughout book viii: Ach. Tat. viii.1.2, 6.14–15, 12.5–7, and 13.2. Morales (2004), 204–5 for a reading of the resistance to rape by Thersandros. Virginity in both 'pagan' and Christian novels is fundamental to themes of identity, social authority, and resistance: Burrus (2005).

[10] Morales (2004), ix.

[11] For a general overview of *ekphrasis* in the novels: Billault (1979). For Akhilleus Tatios specifically: Harlan (1965) and D'Alconzo (2014a), esp. 107–70. For the suggestion that Akhilleus Tatios was important for the development of the genre of *ekphrasis* of works of art, see D'Alconzo (2014a), 13–14. For the relationship between art and novelistic conceit, cf. Longus *D&C. praef.*

[12] Bartsch (1989), 41–2. The importance of the description of Europa on the bull which opens the novel has been discussed extensively: Reeves (2007) and Morales (2004), 36–48 for its programmatic status as a riddle of the entire novel.

[13] Ballengee (2009), 65–90 for a critical reading of the contemporary approach to gender.

the object of a sexualized and aggressive male gaze. Morales's and Ballengee's (different) arguments stress, broadly, the connection between viewing trauma and the pleasurable consumption of the female body through the masculine gaze; as a consequence, trauma is seen as something which is viewed pleasurably (and often erotically) by viewers inside the text as well as external readers.

I contribute to this debate in two principal ways. Firstly, I complicate the model of pleasant or erotic viewing. Trauma is not always presented as a pleasing sight. Indeed, the complex emotional responses developed throughout this novel concatenate a range of different modes of affective engagement. These stretch from distress through to emotional stupefaction and pity. In so doing, they situate the viewing (and experience) of trauma within a complex cultural landscape. Secondly, these emotional responses are often developed in contexts which knowingly distance or ironize the extra-diegetic reader. Akhilleus Tatios' narrative constructs emotional responses through a highly self-aware rhetorical ego-narrative which is recounted in tranquil retrospect to an internal narratee by the novel's protagonist, Kleitophon. For the external reader, it is (at best) difficult to separate affective reactions to events from an awareness of the focalizing structure and self-aware qualities of the narrative as a whole. As a consequence, the text dramatizes multiple viewing positions, ranging from Kleitophon's immediately pathetic responses to trauma through to more knowing, 'ironized' viewing positions of the extra-diegetic reader. How one views trauma, how one understands its link with pain, and how one reacts to it are dependent upon how one views the body. If Akhilleus Tatios does not seem to be committed to one single way of seeing trauma and pain, then he is, at least, devoted to the idea that trauma and pain shape relationships between the pained and the other, and have a capacity to shape emotional and cognitive relationships between people and their bodies.

There are two further aspects of the novel which are fundamental to the author's treatment of trauma and pain: the (knowing) use of rhetoric and tragedy and the focalizing structure of the novel's narrative. The rhetorical texture of the work has long been recognized. It is saturated with themes and set pieces that are common to rhetorical training schools (and the rhetorical handbooks, the *Progymnasmata*), such as the storms at sea or the description of visual wonders;[14] the

---

[14] Storms: (Ps.-)Longin. *Subl.* 9.14; Hermog. *Id.* 1.6.45–9 for Aristeides' use of an *ekphrasis* of a storm and the creation of *semnotēs*. For a full discussion of the subject matter of rhetorical description, see Webb (2009), 147.

use of *ekphrasis* is built upon the author's training within the rhetorical schools (and, according to some critics, reflects cultural interest in the rhetorical description of visual scenes).[15] Rhetorical culture and theory also stand behind a considerable amount of Akhilleus Tatios' interest in the power and nature of language and narrative—as we shall see, the impact of *logos* and *muthos* on the listener is phrased through concepts and terminology consistently drawn from the rhetorical tradition. Rhetorical language and tropes like *ekplēxis* help to conceptualize the process of both looking at the body and listening to stories about it. The relationship between rhetoric and the emotional complexity of the novel is also layered with elements drawn from other generic traditions, such as tragedy or mime.[16] Events throughout the novel are represented as dramatic performances and the act of viewing is linked with spectatorship in the theatre; this is further complicated by the use of tragic language and lamentation by the author to recount certain events or by the protagonists to express their feelings about such events.[17] Recourse to rhetorical language or the use of tragic elements is also highly self-aware, caught between its use to represent the emotional reactions of the protagonists to events and readers' awareness of the highly troped nature of such bombastic forms. Readers are caught between the types of reaction that Kleitophon demonstrates—the type of reaction that is phrased in deeply familiar cultural terms—and the reaction of a knowing, cynical reader who is accustomed to rhetorical and tragic tropes and mythic themes. By asking readers to navigate these two levels of reaction, Akhilleus Tatios asks them to navigate what it means to view trauma in ways that are familiar, known, *clichéd*.

The second aspect of the novel which, famously, inflects the construction of the reader's viewing position is the focalizing structure of the novel. *Leukippe and Kleitophon* is unique among the 'ideal' Greek novels for being told from a first-person perspective to an internal narratee.[18] The problematics of viewing throughout the novel are heightened precisely because the spectacles and *theamata* are focalized through Kleitophon's gaze. Such focalization shapes the way that others (either the internal narratee or extra-diegetic readers) view the

---

[15] Rohde (1876), 348, 360, and 512. See also Harlan (1965) (esp. the first two chapters).
[16] On mime, see Mignogna (1997).
[17] On tragic lamentation in the novels, see Fusillo (1989), 36–40. For further discussion of the 'tragic mode': Whitmarsh (2011), 225–32, esp. 225 for further references to the discussion in other novels.
[18] Reardon (1994).

scenes described by Kleitophon: readers are forced, at one level, to become viewers like Kleitophon—we, like him, see certain elements of the scene and cannot see what he chooses to occlude. The focalizing structure of the novel often breaks down when Kleitophon describes traumatic events; it is at these moments that Akhilleus Tatios undermines the distance provided by the narrative frames that separate the action of the novel from different audiences. Viewing pain collapses potential boundaries between the viewer and those who are traumatized. This process problematizes the perspective that readers have on trauma. Are the meaning and significance of trauma created solely through the eyes of Kleitophon (and to satisfy his agenda), or are there times when Leukippe herself is able to shape the meaning and reactions to pain? Thinking about the view almost always involves thinking about what it means to present *a*, or *the*, view of events recounted to an internal narratee.

1. VIEWING PROMETHEUS

Let us begin with the detailed *ekphrasis* of a painting of Prometheus' punishment by an eagle. Upon leaving a temple in Pelousion at the mouth of the Nile, the protagonists encounter a painting of two subjects—the first, the incarceration of Andromeda; the second, the torture of Prometheus—which is attributed to a painter called Euanthes. The description of the painting has attracted interest as the only reference in the novels to a painting which has the painter's name inscribed and as a unique diptych.[19] A considerable amount of scholarly literature has, consequently, discussed whether or not Akhilleus Tatios' reference to Euanthes refers to a historical artist and, therefore, whether or not the description is based on a historical painting.[20] I am less interested in such historical questions, which, to my mind, are secondary to those concerned with the ways in which Akhilleus Tatios figures the process of viewing trauma.

---

[19] D'Alconzo (2014b), 76 with n. 4 on the naming of Euanthes in this passage. For its unique status as a diptych: Goldhill (1995), 72.
[20] Cf. D'Alconzo (2014b), 77. For other treatments (historical and fictional) of the Perseus and Andromeda theme: Elsner (2000), 46–52. For the connections between the description of Prometheus and contemporary presentations of his body, see the text to nn. 24–5 below.

Both elements of this painting recall earlier moments within the novel where Leukippe is imagined to be the subject of physical abuse by a rapist (ii.23) and anticipate later events in which she is thought to be ritually disembowelled by a series of bandits (iii.16).[21] Morales argues that this passage, in helping both to recall and to prefigure Leukippe's rape, is part of the process that accentuates the male gaze and sexuality as both predatory and aggressive.[22] I want to suggest a slightly divergent reading of the *tableau*. There are common elements to the two images in the diptych—as indeed Kleitophon points out—which invite reading these two scenes together. There are, however, also critical differences between the images which accentuate and emphasize, to my mind, differing viewing and readerly experiences. The first of the two images—the description of Andromeda—focuses heavily on her beauty. The description lingers over her body, stressing its erotic qualities.[23] Even though she is presented as feeling fear towards the monster that has been sent to sacrifice her, this does not diminish her beauty, her *eidos*. In the second image, however, the focus on beauty is replaced by a more sustained (and more determined) focus on the physical destruction and rupture of Prometheus' body. There is a sense in which these two halves, through their alternate foci, juxtapose different ways of looking at the body; that juxtaposition emphasizes the ways in which one looks at pain and (/as opposed to?) beauty.

This pain is most clearly emphasized in the intense and evocative description of the body of Prometheus:

ὄρνις ἐς τὴν Προμηθέως γαστέρα τρυφᾷ· ἔστηκε γὰρ αὐτὴν ἀνοίγων, ἤδη μὲν οὖν ἀνεῳγμένην, ἀλλὰ τὸ ῥάμφος ἐς τὸ ὄρυγμα κεῖται, καὶ ἔοικεν ἐπορύττειν τὸ τραῦμα καὶ ζητεῖν τὸ ἧπαρ· τὸ δὲ ἐκφαίνεται τοσοῦτον, ὅσον ἠνέῳξεν ὁ γραφεὺς τὸ διόρυγμα τοῦ τραύματος· ἐρείδει τῷ μηρῷ τῷ τοῦ Προμηθέως τὰς τῶν ὀνύχων ἀκμάς. ὁ δὲ ἀλγῶν ταύτῃ συνέσταλται καὶ τὴν πλευρὰν συνέσπασται καὶ τὸν μηρὸν ἐγείρει καθ'αὑτοῦ· εἰς γὰρ τὸ ἧπαρ συνάγει τὸν ὄρνιν· ὁ δὲ ἕτερος αὐτῷ τοῖν ποδοῖν τὸν σπασμὸν ὄρθιον ἀντιτείνει κάτω καὶ εἰς τοὺς δακτύλους ἀποξύνεται. τὸ δὲ ἄλλο σχῆμα

---

[21] For this scene as proleptic: Bartsch (1989), 55. For an alternative reading of the prolepsis in this episode: Anderson (1979b), 517, who associates it with the statue of Zeus in the same temple. For further discussion of the integration of this scene into both proleptic and analeptic modes of reading: Morales (2004), 176-7.

[22] Morales (2004), 177.

[23] Such as the 'beauty' (κάλλος) and 'fear' (δέος) in her cheeks; and 'the beauty that blooms in her eyes' (ἐκ δὲ τῶν ὀφθαλμῶν ἀνθεῖ τὸ κάλλος): Ach. Tat. iii.7.2-3.

δείκνυσι τὸν πόνον· κεκύρτωται τὰς ὀφρῦς, συνέσταλται τὸ χεῖλος, φαίνει τοὺς ὀδόντας. ἠλέησας ἂν ὡς ἀλγοῦσαν τὴν γραφήν. ἀναφέρει δὲ λυπούμενον Ἡρακλῆς.

The bird feeds on the stomach of Prometheus. She stands there, opening it; indeed, it is already opened. The beak dives into the canal and it seems to dig into the wound and to search for the liver; this is visible to the extent that the artist had opened up the canal of the wound. And she plants the points of her talons in the thigh of Prometheus. He, since he feels pain at this, is contracted and is doubled over on his side and lifts up his thigh towards himself. In this way, he leads the bird to his liver. The other leg is stretched straight out in the opposite direction down to his feet in a spasm and is brought to a point at his toes. The rest of his arrangement displays his pain; his eyebrows are arched, his lips drawn up, he shows his teeth; you would feel pity for the portrayal as if it were in pain. And Herakles is raising him up in his distress.

Ach. Tat. iii.8.1–5

Kleitophon's description of the picture presents bodily rupture in particularly vivid language. The actions, and physical details, of the bird direct the viewers' attention to the ways in which Prometheus' body has been violated. The beak plunges 'into the canal', that is the wound it has created; the beak gouges out the wound and searches for the liver. In a similar fashion, she does not just hold onto the leg of the victim, but 'she plants the points of her talons in' the flesh of his thigh. The use of 'search' (ζητεῖν), here, forces the viewers themselves to search for the missing organ, peering deep into the opened body of the Titan; the use of 'dig' (ὀρύττω) emphasizes the physical violence of the process. Here, the internal body has been revealed by the eagle's beak, the body's normal closed form violated, its hidden internal state revealed for the eyes of viewers in the temple, the internal narratee, and those outside the story entirely. The description has some parallels in contemporary iconography, which during the Roman period increasingly portrayed Prometheus standing erect in the manner he is described by Kleitophon.[24] At the same time, the concern with the exposure of the internal spaces of the body is reminiscent of contemporary approaches to the body driven by anatomy in which the internal *sōma* is literally 'revealed' or 'displayed' to the viewing and

---

[24] D'Alconzo (2014b), 81–2, for comparison with the depiction of Prometheus in a fresco in the Casa dei Capitelli Colorati at Pompeii; cf. *LIMC* VII.1.531–53, esp. nos. 59 and 64–5.

reading audience.[25] Akhilleus Tatios chooses a familiar posture and draws links with the contemporary culture of anatomy to visualize and express the fundamentally unfamiliar other of the internal body.

Kleitophon's description reads into the *schēma* of the painting the visceral reactions of Prometheus—his feelings of pain—and his emotional responses to his situation. Kleitophon, in narrating or describing this image, engages in a critical act of constructing the meaning of Prometheus' physical form and expressions in order to interpret what he feels: trauma is read, (re)viewed, as a physically painful experience. The act of drawing together parts of the body and his spasms are read in terms of his perception; he does these things 'since he feels pain' or 'being pained' (ἀλγῶν). The sentiment that 'the rest of his arrangement displays his pain' provides a hermeneutic framework for reading the 'signs' of his physique and his *mien*; the *minutiae* of his physical contortion become, on this level, signs of physical pain. The language of showing and revelation seems also to play up the importance of visualization or visual engagement. All that is required to understand that Prometheus is in pain is 'to see' the signs of his contortions. The choice of *deiknumi* downplays the viewer's, or the reader's, act of interpretation—it is the contortions that *show*, rather than the reader's hermeneutic activity which *interprets*. In a rhetorical move familiar from anatomical contexts, it naturalizes the connection between the trauma, the body's spasms, and the interpretation of his pain: the evidence reveals for itself! If Kleitophon's act of viewing stresses Prometheus' pain, it also structures how viewers or readers outside of his narrative view the experience. The focalizing structure means that we see in this painting what Kleitophon wants readers to see; there is little possibility of reading this picture differently; we cannot help but see Prometheus as a figure in pain.

The account is also concerned to guide how and where one looks; the description continually plays up the wound's (and pain's?) capacity to arrest the gaze. The first half of the passage describes the contortions of the body, while the second shifts to the almost serene gentleness of the rescuer, Herakles. In the final sections, Kleitophon

---

[25] For the contemporary culture of anatomical display: Debru (1995), and von Staden (1995b), for its connection with rhetoric. More relevant, here, is perhaps the work of Gleason on the 'shock and awe' tactics of Galen's anatomical demonstrations: Gleason (2009), with the Introduction (text to nn. 35–9), and for anatomical display and looking inside the body, see Introduction (text nn. 39–40). Zeitlin (2012) sees this as part of Akhilleus Tatios' fascination with 'inner and outer' (106–7) experience.

reports that Prometheus has a look 'full of... hope and at the same time fear' (μεστός... ἐλπίδος ἅμα καὶ φόβου). He looks, both towards 'the wound' (τὸ ἕλκος) and to Herakles as well; although 'he desires to look towards Herakles with his eyes' (θέλει μὲν αὐτὸν τοῖς ὀφθαλμοῖς ἰδεῖν), 'the pain draws half his vision to itself' (ἕλκει δὲ τὸ ἥμισυ τοῦ βλέμματος ὁ πόνος, iii.8.7). Prometheus' vision guides that of the viewers, and, in so doing, stresses the ways in which pain draws upon our sight: the pun on *helkos* plays up the relationship between pain, its arresting capacity, and the wound; pain's effect on the gaze is a type of wound, a tearing away from what Prometheus desires to look at; pain arises from, and effects, violence upon the body.[26] Prometheus' pain is, furthermore, navigated between competing emotions of fear, hope, and desire: his desiring gaze is (re)directed by the power of the wound and his *ponos*. Kleitophon's, and the external viewer's, eyes navigate between competing objects and viewing motivations: we, following Prometheus, look at both, divided between the gentler aspects of the painting and its more distressing ones; we are, like Prometheus, ineluctably drawn to the viewing of the *minutiae* of the Titan's painful trauma. For all the desire—figured by *thelein*—to look away, to avert the gaze to the more serene and pleasant aspects of the picture, the wound forces the viewer to confront pain: the wound controls the gaze, forcing us to engage with the damage to the body.

This elaboration of graphic control of, and power over, the gaze of the external other, compounds Kleitophon's description of Prometheus' torture and helps to shape the reader's emotional reaction to the entire scene as one of pity: 'you would feel pity for the portrayal as if it were in pain' (ἠλέησας ἂν ὡς ἀλγοῦσαν τὴν γραφήν). The grammatical structure of the sentence stresses pity: the indicative plus ἄν structure lends an element of expectation to the sentence. The expectation of piteous feelings on behalf of the reader is linked with the pain that Kleitophon reads into the scene. Indeed, the connection between pity and pain is underlined by the final half of the clause, which draws even closer links between the portrayal and pain.

The final line of the description—with its second-person singular verb—is particularly telling for another reason. At the moment when Akhilleus Tatios' protagonist figures the way that the viewer should

---

[26] See Gal. *MM*. x.232K. For further discussions of the link between pain and the wound, see Chapter 9 (text with nn. 16–20).

react, he chooses a verb form which collapses the distance between his unnamed interlocutor of the narrative frame and the reader outside of the text. Akhilleus plays upon the power of the *ekphrasis* to transcend the narrative frames of the novel and speak directly to the listener and the reader. That process is also figured by the play on the word *graphē*. At the precise moment that we encounter a text that ekphrasticly produces a painting before readers' eyes, Akhilleus chooses to play on the polysemy of *graphein*.[27] Do we feel pity at the painting, or Akhilleus' Tatios' narrative, his *graphē*? At the moment when the reader is asked to contemplate explicitly what they feel about this painful scene, the distance between trauma, the text, the listener, and the external reader disappears. Significantly, any hope that the reader might have of maintaining a safe, emotionally detached distance from the events being described is undercut, asking them to engage affectively with what Prometheus feels.

Kleitophon, then, reads into the depiction of Prometheus' body the Titan's pain at his punishment. It links that reading of pain to the ways he sees or interprets the presentation of Prometheus' body. Here, readers see through Kleitophon's eyes and his act of reading: that process of reading and viewing figures our reaction to the wounds of Prometheus. Prometheus', Kleitophon's, and the reader's gaze are all drawn to the wound itself. This dramatizes the emotional reactions that one might feel towards those in pain. Not only are we, like the pained, caught by the need to look at the wound, but we are forced also to feel what Prometheus feels.

2. DISPLAYING LEUKIPPE'S TORTURES

I want now to turn to the treatment of Leukippe's body. The female body, and Leukippe's in particular, is the focus of much of the novel's energy; its violent treatment is particularly eloquent in articulating broader issues of trauma, pain, and viewing perspectives. There are a number of scenes in which the physical torture, abuse, and rape of Leukippe are either alluded to, anticipated, or described. Here, I focus

---

[27] The play on the multiple meanings of *graphē* is well known. Two recent treatments are: Newby (2009), 324–5 and Squire (2013), 106–7. For the novelistic context: Longus *D&C. praef.*, along with Whitmarsh (2011), 94.

on two moments—the ritual disembowelling of Leukippe and her own epistolary description of her treatment as a slave—in which her body is presented as a traumatized corpus for readers to view. In some respects, it is possible to approach these *tableaux* through a model of fetishistic viewing, in which the female body is pleasurably devoured (metaphorically and literally) by a sexualized and consumptive male gaze.[28] Indeed, a number of scholars have stressed the way that these scenes are constructed for the aesthetic pleasure of the reader/viewer. While the sexual undercurrents of such scenes are never far from the surface, there are also less pleasant viewing positions and experiences developed at these points. Indeed, their complexity argues against any one reading of the ways in which the gaze of the reader is directed. By developing—and juxtaposing—multiple viewing positions, Akhilleus Tatios asks readers to re-evaluate not only how they react to her trauma, but also how the body's experiences can be understood through different cultural frameworks of meaning and engagement. If the Prometheus passage could be seen in explicitly painful terms, the treatment of Leukippe is presented in slightly different ways which do not always stress her perception of pain.

The first scene that I wish to discuss is Leukippe's ritual disembowelling at *Leukippe and Kleitophon* iii.16. This scene presents one of a number of *Scheintode* throughout this and other novelistic texts.[29] Brian Reardon, along with other critics, has argued that this scene is constructed for the reader's pleasure.[30] What has been less discussed is the ways in which the viewer is asked to navigate between multiple ways of understanding and viewing trauma. At one level, the viewing experience is characterized by the emotional impact and distress caused by the event and figured through references to powerful, impactful language and ideas drawn from rhetorical theory, tragedy, and myth.[31] For the external reader, however, the knowingness of these tropes helps to figure a slightly different, more aware (and distanced?/detached?) viewing experience in which they are

---

[28] Morales (2004), 166–7.
[29] Bowersock (1994), 99 for the common theme of 'resurrection' after death. See, e.g., Chariton i.4.12, X. Eph. iii.5.11, and Hld. ii.3.5 and viii.7.7. Létoublon (1993), 74–80 and Morales (2004), 167–9, with further references to the other novels; cf. Whitmarsh (2011), 208–9 for the *naïveté* of Kleitophon's reading of this generic commonplace.
[30] Reardon (1994), 83 for the 'relish' with which we view these scenes.
[31] For the complexity of the allusions: Mignogna (1997), who stresses the connection with *Iphigenia at Tauris*. On theatricality in this scene: Liviabella Furiani (1985).

exposed to both the contextualizing frameworks and language and aware of their status as troped *clichés* of the novelistic genre.

Leukippe's sacrifice is described far more cursorily than that of Prometheus. The bandits lead her up to the altar, and although Kleitophon does not know who they are, he is immediately able to recognize Leukippe. They pour libations over her head; the priest sings what Kleitophon assumes to be an Egyptian chant (iii.15.4). Then one of the attendants ties their victim down in a manner reminiscent of Marsyas:

> ἔδησεν ἐκ παττάλων ἐπὶ τῆς γῆς ἐρηρεισμένων, οἷον ποιοῦσιν οἱ κοροπλάθοι τὸν Μαρσύαν ἐκ τοῦ φυτοῦ δεδεμένον. εἶτα λαβὼν ξίφος βάπτει κατὰ τῆς καρδίας καὶ διελκύσας τὸ ξίφος εἰς τὴν κάτω γαστέρα ῥήγνυσι· τὰ σπλάγχνα δὲ εὐθὺς ἐξεπήδησεν, ἃ ταῖς χερσὶν ἐξελκύσαντες ἐπιτιθέασι τῷ βωμῷ, καὶ ἐπεὶ ὠπτήθη, κατατεμόντες ἅπαντες εἰς μοίρας ἔφαγον.

He bound her to pegs which had been fixed in the ground, just as those who make images represent Marsyas bound to the tree; then, taking a sword, plunged it in below the heart and, having dragged the sword down to the area below her stomach, opened her up; the innards jumped out immediately, and these they placed on the altar, having first torn them out with their hands, and, when they were roasted, everyone cut them up into shares and ate them.

Ach. Tat. iii.15.4–5

Binding, here, obviously connects the scene with both the painting of Andromeda and that of Prometheus; the reference to Marsyas connects the image with visual culture and mythical torture and punishment, especially that carried out by Apollo. While these connections carry the threat of great violence—torture even—such implications remain underdeveloped in terms of elaborating her sense of pain. The act of bodily mutilation is, moreover, glossed over. There are moments when the narrative is vivid: the description of plunging the sword into the body of Leukippe and dragging it through her stomach brings the scene almost before the readers' eyes. But, having said this, there is a conspicuous absence of the ways in which Leukippe's body is contorted or reacts to pain; there is far less visual engagement with the ways in which the internal condition of Leukippe's body might be viewed. Compounding this, there is a critical absence of references to, or interest in, Leukippe's pain. If the Prometheus account accentuated Kleitophon's (external) reading of the body's *ponos* or *algos*, then the depiction of Leukippe's disembowelling seems remarkably unconcerned with it or the *minutiae* of the event.

If the scene itself is less extensive than its Promethean counterpart, Kleitophon does focus closely on the possibilities of readerly and viewer reactions. In contrast to the gaze which analysed the signs of Prometheus' body—which viewed it with an almost scientific eye—Kleitophon's reaction figures what trauma means for the pathetic engagement of the other:

> ταῦτα δὲ ὁρῶντες οἱ στρατιῶται καὶ ὁ στρατηγὸς καθ' ἕν τῶν πραττομένων ἀνεβόων καὶ τὰς ὄψεις ἀπέστρεφον τῆς θέας, ἐγὼ δὲ ἐκ παραλόγου καθήμενος ἐθεώμην. τὸ δὲ ἦν ἔκπληξις· μέτρον γὰρ οὐκ ἔχον τὸ κακὸν ἐνεβρόντησέ με. καὶ τάχα ὁ τῆς Νιόβης μῦθος οὐκ ἦν ψευδής, ἀλλὰ κἀκείνη τοιοῦτόν τι παθοῦσα ἐπὶ τῇ τῶν παίδων ἀπωλείᾳ δόξαν παρέσχεν ἐκ τῆς ἀκινησίας ὡσεὶ λίθος γενομένη.

When the army and the general saw these very things, they screamed out at each one of the acts and turned their eyes from the spectacle, but I, irrationally, sat there and continued to gaze. The event was shocking! For the extreme horror struck me like a lightning bolt. Probably, the myth of Niobe is not false, but that woman too, suffering so greatly in some way at the destruction of her children gave the impression, from her immobility, that she had become stone.

Ach. Tat. iii.15.5–6

The most obvious development of divergent viewing positions lies in the alternate reactions of the army who 'screamed out' and 'turned their eyes'—choosing not to look, through either some feeling of disgust or other motivation, is one way of (not) viewing the traumatic. Kleitophon, however, is glued to the scene in an act of continued gazing marked by the imperfect form ἐθεώμην. That act of gazing, more importantly, is figured in telling terms. He sits, unable to look away, because of the power the scene has over him: ἐκ παραλόγου suggests that his vision is underpinned by some irrational force. As the passage continues, the emotional impact is developed in terms which are reminiscent of discussions of the capacity of sublime rhetoric for emotional impact: 'the extreme horror struck [him] like a lightning bolt [ἐνεβρόντησέ]', and 'the event was shocking', literally ekplectic (τὸ δὲ ἦν ἔκπληξις). As with the Prometheus scene, the wound ineluctably holds his (and our) attention. We have already seen that ἔκπληξις was regarded as an effect of language which rhetorical and literary theorists considered to be particularly powerful.

Pseudo-Longinos, for instance, often compares the language of great speakers (such as Demosthenes) to a lightning bolt which shocks but also exercises an irrational hold over the listener.[32] Akhilleus Tatios chooses terminology which aligns Kleitophon's viewing with the power of rhetorical language to control and shape the reactions of the listener or reader.

The use of *ekplēxis*, here, recalls other scenes throughout the novel where looking at Leukippe is conceptualized in similar terms: when Kleitophon first sets eyes on the girl, her beauty strikes him like a lightning bolt, it 'destroys' him.[33] The reference to Niobe and her grief at the destruction of her children, which underpins the way in which Kleitophon initially makes sense of the sight, separates this viewing scene from others earlier (and later) in the novel. The event drives Kleitophon to make sense of what he feels; he does so by offering a mythical account of his inability to move. The story of Niobe's petrification has been seen as one which carries connotations of eroticism.[34] While this reading is certainly valid, it seems to me that the reference plays up what is at stake in the loss of loved ones. The Niobe story takes a number of different forms in tragedy and other contexts. The story of *Iliad* 24, however, dramatizes the effect of extreme personal loss and its resultant emotive effect on the viewer. Niobe and Kleitophon are connected by the proximity that they feel to the events described, and the sense of loss that ensues. The suggestion that it is 'not false' is also telling. It looks towards philosophical debates about the truth content of such *muthoi*—a point that seems to be a particularly important issue for contemporary literary critics, such as Plutarch.[35] It also recalls Kleitophon's own opening

---

[32] (Ps.-)Longin. *Subl.* 12.3. For the power of *ekplēxis* over the listener: 1.4, and esp. 15.11. See also Goldhill (2007).

[33] For references to ἔκπληξις and the experience of looking: e.g. Ach. Tat. i.4.5 and i.10.4. For the connection with events that are παράλογος ('unexpected' or 'inexplicable'): e.g. Ach. Tat. iii.15.6, iv.14.5, v.23.5, and vii.8.1. For the theorization of the process of looking at beauty: i.4. For the destructive qualities of Leukippe's beauty: ἀπωλώλειν at i.4.4. The connection between shock and the 'unexpected', see Plut. *Quomodo Adulesc.* 25d.

[34] Morales (2004), 165–71, on this scene and the 'consumptive gaze'. For the erotics of the scene, see 171: 'the dual possibilities implied by petrifaction complicate a straightforward reading of Kleitophon's reaction and create an undercurrent of eroticism in the audience's reception of the *Scheintod*'.

[35] For the (famous) connection between mythic stories and falsehood, see, e.g., Plut. *Quomodo Adulesc.* 16b–d.

gambit—that his experiences 'are appropriate for myth' (τὰ γὰρ ἐμὰ μύθοις ἔοικε)—in the initial meeting with his unnamed narrator.[36] One way to read Kleitophon's experiences, he claims then and now, is through myth. If Kleitophon's inability to move immediately helps us to read or understand Niobe's story as something that is 'not false', it also helps us to understand Kleitophon's position as a viewer of traumatic events. The scene drives a search for interpretation and explanation through an act of mythic narrativizing in which myth and reality are reinterpreted in the light of each other. Scholars have commonly emphasized the importance of thinking about the myths of Andromeda and Prometheus as frameworks for understanding the destruction of Leukippe's body, but it is important, too, to note that this story also figures the emotional impact of trauma on those around Leukippe.[37]

The impact of her destruction on those who view it continues to reverberate throughout the following chapters of the narrative. In the following lines, the general attempts 'to console [Kleitophon] as he is distressed' (με παρηγορεῖν ἀνιαρῶς ἔχοντα, iii.16.1). The choice of παρηγορεῖν to represent the general's actions looks towards the tradition of philosophical consolation developed in near-contemporary authors such as Plutarch and Dio of Prusa.[38] At the same time, the suggestion that Kleitophon is ἀνιαρῶς ἔχοντα underscores his own feelings of distress at the treatment of Leukippe. It is worth recalling that ἀνιαρῶς is precisely the term used by Plutarch in book five of his *Sympotic Questions* to describe the distressed feelings when we view the bodies of the sick and deformed. According to iii.17, when he sees his travelling companions, Satyros and Menelaos (who escape from the bandits unexpectedly), he recounts that neither is he able to embrace them nor is he 'amazed by pleasure' when they arrive (ἐξεπλάγην ὑφ' ἡδονῆς) since 'the grief of the disaster had stupefied him' (τοσοῦτον ἡ λύπη με τῆς συμφορᾶς ἐξεκώφησε, iii.17.2). Both

---

[36] Cf. the repetition of the phrase by Kleitophon's interlocutor at Ach. Tat. i.2.2: 'in the name of Zeus, and Eros himself, to speak about them more in this way, if, indeed, they are like myth' (πρὸς τοῦ Διὸς καὶ τοῦ Ἔρωτος αὐτοῦ, ταύτῃ μᾶλλον ᾔσειν, εἰ καὶ μύθοις ἔοικε).

[37] On emotional stupefaction in the novels: Fusillo (1999). For examples of types of emotional 'aporia', see X. Eph. i.7 when Anthia's and Habrokomes' parents encounter the oracle's account of the protagonists' fate and, on this passage, Whitmarsh (2011), 179–83. Cf., e.g., Ach. Tat. iii.11.1.

[38] For παρηγορεῖν and consolation, see E. *Ph.* 1449.

ἀνιαρῶς and λύπη speak to high degrees of emotional distress at what he has seen. Kleitophon's reaction to the image of his girlfriend being sacrificed runs the gamut of emotional responses from stupefaction through to distress and grief which are familiar throughout Imperial literary and art-criticism.

These two references to distress bookend a long, hyperbolic tragic-style lament in which Kleitophon expresses his horror at what has happened.[39] He claims that he 'laments not only her death' (οὐ τὸν θάνατον ὀδύρομαί σου μόνον, iii.16.3), but also the circumstances in which it occurred. It is in this context that the viewer is given the opportunity not only to consider what is seen as significant by Kleitophon (that she died in a foreign land, that the purity of her body was preserved only to become a sacrifice, etc.), but to understand what it means for him (or, at least, what he would like his listeners and readers to think what it means for him). His language stresses the emotionality of the event by linking his reaction to familiar forms of grief expression within the Greek literary tradition. If that gives greater context and meaning to the sight of Leukippe, it is also at this stage that we are asked to consider further consequences of her physical destruction, such as the separation of her bodily parts and the revelation of the mysteries of her internal body. He laments that she had been 'cut up while she still lived' (ζῶσαν ἀνέτεμον), that she had watched 'the entire dissection' (ὅλην τὴν ἀνατομήν), and that 'the mysteries of her stomach were dispersed' (τῆς γαστρὸς τὰ μυστήρια ἐμέρισαν, iii.16.3); he stresses the exposure of her inner body, and its separation from her external *sōma*. Kleitophon's lament rephrases the experience in a number of different ways, especially in terms of ritual sacrifice in which the mysteries of the body are laid bare. It is worth recalling that the language Kleitophon uses at this point also looks to themes of anatomy and the display of the internal body being developed in contemporary medical culture. Elisa Mignogna, in particular, argues that the entire account of Leukippe's disembowelling is predicated on pantomimic and mimic versions of *Iphigenia at Tauris*.[40] There are certainly elements of this cultural practice which have been incorporated into this scene. It is also worth pointing out

---

[39] For further implications for a tragic reading: Ach. Tat. iii.11.1; ταῦτα μὲν ἐθρήνουν ἡσυχῇ ('I lamented these things in silence') in relation to their capture by pirates at iii.10. cf. its use throughout iii.10. For its use in tragic contexts: A. *Ch.* 926 and S. *Aj.* 632.

[40] Mignogna (1997).

that Kleitophon's description of the event gestures in a number of different directions. Kleitophon navigates and reads his viewing experience through frameworks drawn from tragedy and contemporary rhetorical culture, which figure both the emotional impact of the sight and its broader emotional meanings in terms of the distress of loss.

At one level, then, Kleitophon phrases the impact of the event in terms of contemporary ideas about emotional impact and stupefaction and the language and emotionality of tragedy. How might the external reader of the novel view such language or contextualization? Some aspects of the entire episode suggest that this scene might be a 'false death', a common theme within the novelistic genre.[41] Moreover, the treatment of the body in the initial description of her disembowelling is so superficial as to downplay the emotionally impactful elements of the scene for those who are familiar with the tropes of the genre. Furthermore, the way in which Akhilleus Tatios figures Kleitophon's lament continues to undermine our secure emotional readings of this passage. To speak in tragic language, τραγῳδεῖν, was commonly assumed to mean 'to exaggerate' or 'to speak bombastically'[42] and the tragic-style lament is a common motif adopted throughout the genre.[43] What interests me is the mixing that occurs between the heavy implications of the sublimated viewing practices represented by the power of the image and the author's knowing game with the scene's—and the reaction's—troped quality. How we view—and react to the sight of—Leukippe's dissection becomes a question of how readers navigate these two competing readerly positions. Do readers react as Kleitophon does to the emotional force of the event? Or do readers interpret his attempt to make sense of the trauma cynically (or ironically) as a *cliché*? Or, on seeing both ways of viewing, do they think consciously about where we might be positioned as viewers? If we are meant to feel pity at the fate of Prometheus, then the image of Leukippe presents very different problems for the viewer and their engagement with what they see.

The second example of Leukippe's tortured body that I wish to consider concerns the strategic revelation of her scars to Melite and Kleitophon in book five. In the final stages of the novel, Leukippe, who has been captured by pirates and sold as a slave, is transported by a series

---

[41] For other false deaths in the five 'ideal' novels, see Chariton i.4.12; X. Eph. iii.5.11 and iii.7; Hld. ii.3.5 and viii.7.7; and Létoublon (1993), 74–80.

[42] Cf. Gal. *UP.* iv.286K: τραγῳδεῖν ἂν δόξειε μᾶλλον ἢ ἀληθεύειν ('he would seem to be speaking bombastically rather than honestly'). For exaggeration: Epict. 4.7.17, who contrasts it with speaking about matters 'as they really are'. Whitmarsh (2011), 208–9.

[43] Fusillo (1989), 56–66 and Birchall (1996).

of events to an estate near Ephesos where she happens upon Kleitophon and his new mistress, Melite. As with the last scene, she becomes the sight and the site at which pain and trauma are contextualized.

At her first meeting with Kleitophon and Melite, Leukippe throws herself at the feet of Melite and begs to be taken into her care. She begins by entreating Melite as a woman who has suffered great reversals: 'Mistress, pity me, she said, a woman to a woman, a free one, as I was born, who is now a slave' (ἐλέησόν, ἔφη, δέσποινα, γυνὴ γυναῖκα, ἐλευθέραν μέν, ὡς ἔφυν, δούλην δὲ νῦν', Ach. Tat. v.17.3). The use of pity is directly linked to the reversals that the character has suffered at the hands of fortune. But, it also sets up the scene as one in which the revelation of the body is designed to evoke emotional responses from those who view her harsh treatment. As the encounter proceeds, the revelation of her body and its construction as a *theama* is made more explicit:

'ὁρᾷς δὲ καὶ πληγαῖς ὡς ἔξανέ με πολλαῖς.' καὶ ἅμα διανοίξασα τὸν χιτῶνα δείκνυσι τὰ νῶτα διαγεγραμμένα ἔτι οἰκτρότερον. ὡς οὖν ταῦτα ἠκούσαμεν, ἐγὼ μὲν συνεχύθην· καὶ γάρ τι ἐδόκει Λευκίππης ἔχειν.

'You see, too, how he carded me many times with blows.' And at the same time, having opened her chiton, she revealed the back which had been inscribed even more pitiably. When we heard these things, I [Kleitophon] was confounded, for she also seemed to have something of Leukippe about her.

Ach. Tat. v.17.6–7

In some ways, the scene reads like a titillating striptease in which we get to see inside Leukippe's chiton—a view which is normally concealed. But the pre-emptive explanation seems to structure the experience of viewing in terms less pleasurable. This scene does not direct our gaze to the pain of the body specifically and is certainly a long way removed from the intense focus on the body in the Prometheus narrative. There are, nevertheless, some clues as to how we might read the bodily experiences of Leukippe. The reference to things which had been written on her back suggests that her scars or bruising have become a kind of script available for reading her corporeal abuse. Scars, in particular, often hold a privileged status as signs that attest to the nature of past experience, hardship, or endurance of difficulty.[44] Kleitophon's reading of her body, his act of viewing and interpretation, is marked by the immediacy of his pity.

---

[44] King (2012), 150–1, Leigh (1995), and Gleason (2001). The semiology of scars goes back to the οὐλή at Hom. *Od.* 19.391 and 393. For the paradigmatic status of the scar for the novels: Ach. Tat. viii.5.14; Cf. Aristid. 47.68K with Holmes (2008), 104–5.

The representation of her past experiences, to which her body attests, is explained further in a letter that she writes to Kleitophon in the hours following their meeting. Here, her experiences are explicitly presented in terms of prolonged difficulty and pain. Leukippe's letter is carefully framed so as to remind Kleitophon of all that she has undergone: 'such things I have suffered because of you, you know, but it is now necessary to remind you' (ὅσα μὲν διὰ σὲ πέπονθα, οἶδας· ἀνάγκη δὲ νῦν ὑπομνῆσαί σε, v.18.3).[45] This language of 'suffering', figured by *paschein*, is repeated throughout the epistolary list of experiences: she 'suffered' (πέπονθα, 18.4) shipwreck, she 'was scourged' (ἐμαστιγώθην), she 'endured patiently' (διεκαρτέρησα, 18.5) all of these pains, and feels she is deserving of 'some thanks' (τις . . . χάρις) for the 'things that have been endured' (τῶν πεπονημένων, 18.5) on behalf of Kleitophon; she closes her letter by repeating her constant refrain that she suffered these pains on behalf of him.[46] Aside from the emotional blackmail which obtains in the letter, it is telling for the ways in which it figures experiences as hardships which are endured. '*Ponōn*', translated as 'pains', points to a sense of physical pain, but also integrates the perception into a broader sense of difficulty, harsh experiences, and *pathēmata*: if it is physical pain to which she refers, it is part of a long list (and just one?) of endured hardships. Leukippe's letter presents a more holistic view of her pain, and the things that have been written on her back. If Kleitophon and she both stressed the need to feel pity at her body, then Leukippe's letter goes further by linking her scars and her pain (and their capacity to evoke pity) to other examples of her endurance, her patience, and her loyalty. What the scars and the pain mean for Kleitophon and Leukippe appears to be very different.

Leukippe's letter wreaks emotional havoc.[47] Even before Kleitophon begins to read the letter, he is thunderstruck (κατεπλάγην, v.18.2). As he proceeds, however, he 'recognized the words of Leukippe' (ἐγνώρισα γὰρ Λευκίππης τὰ γράμματα, v.18.2). The contents of the letter also appear to have a particular effect on their reader. When he rereads the letter in the following chapter, he claims that he experienced everything

---

[45] Cf. Anthia's lament that she does not experience suffering similar to that of Habrokomes (X. Eph. iii.5).
[46] Ach. Tat. v.18.6: . . . νόμιζε μισθόν μοι δεδωκέναι τῶν ὑπὲρ σοῦ πόνων. ('consider it granted to me as a payment for my sufferings on your behalf').
[47] For the emotional power of the letter, see Repath (2013), 244–5.

at the same time (πάντα ἐγινόμην ὁμοῦ, v.19.6): indeed, he was inflamed (ἀνεφλεγόμην), he turned pale (ὠχρίων), he wondered (ἐθαύμαζον), he disbelieved (ἠπίστουν), he was pleased (ἔχαιρον), and he was distressed (ἠχθόμην). The spectrum of emotional and intellectual responses to the letter is partly because he thought that she was dead (again!), but they also dramatize the ways in which we navigate exposure to the sufferings and experiences of others. As his reaction is recounted further, he explores the way in which the spectacle of Leukippe's tortures moves him especially. Forcefully reminding the reader of the experiences of the other involves ensuring Kleitophon encounters her trauma as if he were an eyewitness of the events that she has endured:

> ὡς δὲ εἰς τὰς μάστιγας καὶ εἰς τὰς βασάνους ἐγενόμην, ἃς ὁ Σωσθένης αὐτῇ παρετρίψατο, ἔκλαον ὥσπερ αὐτὰς τὰς βασάνους βλέπων αὐτῆς· ὁ γὰρ λογισμός, πέμπων τῆς ψυχῆς τὰ ὄμματα πρὸς τὴν ἀπαγγελίαν τῶν γραμμάτων, ἐδείκνυε τὰ ὁρώμενα ὡς δρώμενα... οὕτως ᾐσχυνόμην καὶ τὰ γράμματα.

And when I read the part about the whips and the tortures which Sosthenes had inflicted upon her, I wept as if I was watching her tortures themselves; for consideration, directing the eyes of my soul to the message of the letter, revealed what I was seeing as if they were actions... so in this way I was shamed by even the letter.

Ach. Tat. v.19.6

The emotive responses of Kleitophon are, on this rhetorical reading of the passage, manipulated through a process in which the description of suffering literally transports him in time and space back to those events. On one level, Kleitophon's response is specifically associated with an emotive reaction (note the use of ἔκλαον, 'I wept'), which is connected with the letter's capacity to transform distant events into ones which occur before his eyes.[48] In documenting his emotional response to vivid description, Kleitophon's reference to the interplay between the 'eyes of his soul' (τῆς ψυχῆς τὰ ὄμματα) and his reception of visual phenomena (ἐδείκνυε τὰ ὁρώμενα ὡς δρώμενα) tap into a particular aspect of ekphrastic theory which stresses the way that language

---

[48] For the listener or reader as an eyewitness, see the discussion of the rhetorical techniques of 'transference', 'metastasis', or 'metathesis' in Webb (2009), esp. at 100 and n. 34. The letter appears to be particularly efficacious at transporting the reader because of its ability to play on the dynamic between presence and absence: Robiano (2007), esp. 203-4. On the scenes of letter reception in general: Koskenniemi (1956), 172-86. See also the chapters in Hodkinson, Rosenmeyer, and Bracke (2013).

exposes individuals to events. Ruth Webb has pointed to how rhetorical theorists' discussions of *ekphrasis* start from a conception of language in which words operate as a powerful physical force which penetrate the readers' (or listeners') bodies and appeal to the eyes of the soul, and in so doing construct them as a type of eyewitness of the events described.[49] For rhetorical theorists, it seems that this ability to penetrate the body of the listener is central to vivid description's capacity to induce an emotional effect (pleasure, indignation, pity, etc.) in the reader.[50]

One important factor about this letter concerns the way in which it fits with the focalizing structure of the novel as a whole. As some scholars have noted, the letter offers one of the few occasions when the voice of Leukippe can be heard.[51] It is worth noting that the letter is, of course, narrated through the eyes of Kleitophon. Does the letter represent Leukippe's understanding of her experiences, and her interpretation of the 'pitiable' writing on her back, or Kleitophon's focalization of that view? Akhilleus Tatios asks us to confront exactly who speaks about the body, what readers see or read in the body, through whose focalization, and on whose terms. On one reading, Kleitophon's account of the letter constitutes yet another act of reading into another's body his understanding of their experiences; on another, it seems to constitute one moment in the text where the process of understanding pain and suffering is dependent on Leukippe's views about her own body. How one sees pain, here, seems inextricably linked to how one positions oneself in relation to the body and its narration by either Leukippe or Kleitophon. The multiple focalizations of the letter, at some levels, force readers to view Leukippe's letter, and her experiences, through the male perspective. Kleitophon's emotional reactions help to define and, indeed, are inseparable from his narration of such events. But at the same time, there appear to be, at this point, important fissures in the security of that perspective. The letter critically explores how audiences see or understand pain by problematizing the position from which audiences view pain.

There are few texts which are quite so concerned with the permutations of the gaze and the experiences of the viewer as the *Leukippe*

---

[49] Webb (2009), 98–9. See especially her discussion of the rhetorical theories of Quintilian and Pseudo-Longinos.
[50] Webb (2009), 99–100. [51] Repath (2013), 246–7 with n. 30.

and Kleitophon. In the context of pain, there are several important themes. Akhilleus Tatios creates a number of different *tableaux*, all of which figure viewing from a number of different perspectives. Each of these perspectives entails slightly different readings of what constitutes pain and how the viewer or other might react to, or engage with, it. There are several themes which emerge from this process. Firstly, the wound, as in Philostratos' *Imagines*, has the capacity to transfix the viewer's gaze. Whatever they may desire to look at, the wound forces individuals to return to the site of physical damage: the wound has arresting qualities that mean one (very often) cannot look away. Secondly, the reaction of viewers is often mediated through an ambivalent emotional reaction to that site. On the one hand, many of the scenes in which the wound is displayed carry implications of erotic and viewerly desire, developed either through their context or through the explicit allusions to the emotional reactions of some viewers. On the other hand, such potentially pleasurable reactions seem to sit alongside a conscious effort to think about the ways in which trauma evokes more problematic emotional responses. It evokes feelings of pity (or at least the assumption that we should feel such emotions). At other times, it speaks to an emotional stupefaction or an emotionally conflicted response such as distress and pleasure. When viewed in relation to Philostratos, it seems that Akhilleus Tatios is far more concerned with developing both elements such as pity in relation to pain itself and other aspects of a conflicted emotional (or quasi-emotional) response.

The variety and diversity of Akhilleus Tatios' treatment of trauma and viewing lead to two further points. As has been acknowledged, the text is characterized by the self-conscious play on its status as a retrospective ego-narrative. While Kleitophon dramatizes one way of reacting to trauma within the narrative, it is also clear that the reader is positioned in a slightly different way from such reactions within the storyworld of the romance. Akhilleus Tatios constantly asks readers to negotiate both the *naïve* reactions of Kleitophon and a more knowing, extra-diegetic reaction to events and the experiences of the other. In so positioning the reader—interminably caught between these two viewing positions—Akhilleus Tatios phrases one of the more important points to emerge from his novel. The ways in which we react to pain and trauma are consequences of the ways in which we are implicated in events; the types of viewers we are, or choose to be; the relationships we have, or choose to have, with those who feel trauma.

12

Viewing Trauma in Plutarch

I want to close the discussion of viewing trauma by turning to a text which might be considered unusual in this context: Plutarch's *On Flesh-Eating*. Plutarch's treatise presents, over two lacunose *logoi*, a highly rhetorical argument for the adoption of a restrained practice of meat-eating among humans. Little is certainly known about this work and it has held an ambivalent position in modern scholarly discussion. It is not known when it was produced; although it is often connected with treatises focused on animal intelligence, principally *Animals are Rational* and *On Whether Land or Sea Animals are Cleverer,* its literary context is unclear; the text itself is highly problematic.[1] It has been taken as an expression of Plutarch's (highly unusual) concern with, and advocation of, animal rights and vegetarianism.[2] Outside discussions of animal rights and dietary practices, *On Flesh-Eating* has been less well received. It has been traditionally dismissed as both indicative of a youthful interest and as a 'highly rhetorical' and 'emotive' piece.[3] The rhetoric of Plutarch's treatise is hard to miss, but such characterization (which also functions as a

---

[1] For the connection with other texts on animals, see *Brut. Anim.* and *de Sollert. Anim.* Although they are often taken together, and as representative of Plutarch's view of animals, the relationship between these texts is not certain: on these two texts' connection with *de Esu Carn.*, see Newmyer (1992), 38-54. The text of *de Esu Carn.* is badly mutilated: multiple *lacunae* are indicated throughout the Teubner edition. I will discuss them at moments when they directly influence my interpretation. Finally, both *logoi* appear to end with the promise of more material: 996c and 999b.
[2] Barrow (1967), 112 for Plutarch's 'sympathy' towards animals. See also Newmyer (1992), 40, (1995), and (2005), and Beer (2009).
[3] 'Highly rhetorical': Krauss (1912), 77. For a 'youthful fancy': Russell (1968), 131, and Brenk (1977), 70 for a typically dismissive (and to my mind internally inconsistent!) view of the treatise.

dismissal of the intellectual or 'serious' qualities of the material) misses, to my mind, some of the point of the author's use of rhetoric. Indeed, a significant part of the treatise's point is to explore the ways in which rhetoric can effectively represent others' experiences, and to use that rhetoric to construct and figure the ways in which readers imagine, and emotively engage with, the suffering of others. Although Plutarch rarely refers explicitly to the concepts of *ekplēxis* and *enargeia,* it is clear that he adopts and adapts a number of rhetorical techniques in order to shape the way in which animal suffering might impact on the reader or viewer. As with Akhilleus Tatios, affective engagement is inherently conflicted—it combines empathy, sympathy, and distress with a complex renegotiation of the pleasure one feels at viewing (and consuming) destroyed animals.

Plutarch's work offers the opportunity to view suffering. It is immediately clear from Plutarch's *logoi* that his concern with visual culture is very different from that which we encountered in Akhilleus Tatios. Nevertheless, it is worth pursuing as an example of ancient viewing culture for a number of reasons. The treatise is predicated on the ways in which rhetorical strategies such as *enargeia* and *ekphrasis* transform the reader into an eyewitness of the traumatic experiences of animals. The two *logoi* are littered with intense descriptions of the acts of torture and corporeal destruction which function as *ekphraseis* and are allied to the ways in which Plutarch shapes the viewing experience: *ekphrasis* emerges, in this context, as a technique to regulate the conflicted ways audiences engage with animal suffering. As I shall discuss, one common theme in this discussion is the way in which the sensory processes operate and how they are harmed by viewing the violent treatment of the body. Looking at the spectacle (*theama*) of violence changes the way audiences see, recognize, and feel about pain. Plutarch's texts aim to (re)teach how to see and engage with suffering through his manipulation of rhetorical vividness and its subsequent effect on readers' *pathē*. Plutarch continually oscillates between the alternate viewing positions and emotional experiences of those who consume animals wantonly for pleasure and those who do so with (in Plutarch's view) more humane sentiments. In so doing, he problematizes the ways in which pain is constructed as a visual and rhetorical subject and how audiences might engage with it.

The interest in the way in which the viewer is positioned is underscored by the marked use of animals to phrase questions about, and discussions of, human experiences. Scholars have been particularly awake to the importance of animals in ancient thought and their role in helping to raise and answer questions about the human body and what it means to be human.[4] This has been particularly true in relation to the nature of physical perceptions and emotional experiences of different animals. Richard Sorabji has shown that a number of ancient philosophical views of animals distinguished definitively between the sensorial experiences of humans and non-humans.[5] Due to different degrees of natural reason, animals' sensorial experiences—pleasure, pain, etc.—and other emotions were of a fundamentally lesser quality than those of higher animals, principally humans.[6] The fact that animals lack the linguistic capacity to express their claims to justice or describe their treatment underpinned a philosophical debate about whether or not animals did in fact experience pain in a similar manner to humans. The critical lack of linguistic capacity justified (in Stoic thought at least) the idea that animals could be mistreated on the basis that their experiences were of a fundamentally lesser nature than ours.[7] As such, it was possible to exclude animals from the ethical and moral community that defines human interaction because they were utterly unlike 'us' in nature. Indeed, these questions seem particularly acute in Plutarch's treatise, where approaching violence towards animals explicitly raises questions about man's capacity to understand and imagine others' pain. Questions about one's empathy for animals and the extension of the claims of justice to them are exacerbated precisely because they lack the capacity to communicate with us. By focusing on the traumatic destruction of the body, he both speaks to, and ask readers to reconsider, traditional ancient arguments for the distinctions between

---

[4] Cassin, Labarrière, and Dherbey (1997) for an overview of the main issues. Lloyd (1997) and Ayache (1997) on the role of animals in medical thought. In anatomy specifically: Hankinson (1997).

[5] Sorabji (1993b), 7-16, 78-96 (on animal reason and speech), and 107-33 (on animal claims to justice). For these claims in relation to Plutarch's own *Moralia*, see Newmyer (1999) and (2006), 85-102.

[6] For distinctions between the Stoic and the Academic view: Labarrière (1997). On the evolution of views about animals' capacity for perception, but the denial of belief and reason: Sorabji (1993b), 16-20 and Newmyer (2006), 17-30. A number of texts in Plutarch's corpus deal explicitly with animal communication and their perception of pleasure and pain: Plut. *Brut. Anim.* (which contains a sustained argument for the superiority of animal virtue, and the intensity of their sensorial experiences, especially pleasure) and *de Sollert. Anim.* Of particular interest in this regard is the attribution of perceptual soul and mental impressions which must allow them to flee from pain or distress at Plut. *de Sollert. Anim.* 959d–961a.

[7] Sorabji (1993b), at 80-5.

man and beast; he confronts the notion of the 'other' and refigures what it means to engage—visually, emotively, and ethically—with the pain and trauma of both the ultimate 'other' and other humans.

This concern is most eloquently expressed towards the close of the second *logos*, where he stresses the need for the emotional consideration of animals. At 999b, he turns explicitly to the Stoic interlocutors that he imagines himself arguing with. He points out that there is no good to come from meat-eating or that such practices are hardly appropriate to that sect's concern with the extirpation of pleasures in other fields of life.[8] He sums this up with a final plea to the reader:

οὐ μὴν ἀλλὰ καὶ τοῦτ' ἤδη σκεψώμεθα, τὸ μηδὲν εἶναι πρὸς τὰ ζῷα δίκαιον ἡμῖν, μήτε τεχνικῶς μήτε σοφιστικῶς, ἀλλὰ τοῖς πάθεσιν ἐμβλέψαντες τοῖς ἑαυτῶν καὶ πρὸς ἑαυτοὺς ἀνθρωπικῶς λαλήσαντες καὶ ἀνακρίναντες...

But, let us examine this now, the question of whether we are just towards animals, not technically or sophistically, but considering our emotions and conversing and making judgements with ourselves as humans....

Plut. *de Esu Carn.* 999b[9]

Plutarch's words speak explicitly to what it means to be human: judging and speaking '*anthropically*' regarding the question of justice towards animals. The passage is, on one reading, defined by its interest in critical, rational judgement: σκεψώμεθα and ἀνακρίναντες both convey a sense of the intellectual consideration of logical debates. But the emotions are also a key element in the act of consideration—the question of justice towards animals is one that is to be decided by combining emotional and intellectual considerations. Plutarch's treatise trails off after these lines and it might be that they refer to an ensuing discussion which is now lost. They also, however, sum up effectively much of the focus on our emotional engagement with the pain and suffering of animals throughout the treatise. As a final comment on *On Flesh-Eating*, these words bring home just what his two *logoi* have focused on.

---

[8] Plut. *de Esu Carn.* 999a: ... ὁ ἀγὼν τοῖς Στωικοῖς ὑπὲρ τῆς σαρκοφαγίας ('... the argument against the Stoics concerning meat-eating'). For the relationship between Stoic ideas and Plutarch's thought, generally, see Babut (1969).

[9] The treatise tails off at this point.

1. DESENSITIZATION AND THE ETHICAL FAILURES OF MAN

Plutarch's attempt to refigure the emotional hardwiring of his readers involves shocking the reader out of an emotional and sensorial malaise. The reader is asked to navigate between the pleasures of meat-eating and more problematic, distressing emotional responses to the subject matter and the text itself. Throughout his treatise, Plutarch uses a direct correlation between flesh-eating and textual consumption to conceptualize the objectives of his work. The suggestion that eating could operate as a metaphor for textual consumption is well established within rhetorical and literary theory.[10] In Plutarch's hands, this correlation is used to explore the discordance between alimentary pleasure and disgust and the powerful and discomforting message of his treatise.

At one point, he tells us that his aim is to speak to the belly, although this objective is not an easy one: 'for it is a difficult thing, as Cato said, to speak to the belly, as it has no ears' (χαλεπὸν μὲν γάρ, ὥσπερ Κάτων ἔφησε, λέγειν πρὸς γαστέρας ὦτα μὴ ἐχούσας, 996d). The interplay between the belly and its lack of aural equipment plays up precisely Plutarch's attempt to negotiate between the various modes of the audience's consumption. Even more so, because his listeners, he claims, 'have drunk the mixture of habitual practice' (πέποται ὁ τῆς συνηθείας κυκεών), which, like the mixture of Kirke, combines 'pains and pangs and deceit and wailing' (ὠδῖνας τ' ὀδύνας τε... ἀπάτας τε γόους τε, 996e).[11] Plutarch's reference to Kirke's potion is eloquent. At first reading, it alludes to the transformation of humans into animals by their carnivorous practices—men have been reduced to subhuman beasts. It also speaks directly to the conceptualization of man's habitual (and pleasurable) practices: not only does it involve deceit, but it combines the pains and groans of those who are consumed. Like the consumption of Kirke's mixture, eating meat is an ambivalent process, facilitating pleasure and its opposites. Plutarch is playing, here, on the different perspectives of

---

[10] Rimell (2002), esp. 9-13 and 20-3 on the relationship between body and text, and reading and eating as comparable models for textual consumption in Petronius' *Satyricon*. Plutarch's own views on the connection can be found at, e.g., Plut. *Quomodo Adulesc.* 14d-f and 15b.

[11] Perhaps a quote from Empedokles: Empedokles Frag. 154a (DK).

those involved in meat-eating. For one party, this habitual practice involves pleasure, while for those who are consumed it involves pain and wailing.

Extending these culinary references, Plutarch tells us that his aim is 'to extract the "fish-hook" of meat-eating' (τὸ ἄγκιστρον ἐκβάλλειν τῆς σαρκοφαγίας) which is 'embedded in and driven through the love of pleasure' (ἐμπεπηγμένον τῇ φιληδονίᾳ καὶ διαπεπαρμένον, 996e). The metaphorical presentation of his aims reverses the ordinary relationship between the reader and his meal: reference to the 'fish-hook' (τὸ ἄγκιστρον) casts the reader as the passive victim of the process of hunting; it is the reader who has been caught and trapped and who will be the subject of violent treatment. It also suggests that our normal pleasurable practices will be reversed by the rhetorical success of Plutarch's treatise and that the reader will get to see what it is like to be on the plate. Plutarch's text, then, is presented as talking directly to the process of bodily consumption and also violently destroying the reader's corporeal integrity. In so doing, it effects a shift in their perspective and understanding of others' pain. Plutarch's metaphors at this point suggest that process will be inherently distressing.

The first *logos* opens with rhetorical questions about how man could endure the pollution of eating, or how his sensory organs could endure the sight, smells, and sounds associated with animal slaughter.[12] Plutarch answers his own question by developing a model of desensitization in which the search for pleasure and the continual exposure to deleterious sights have rendered man callous and unable to imagine the pain of others. According to Plutarch, man's desensitization starts from his pursuit of pleasure:

εἶθ' ὥσπερ ἐν γυναιξὶν κόρον ἡδονῆς οὐκ ἐχούσαις ἀποπειρώμενος πάντα καὶ πλανώμενος ὁ ἀκολασταίνων ἐξέπεσεν εἰς τὰ ἄρρητα, οὕτως αἱ περὶ τὴν ἐδωδὴν ἀκρασίαι τὸ φυσικὸν παρελθοῦσαι καὶ ἀναγκαῖον τέλος ἐν ὠμότητι καὶ παρανομίᾳ ποικίλλουσι τὴν ὄρεξιν.

If, just as among women who do not achieve satisfaction in pleasure, the one who is licentious, trying everything and wandering, comes to unspeakable acts, in this way those who are intemperate concerning food transgress what is natural and the appropriate boundary and diversify their appetites in savagery and lawlessness.

Plut. *de Esu Carn.* 997b

---

[12] Plut. *de Esu Carn.* 993a-b.

When Plutarch imagines the incontinent 'trying everything' and 'wandering', he figures the achievement of pleasure as an endless quest. The repeated markers of liminality and transcendence are significant here (note, for example, τὸ φυσικὸν παρελθοῦσαι καὶ ἀναγκαῖον τέλος; ἐξέπεσεν), painting achievement of satiety not only as a never-ending transcendence of the 'natural limit', but also as an endless journey of one who goes beyond in the ineluctable search for variety. This quest has important corporeal implications. He continues his social analysis by reminding his reader that the 'sensory organs' (τὰ αἰσθητήρια, 997b) 'become sick' (συννοσεῖ) and cease to be governed by proper limits when they are presented with excess in other areas; exposure to shameful music, for instance, engendered illness in the sense of hearing, which in turn fostered 'yearning' (ποθεῖ) for effeminate gropes and pleasures; 'foreign' or 'inappropriate sights' (θέατρα ἔκφυλα) follow shameful dances and music; and 'wild images induce insensitivity and savagery towards man' (θεάμασιν ἀνημέροις ἀπάθεια πρὸς ἀνθρώπους καὶ ὠμότης, 997c). The torture of animals to produce alimentary delicacies is, so Plutarch argues, a direct consequence of man's sensorial deterioration.

Plutarch's vision of this malaise singles out the way in which exposure to inappropriate stimuli alters the way that the senses operate. Encountering acts of savagery actually changes the way that different phenomena are seen: such spectacles of violence 'taught sight not to take pleasure in warlike exercises, pantomimic gestures or refined dances or statues or paintings' (τὴν ὄψιν ἐδίδαξε μὴ πυρρίχαις χαίρειν μηδὲ χειρονομίαις μηδ᾽ ὀρχήμασι γλαφυροῖς μηδ᾽ ἀγάλμασι καὶ γραφαῖς), 'but to make slaughter and the death of men, wounds, and war the most-valued spectacle' (ἀλλὰ φόνον καὶ θάνατον ἀνθρώπων καὶ τραύματα καὶ μάχας θέαμα ποιεῖσθαι πολυτελέστατον, 997c). Plutarch's language offers a methodology for thinking about the culture of viewing that we have been tracing over the last two chapters. If pleasure in the deaths of men and wounds were subjects of viewing pleasure, then Plutarch offers both an alternative view and a way of explaining that type of viewing. The sheer volume of exposure is the critical matter in Plutarch's model. The language, here, seems well suited to the critique of a society where the spectacular images of pain, violence, and torture saturated the cultural fabric. Indeed, Plutarch's argument attempts to extrapolate from the treatment of animals to the fundamentally violent, bellicose nature of ancient society. It is through gradual exposure to violence, he claims, that, 'being hardened' (στομώσαντες), people developed 'the appetite' (τὴν ἀπληστίαν) 'for the slaughter of men, war, and death' (ἐπὶ σφαγὰς ἀνθρώπων καὶ πολέμους καὶ φόνους, 998b). Pleasure in the pain of others is taken to be a result of a certain kind of perceptual reconditioning induced by long exposure to similarly deleterious spectacles and characterized by the failure to be governed by natural limits. Viewing pain has the potential to harden the viewer to that very subject.

As he goes on, he returns this general social criticism to the specific question of the treatment of animals: '[n]othing', Plutarch admonishes his readers, 'shames us, not the brilliant colour of their body, nor the convincing harmony of their voice' (οὐδὲν ἡμᾶς δυσωπεῖ, οὐ χρόας ἀνθηρὸν εἶδος, οὐ φωνῆς ἐμμελοῦς πιθανότης, 994e). In this instance, δυσωπεῖ appears to refer directly to the experience of shame. It also suggests, however, problematic direct sensorial engagement: the act of looking at animals has been readjusted by the pursuit of pleasure. In this situation, we imagine their voices to be inarticulate cries: 'we consider what they utter or squeak to be inarticulate sounds' (εἶθ' ἃς φθέγγεται καὶ διατρίζει φωνὰς ἀνάρθρους εἶναι δοκοῦμεν, 994e). In the immediate context of Plutarch's polemic, his point might be read as a criticism of Stoic views about the linguistic capacity of animals. Against the broader backdrop of discussions of pain across the Imperial period, however, there is a further implication. We have already learnt that, in a range of contexts, the ways in which others' pains could be recognized and then affectively engaged with on either an emotional level or a social one was dependent on language: the types of language used to convey pain perceptions and experiences moulded the ways in which pain was given meaning by individuals and within their social contexts. Here, the critical failure to understand language—or rather to dismiss it as inarticulate and, therefore, without meaning—makes a more substantial point about the inability to imagine others' pain, to give those experiences context and meaning, and to engage affectively with them.

2. SHOCKING THE READER

On Flesh-Eating creates a model of desensitization in which the metaphor of the hardened body figures the inability to understand and empathize with the pain of others (animal and human). Plutarch's engagement with that sensorial malaise is primarily motivated towards shocking the reader out of their hardness. The process by which he achieves that involves manipulating different rhetorical qualities. This manipulation is encapsulated, I argue, in the way that the reader is forced to engage psychosomatically with the subject matter of the treatise and the image of the destroyed animal body. The representation of pain forces the reader to recognize and to understand others' experiences by moving their emotions and eliding the distance between the traumatic subject matter and the external viewer.

The primary method by which Plutarch achieves this is the mobilization of emotionally powerful language which forces the reader to experience more vividly the practices that man engages in. At 993b, Plutarch asks, provocatively, how sight (ἡ ὄψις) could endure 'the death of those who have been slaughtered, flayed, dismembered' (τὸν φόνον σφαζομένων δερομένων διαμελιζομένων). Plutarch's use of σφαζομένων carries implications of ritualistic slaughter (of both human and animal victims), while his references to flaying or skinning insinuate wanton violence, punishment, and even torture.[13] He continues by confronting readers with a series of powerful images. In what state, Plutarch wonders, 'did the first man touch with his mouth the gore of a dead animal and take to his lips the flesh and the body of a corpse' (ὁ πρῶτος ἄνθρωπος ἥψατο φόνου στόματι καὶ τεθνηκότος ζώου χείλεσι προσήψατο σαρκὸς καὶ νεκρῶν σωμάτων, 993b), 'portions' (τὰ μέρη) which not long before had 'mooed and cried and moved and seen' (βρυχώμενα ... καὶ φθεγγόμενα καὶ κινούμενα καὶ βλέποντα, 993b); meat-eating involves 'touching foreign bodies and taking the juice and ichor from their mortal wounds' (ψαύουσαν ἀλλοτρίων καὶ τραυμάτων θανασίμων χυμοὺς καὶ ἰχῶρας ἀπολαμβάνουσαν, 993b). For Plutarch, clearly, meat-eating is mired in the bloody, gory, wounding of animals, and the pollution of the human body with the carcasses of the dead.

These early sections of the treatise mobilize powerful rhetorical imagery and language which help to develop awareness of the viciousness of our carnivorous practices. Note the *onomatopoeias* ('βρυχώμενα ... καὶ φθεγγόμενα') which imbue the passage with a

---

[13] Cf. the use of ἐκδείραντι at 996a, which continues to strengthen the implications of torture. On the implications of ἐκδέρω, see Hom. *Od.* 10.19, E. *El.* 824, or X. *An.* 1.2.8. δέρω: Hom. *Il.* 2.422. On the implications of σφάζω, see Chapter 2 (text and nn. 37–8).

degree of vividness.[14] The effect of the *onomatopoeias* is literally to bring the sounds of the erstwhile animal into the treatise itself: to make the reader hear its voice. Also significant is the use of the accumulative strategies of *polysyndeton* (βρυχώμενα ... καὶ φθεγγόμενα καὶ κινούμενα καὶ βλέποντα) and *asyndeton* (σφαζομένων δερομένων διαμελιζομένων). Rhetorical theory associates these strategies with the achievement of character and grandeur in rhetorical narrative. The treatise *Concerning the Pursuit of Intensity*, attributed to Hermogenes of Tarsos,[15] suggests that the appropriate use of these respective tropes creates 'grandeur' (μέγεθος) and 'character' (ἦθος). For Hermogenes, in particular, these tropes appear to be critical for the creation of the quality of 'intensity' or δεινότης.[16] Plutarch's text confronts the reader with animals' suffering through the employment of rhetorical language which is designed to have an impact on the emotional constitution of the reader.

The second strategy that Plutarch employs to force the reader to confront animal suffering involves the use of the animal voice. Plutarch's treatise refers to the animal voice on a number of occasions (recall the use of *onomatopoeias*). Importantly, it also makes use of the strategy of *prosopopoeia*, in which animals are explicitly represented as pleading for justice before the listener. This strategy was common throughout ancient rhetorical practice as a technique for forcing the audience to imagine inarticulate beings such as animals or inanimate objects such as the dead. Quintilian notes that it is particularly effective for making the audience see the speaker as both possessed of human qualities and being present before them.[17] In this context, it humanizes the animal, eliding the ethical bridge that exists between man and animal and forcing humans to confront their torture in visceral and emotional terms. It literally asks the reader to imagine them speaking or pleading before one: to see them with the mind's eye. At a second level, however, it rhetorically undoes the traditional argument that their sensorial experiences are less than others' because they do not express them in a language.

---

[14] The use of φθεγγόμενα here appears to imply human speech. For the term in connection with human language, see Hdt. 2.57; cf. LSJ s.v. φθέγγομαι.

[15] The dates of Hermogenes' life are contested, though it is likely that he worked in the second half of the second century CE; on his life, see Phil. *VS.* 577 (250K).

[16] Hermog. *Meth.* 11.1-4. For the connection between *megethos,* the use of *phantasia*, and the achievement of the sublime in Euripides: (Ps.-)Longin. *Subl.* 15.3.

[17] On *prosopopoeia*: Quint. *Inst.* 9.3.30-4, esp. 34.

The first example of this is played out in a provocative scene from early in the first *logos*. In the middle of this emotive passage, Plutarch turns to Homer to provide another image for the mistreatment of animals:

εἷρπον μὲν ῥινοί, κρέα δ' ἀμφ' ὀβελοῖς ἐμεμύκει ὀπταλέα τε καὶ ὠμά, βοῶν δ' ὣς γίγνετο φωνή· τοῦτο πλάσμα καὶ μῦθός ἐστι, τὸ δέ γε δεῖπνον ἀληθῶς τερατῶδες.

The hides crawl, and the meat bellowed about the spits, both the cooked and the raw, and so the voice of the oxen arose. This is a fabricated story and a myth, but the dinner is truly monstrous.

Plut. *de Esu Carn.* 993c (quoting Hom. *Od.* 12.395-6).

On one reading, the textual strategy seems to distance the reader. Plutarch's description of the passage as 'a fabricated story and a myth' (πλάσμα καὶ μῦθος) neatly brackets off the reference to the animal voice by highlighting the mythical nature of the quotation. At one level, Plutarch might be seen to protect the reader from direct engagement with the sound of the animal voice as the beasts burn on the spit. Yet what seems to matter in this context is the way in which the potential poetic fabrication is contrasted with the reality of practice: the meal that the poetic line speaks about is 'truly monstrous'. The choice of τερατῶδες is particularly compelling because it can be used of visual wonders that are pleasing on the eye, such as wondrous works of art, or monstrosities that produce a very different reaction.[18] On another reading, this passage underscores the connection between the treatment of the animals and their voice. The quote from Homer seems to emphasize the close association between the treatment of animals as food and the expression of pain: it is the meat which lows, literally linking the sounds of a live animal with the destructive and traumatic process of food preparation. In this context, the use of *phōnē* seems to take on heightened significance by intimating speech. Plutarch's passage plays up a strategy for making readers think through the effect of animal wounding and the production of voice.

The second example of this process occurs in a context in which Plutarch represents animals literally pleading their case for just and humane treatment:

---

[18] For the associations of τερατῶδες (and τέρας) with visual engagement: Theoc. 1.56 (pleasing marvel) and A. *Ch.* 548 (monstrosity).

εἶθ' ἃς φθέγγεται καὶ διατρίζει φωνὰς ἀνάρθρους εἶναι δοκοῦμεν, οὐ παραιτήσεις καὶ δεήσεις καὶ δικαιολογίας ἑκάστου λέγοντος 'οὐ παραιτοῦμαί σου τὴν ἀνάγκην ἀλλὰ τὴν ὕβριν· ἵνα φάγῃς ἀπόκτεινον, ἵνα δ' ἥδιον φάγῃς μή μ' ἀναίρει.'

We consider what they utter or squeak to be inarticulate sounds, and not supplications, entreaties, and requests for justice, when each one says 'I don't beseech you concerning necessity but hubris; kill me, so that you might eat, but do not destroy me, so that you might eat more pleasantly.'

Plut. *de Esu Carn.* 994e

I quoted the first half of this passage to point to Plutarch's interest in desensitization. Here, I want to explore more fully the implications of the second half in terms of the ways in which Plutarch attempts to overcome man's misrecognition by constructing a framework for understanding animals' speech. The choice of φθέγγεται ('utters'), which is used throughout the treatise to refer to animal voices, intimates a human voice; this intimation is strengthened by Plutarch's choice of παραιτέομαι.[19] Animal cries are transformed from inarticulate cries into powerful and provocative expressions of their objections to unjust treatment. By bringing their voice into the text itself, Plutarch forces the reader to vividly imagine the animal, its torture, and its suffering before their eyes. Just as *prosopopoeia* forces the audience to imagine inanimate objects speaking before them, so too readers are dragooned into imagining the experiences of the other.

3. *EKPHRASIS* AND CONFLICTED CONSUMPTION

The final strategy that I want to turn to is an explicit description of animal torture, which, I hold, functions as an *ekphrasis* of animal destruction. Plutarch's interest in the sensorial malaise caused by luxurious meat-eating made much of the ways in which deleterious or problematic sights (*theamata*) had undermined individuals' capacity to effectively view or see phenomena for what they really were. That interest in the deterioration of sight has important implications

---

[19] For the implications of φθέγγομαι, see above (text with n. 14). For the legalistic implications of παραιτέομαι, see its use in D. 21.58 or Hdt. 3.132 for the sense of 'intercede'.

Viewing Trauma in Plutarch   229

at a number of points throughout the treatise in which the reader is asked to view vivid visual *tableaux*. Much of this process revolves around the practice of explicitly describing how the animal should be treated and nurtured in order to satisfy the tastes of consumers. Early in his first *logos,* he links the production of delicacies with the process of teaching people how to raise and prepare different animals.[20] At other points, especially in his second *logos,* he goes into a great deal more detail, describing specific methods of slaughtering animals for different meals by those who make delicacies:

> οἷα νῦν πολλὰ δρῶσιν οἱ μὲν εἰς σφαγὴν ὑῶν ὠθοῦντες ὀβελοὺς διαπύρους, ἵνα τῇ βαφῇ τοῦ σιδήρου περισβεννύμενον τὸ αἷμα καὶ διαχεόμενον τὴν σάρκα θρύψῃ καὶ μαλάξῃ· οἱ δ' οὔθασι συῶν ἐπιτόκων ἐναλλόμενοι καὶ λακτίζοντες, ἵν' αἷμα καὶ γάλα καὶ λύθρον ἐμβρύων ὁμοῦ συμφθαρέντων ἐν ὠδῖσιν ἀναδόντος, ὦ Ζεῦ καθάρσιε, φάγωσι τοῦ ζῴου τὸ μάλιστα φλεγμαῖνον· ἄλλοι γεράνων ὄμματα καὶ κύκνων ἀπορράψαντες καὶ ἀποκλείσαντες ἐν σκότει πιαίνουσιν...[21] ἀλλοκότοις μίγμασι καὶ καρυκείαις τισὶν αὐτῶν τὴν σάρκα ὀψοποιοῦντες.

> Many such things people now do, while some push very hot spits into the wounds of pigs, so that by dipping the iron in, the blood is held in check and pours through the flesh, and tenderizes and softens it. Others jump and stamp upon the udders of pregnant sows, so that, having combined the blood, milk, and the gore of the embryos which were destroyed at the same time as childbirth, O Zeus Purifier, they might eat the most inflamed part of the animal; others having sewn up the eyes of cranes and swans, shut them up in darkness and fatten them...and then refine their flesh with foreign mixtures and some rich sauces.
>
> Plut. *de. Esu Carn.* 996f-997a

In this way, then, Plutarch brings home the savagery of our carnivorous diet. A range of possible readings obtains in this passage. On one approach, this scene might be read through a framework associated with the consumptive gaze of the reader.[22] Plutarch's narrative technique obscures the destroyed animals from view, presenting instead a series of disassembled body parts prepared, simply, for their gastronomic consumption. Seen in this light, the reader is asked to engage

---

[20] Plut. *de Esu Carn.* 993c.
[21] Wilamowitz indicates a *lacuna* here. Hubert suggested ἵνα τρυφερῶς ἐσθίωσιν. Although the full meaning of the original passage is unavailable, the general thrust and certainly the ekphrastic qualities of the passage are clear.
[22] Morales (2004), 32-4 and 165-6.

pleasurably with the destruction of the animal body—Plutarch's text fetishizes the animal body for the consuming pleasure of the reader.

Yet the passage is embedded in a particular approach to carnivorous meals which Plutarch has developed throughout the treatise. At one point, he refers to the tables of the rich, laid with carcasses, as a terrible sight;[23] the quotation of *Odyssey* 12.395-6 at 993c stressed the connection between the visual and its capacity for terror: 'but the dinner is truly monstrous' (τὸ δέ γε δεῖπνον ἀληθῶς τερατῶδες). In a more provocative process, he suggests that eating an animal meal can be seen in analogous terms to eating human flesh (997e). These scenes impact on how we approach the presentation of animals and their preparation as meals at 996f-997a: arguably, we are invited to renegotiate our understanding of the pleasurable process of consumption by its continued association with terrible and traumatic images. These intimations are strengthened by the suggestion, in the clause which precedes this *ekphrasis*, that we should eat them 'feeling pity' (οἰκτείροντες) and 'being pained' (ἀλγοῦντες), not 'outraging and torturing them' (οὐχ ὑβρίζοντες οὐδὲ βασανίζοντες, 996f). The suggestion that pity and pain should underpin our consumption of the animal speaks, it seems, directly to the notion of pleasurable indulgence and consumption that Plutarch seeks to eradicate. If this passage seeks to replicate gastronomic pleasure on the level of visual consumption, it does so by dramatically framing that act of visual consumption in terms of distressing emotions. In this scene, then, we are given a particularly poignant example of the way that Plutarch's text speaks to different levels of readerly consumption—rather than figuring the consumption of the animal body in pleasing or luxurious terms, Plutarch emphasizes the shocking and terrible nature of this act of reading, viewing, and eating. In this scene, we may be invited to consume the animal body, but we consume it in ways which undercut any sense of unproblematic pleasure at alimentary, textual, or visual consumption.

Plutarch's *Flesh-Eating* uses a number of techniques to bring the traumatized body of the animal before the eyes of the reader. Like the works of Philostratos and Akhilleus Tatios, *ekphrasis* and other techniques, such as *prosopopoeia*, help to expose the reader to the

---

[23] Cf. the use of δεινός to describe the sight of the tables of the rich adorned with dead bodies and the comparison with the 'more terrible' (δεινότερον) things that are carried away from them at Plut. *de Esu Carn.* 994e.

wound and trauma caused by the violent treatment of other bodies. In so doing, Plutarch attempts to recalibrate the ways in which one sees and understands the pain of others. Readers are asked, indeed forced, to view with their minds' eyes the violence of man's carnivorous diet, his maltreatment of animals in the search of culinary luxury and pleasure. Plutarch's engagement with the wound, its potential for pain, and its consequent impact on the viewer is linked with the works of the earlier authors in terms of his interest in how people see such corporeal damage. Plutarch's text starts from an assumption of a dangerous desensitization of the viewer. One of the problems (Plutarch sees as) characteristic of his contemporary society is that desire and pleasure have inured viewers to the experience of others' pain. His text aims to recalibrate the capacity to imagine and engage with the suffering of others. In this context, exposure to the wound of the animal is used to shock readers out of their pleasurable view, and consumption, of the traumatized bodies of animals. Viewing the pained body of the animal becomes one way in which readers are exposed to the distressing and painful elements of that process in order to shape an affective connection with the victims of trauma. A central part of this process involves coming to understand the nature of their experiences. Plutarch, in focusing on some elements of animal behaviour—especially their communication—stresses their connection with pain. He asks readers to engage in an imaginative act in which they come to understand the experiences of others as painful. The implications of that process are heightened precisely because the other whose pain readers are asked to consider is the ultimate other, the inarticulate, unfeeling animal.

13

What's in a View?

Over the course of this discussion, I have mapped three major authors' interest in the wound. For all the differences that separate these disparate texts in time, space, and cultural context, they speak to a common concern with trauma and wounds; the wound and trauma emerge as important viewing subjects; all these writers use rhetorical techniques (especially *ekphrasis*) to expose the reader to the physical body's violent destruction. In constructing the wound in these terms, these authors expose the body in a particularly provocative way: they facilitate increased access to the internal body, allowing the eyes of the viewer to reach further inside the *sōma* into areas that are normally hidden from view; in this context, aspects that are often left in abeyance are brought to the fore—blood and gore, the bodily postures and contortions of the traumatized body—and phenomena like the scream which (often) attest to trauma offer a viewing of the confronting, disordered, and broken body.

Out of this attention to the traumatized body, several key areas of discussion and a number of consistent themes emerge. In the first instance, these writers are concerned with the relationship between the traumatized body and pain. One might assume the connection to be both natural and consistent: critical work on trauma and violence has sometimes assumed this to be the case and, as a consequence, has left this connection unexamined. These authors explore that imagined link between the presence of pain and the experience of trauma in a number of different ways. Philostratos questions any automatic connection by emphasizing the ways in which pain can be renegotiated or experienced differently on the basis of the internal qualities of the individual who is traumatized. Akhilleus Tatios draws on a number of contexts to construct images in which the link between pain and trauma is renegotiated in different contexts. Plutarch sets himself against (what he sees as) a social malaise which refuses to see the traumatic treatment of animals in terms of their pain; indeed, the conceit of *On Flesh-Eating* is to ensure that that link between the two experiences is understood more precisely. In all three of these cases, the sign language of the body is read in such a way as to interpret (or imagine) what others feel during corporeal violence. That act of interpretation does not lead to an automatic connection between violence and perceptions of pain. Viewing the body—reading its signs—emerges as an important method for examining precisely when writers assume pain to be perceived.

Indeed, in exploring this connection, these authors contribute to a discussion of what constitutes pain experience. They turn consistently to the question of how the experience of pain might be seen or understood within broader emotional and practical contexts. In a number of *tableaux*, Philostratos, for instance, implies that the individual does not feel pain in the face of trauma because of the emotional context of events, or because of their particular internal qualities; indeed, some of his images focus on the internal qualities of calmness and 'happiness' in the face of trauma and their influence on the individual's perception of pain. Akhilleus Tatios, in a slightly different way, underlines not only the ways in which the wound interacts with the desires and hopes of those who are exposed to trauma, but also the ways in which the infliction of trauma might be understood or experienced within broader emotional contexts. Leukippe continues to shape her pain in terms of tragic frameworks of meaning that connect the experience of physical violence with forms of endurance and the long-term 'suffering' of novelistic hardships; her experience is further shaped by the way in which that experience interacts with her beliefs about Kleitophon's behaviour, their relationship, and her devotion to him. Plutarch's view of pain—for all its differences—plays on some of these themes. Animal claims to justice are based on the principle that they should not be killed out of licentious and luxurious desire, but out of necessity. Plutarch's fictional construction of animal pain, and humans' understanding of it, speaks directly to the ways in which pain and trauma are experienced differently on the basis of the context in which they arise.

As well as shaping the relationship between pain and trauma in the individual who is subject to violent physical treatment, these *ekphraseis* explore the reactions and understandings of viewers. In regulating a viewing subject, they speak to the ways in which pain helps to shape relationships between those who are pained and others. Of course, the very recognition of pain in some bodies is a type of intellectual engagement with what is seen; recognition involves an act of intellectual imagination and reading through the visible signs of the body and its deportment. Philostratos' reference to the way that the body or person 'seems' taught us that the visual aspects of the body and their reading allow for the imagination of internal feelings, perceptions, and qualities of the other. Viewing is a critical method for 'seeing' (in its metaphorical sense) pain in others; viewing is one method for substantiating pain at the centre of the nexus of intellectual reactions that define the relationships between people.

In addition to allowing individuals to 'see' pain in others, they also shape the nature of more affective reactions and relationships between those who feel pain and those who view them. In the first instance, one of the major themes of this discussion has been the ways in which the wound interacts with pleasurable emotions and desires in the viewer. As Elsner has pointed out, the question of viewing pain and traumatic experience pleasurably can be traced back to the ideas of Jacques Lacan and Laura Mulvey. There is much in the Philostratean text which supports this approach to the question of viewerly desire and pleasure.[1] Desire is built into the process of gazing at the destroyed body and contributes to a particular gender relationship between those who view and those who are consumed by such gazing. What emerges from these texts is the way in which the pain of the body is developed in relationship to the beauty of the body—and its concomitant facilitation of desire—and the ways in which the causing of pain is associated with the erotic, pleasurable consumption of the body. Philostratos, in particular, stresses a close relationship between the beauty of the body (and the erotic connotations of the dying youth) and its trauma and pain. He seems particularly concerned with the ways in which the beautiful body stands in opposition to painful experience—the contexts in which beauty and desire are emphasized seem to be those that downplay the presence of pain in the body; pain stands in opposition to beauty, and often to pleasure. Plutarch, conversely, explores a more convoluted engagement with the ways in which pleasure and the satisfaction of desire (in all its forms) impact on and shape the understanding of the pain of others;

[1] Elsner (2004).

since they are hardened against the experiences of others, they literally are unable to 'see' the pain they cause. In his rehabilitative project, the process of viewing and consuming the destroyed body becomes deeply ambivalent, incorporating elements of disgust and distress alongside some intimations of pleasure. Put another way, these texts continually explore a problematic relationship between pain, beauty, and viewerly pleasure. In so doing, they mark out pain's relationship to an important aesthetic criterion and map the status pain holds within the ideology of viewing in Imperial culture. At the same time, they continue to shape viewers' reactions to the experience.

Finally, I want to stress the importance of pity or more distressing reactions to pain. Plutarch and Akhilleus Tatios, in particular, pay close attention to the pity one feels towards the experiences of another. Pity speaks, of course, to the ways in which individuals relate to each other and to the experiences they understand that each other goes through. The traditional Aristotelian model of pity—which is so often the basis for discussions of pity throughout antiquity and particularly in the Christian negotiation of compassion and suffering[2]—seems problematic when considered in this context. Indeed, Plutarch and Akhilleus Tatios seem to develop contexts in which the Aristotelian view of pity is reworked to facilitate greater engagement with the pain of others and its consequences for, and relationship to, the pitier.

---

[2] E.g., Blowers (2010).

Conclusion

Over the preceding chapters, I have elaborated one broad theme in Imperial Greek culture's concern with the body and its pain. Texts from diverse areas of this culture—medical treatises, philosophical texts, and rhetorical works concerned with eating animal meat—are combined, I argue, by a common investment in the perception and navigation of pain. These texts speak to what I have termed 'embodied pain experience' or 'pain experience'. Pain, on this reading, is seen as a phenomenon that begins with the physical corpus, the *sōma,* but connects the physiological process of perception with emotional and psychological elements of the individual's experience and is navigated within—and helps to shape—interpersonal relationships. I touch, briefly, on three strands which are fundamental to this view of pain: the body and physiological pain, language and communication, and the personal and social impact and consequences of pain.

 The notion of pain in this society was underpinned by a fascination with the internal spaces and structure of the body: what I termed in the Introduction the anatomico-aesthetic model of the body. It is difficult to underestimate the importance of anatomy for this culture: in a range of different contexts—literary, rhetorical, and practical—looking at, and inside, the body played a fundamental role in shaping views of pain. This anatomical tenor of the engagement with the body combined not only a precise knowledge of anatomy, but aesthetic and moral views of the individual and their navigation of pain.

 In Part 1, I turned primarily towards rational medical culture in the Imperial period in order to investigate the ways in which scientific concerns for diagnosis and therapy shaped the way doctors approached pain. I should stress that although I started with medical authors, I do not hold that medicine was the only or the most important field of activity concerning pain. Rather, it offered a particularly efficacious starting point for elaborating a particular view of pain's relationship with the body. In this context, the notion of pain is intimately linked with how rational medicine conceptualized the operation and structure of the body. Pain is seen as an *aisthēsis*, a perceptual process, in which individuals are made aware of changes in the nature of the body.

There are two immediate points that emerge from this observation. Firstly, that pain is closely allied with the nature and structure of the body. The different types of pain that an individual might feel are governed by the atomic structure of the body and the texture of internal membranes, nerves, and organs. Diagnosis works, partly, because the relationships between types of pain and different areas of the body or different conditions under which pain is felt can be predicted, discovered, and differentiated. Assumed connections between the anatomical structure of the body and types of pain that the individual reports feeling help to reveal the internal conditions of the body, displaying the hidden internal reality of the individual to the medical diagnostic gaze. The second immediate implication of this approach to pain concerns the way in which pain is individuated at this level. Because of the link with the way the body is structured, pain is assumed, given the same aetiological circumstances and the same corporeal context, to occur in the same way in different individuals. Where individuation does occur is at the higher levels of affective, cognitive, and social responses to, and navigation of, that sensation.

In Parts 2 and 3, I have tried to expand on the model of physiological pain that I discussed in a medical context. I showed how that medical approach to the body was elaborated and contested in a range of different literary *milieux*. In Part 2, I tried to show how physiological approaches to the body and pain were integrated into broader concepts of physical discomfort and hardship. In this context, the boundaries of physiological perceptions and the process of imagining their connection with the internal spaces of the body is reframed through the reception of different literary and representational traditions. In the discussion of viewing trauma, I showed how rhetorical representations of trauma explored what it meant to view violence towards the body. Here, the automatic associations of trauma—physical violation and destruction—and pain were more problematic than scholars steeped in the Foucauldian tradition often assume. Indeed, in many instances, recognizing and understanding the pain of the tortured body are a consequence of the cultural lens through which the violated body is viewed.

A second element to this study has been the ways in which this type of physiological pain is integrated into different relationships. A central facet of this process has been the ways in which pain and language operate together to help shape the socialization of one's physical symptoms and their experiences. It has been a particular mainstay of modern theoretical treatment of pain to emphasize its resistance to language. Elaine Scarry, in particular, has stressed the ways in which pain is 'unshareable' because of its resistance to language.[1] What emerges from the situation in the Imperial period is one in which the experience of pain is intimately related to the ways in which language shapes the communication of the experience as well as the understanding and engagement of others with those who feel pain: pain and language have a difficult, fragile, and intimate relationship. If the relationship between language and pain was highly theorized in this period, it was done in some telling ways. In the first instance, it was fundamentally concerned with the ways in which pain impacts on language and representation. Three fundamental questions were repeatedly phrased and interrogated by writers in this period: (1) How does pain undermine, facilitate, and produce effective and meaningful language? (2) What constitutes meaningful language and why? (3) What are the intellectual, affective, and social effects of certain forms of communication or different linguistic registers?

In Part 1's discussion of the clinical scenario, I was particularly determined to explore the ways in which pain contributed to the diagnostic process through the process of speaking about and communicating pain symptoms. My turn to language in that context was underpinned by a desire to stress the importance of narrative and discussion between doctor and patient for the process of diagnostic recognition, and to explore how this language facilitated an understanding of pain symptoms and perceptions. There are two points which emerged in this context. Firstly, doctors elaborated a precise and intimate connection between the anatomical structure of the body and language. One of the particularly fascinating aspects of this process was the presence in medical contexts of different linguistic registers, the use of which helped to facilitate the understanding the doctor had of others' perceptions. Controlling the language of pain not only allowed the body to be integrated into diagnostic

---

[1] Scarry (1985), 4–5.

systems of understanding, but allowed doctors to navigate the complex relationships that defined the clinical scenario.

At the same time, that language helped to create shared understandings and recognition of pain. It did so because language helped to communicate experiences that many individuals had. In medical contexts, for instance, language helped to communicate the internal conditions of the body because of shared assumptions about the ways in which pain was related to anatomy and to language. In Parts 2 and 3, I questioned the way in which representation approached the issue of communicating pain. Aristeides and Lucian, for instance, both try on different linguistic registers for the communication of pain. In so doing, they interrogate the understandings of pain's effects on language and what constitutes effective communication. Both of these authors investigate how one's language locates the pain-perceiver in different cultural contexts. Indeed, we saw that, in some areas of ancient rhetorical discourse, the focus on coming to understand or imagine the pain of others depended on the capacity of rhetoric to effectively communicate and display the pain felt by those exposed to physical trauma. In Part 3, I showed how the process of rhetorical representation could serve to construct simultaneously different types of internal and external audiences. Pain is integrated into different social relationships through its relationship with language and its susceptibility to the understanding or recognition of the other.

The final aspect of pain experience that I have tried to elaborate concerns the ways in which physical pain produces affective responses in both those who feel pain and those who encounter them. In medical contexts, in particular, the ways in which the individual who feels pain might experience emotional aspects of that was given different emphasis by different writers. Galen's and Aretaios' reaction to the emotional complications of pain were significantly different. What is common to their divergent approaches is their concern to negotiate the ways in which those who are pained feel emotion and the ways in which they emotionally engage with that patient's feelings and pain. How they relate to, feel pity for, or empathize with those emotions was a critical element of the self-definition of different doctors.

In other contexts, the emotional reaction of the pained individual and others to pain is particularly telling. Emotional reactions to painful events shape how one might understand the particular experiences of those who feel pain. They also mark out the ways in which others connect with those who are exposed to pain. In Part 2, the focus on different emotional reactions among audiences (internal viewers, imagined readers, divine interlocutor) is telling for the ways in which Aristeides emphasizes his own particular experiences and separates himself from those who were reading his text or viewing his experiences. In Part 3, we saw that the types of emotional reactions that underpin the act of viewing were far from straightforwardly pleasant. Indeed, in many contexts, they were seen as potentially conflicting—combining both pleasure and other, less pleasant emotions—or highly problematic, involving questions of pity, distress, and shame. My point, here, is that across this culture the emotional element to the experience of pain—the emotions of both those who feel pain and those who encounter those in pain—is something that authors continually return to. Negotiating this aspect of experience is critical to how this society understands the meaning of pain.

In order to delay the pleasure of ending, I wish to draw three implications from this study. The first is that the history of the *aisthēsis* of pain—and other sensory perceptions—and the history of experience need to be integrated into a more holistic understanding of the emotional and social implications of sensation. Writers drew on tools from *ekphrasis,* rhetoric, science, philosophy, and literature to construct a complex sensory experience which impacted on the individual in multiple ways. The (re)emerging history of the body needs to take greater account of the interaction between bodily experiences or sensory perceptions and the affective and social aspects of individual experience: perception of pain is a sociocultural phenomenon. It also needs to take account of the complex and multifaceted discourse which helped to construct that experience.

Secondly, the view of pain that I have elaborated in the preceding chapters cut to the quick of Imperial society. Pain was fundamental to how this society imagined itself (and, by implication, how we should approach it). The people who moved in this world were concerned with pain's capacity to shape and create (and deny) effective and meaningful bonds between individuals. In this light, it is important for scholars to redefine how they understand this society's thinking about itself. The way in which pain is integrated into the cultural fabric of this society is particularly provocative: the pained body stood at the centre of their thinking about affective and social bonds between people. Writers from across the cultural landscape continually rehearse the ways in which individuals imagine others' feelings, perceptions, and experiences; that imaginative act helps writers navigate what it means for others to be in pain, and also to understand and interrogate the implications of that experience for society at large. The traditional view of Imperial Greek society, which holds that there is little place or space given to the experience of pain, does not allow for the full extent of this view.

The final implication concerns how scholars position this community. This book began with a call to re-evaluate the ways in which modern viewers and readers have thought about pain in the ancient world. At one level, this involves thinking about the relationship between pagan antiquity and the emergence of Christianity and the latter's concern with pain. This is especially the case in relation to the importance of martyrdom and violence. The spectacular use of violence against martyrs plays a central role in defining Christian communities: pagan culture's interest in the process of viewing pain asks new questions about the development of that aspect of Christian society. The second important facet of this recalibration concerns the way in which we understand Christian care for, compassion towards, and treatment of the sick and pained individual. When Christianity emerges, it is already embedded in a society which is profoundly concerned with both what it means to be in pain and what others should think, feel, and do about it. At a second level, it also requires recalibrating our relationship with the Classical Tradition. Modern audiences are implicated in the long story of classical pain. They are implicated because of the nature of classical reception, which has often turned to Greek (and Roman) material. They are also implicated because of the way in which these representations seek to explore the capacity of others to imagine and feel. Ancient writers represent and construct a particular experience of pain; they emphasize its social and affective reverberations, and, in so doing, they problematize how modern audiences read, view, imagine, and feel about classical pain.

Bibliography

Agapitos, P. and Reinsch, D. (eds.) (2000), *Der Roman im Byzanz der Komnenenzeit* (Meletemata VIII; Frankfurt am Main: Beerenverlag).
Alexandre, S. (2012), 'Sous les tableaux, l'image: Philostrate et l'invention des images à l'occasion de la peinture antique', in S. Alexandre, N. Philippe, and C. Ribeyrol (eds.), *Inventer la peinture grecque antique* (Lyon: ENS Éditions), 45–70.
Alexandridis, A., Wild, M., and Winkler-Horaček, L. (eds.) (2008), *Mensch und Tier in der Antike: Grenzziehung und Grenzüberschreitung* (Wiesbaden: Reichert).
Allen, E. (2009), 'The Poetics of Pain: Images of Suffering in Archaic and Classical Greek Poetry' (PhD diss.; Harvard University).
Allen, J. (2000), 'Galen as (Mis)informant about the Views of his Predecessors: A Discussion of R. J. Hankinson (ed.), *Galen on Antecedent Causes* (Cambridge, 1998)', *Archiv für Geschichte der Philosophie*, 83 (1), 81–9.
Allen-Hornblower, E. (2013), 'Sounds and Suffering in Sophocles' *Philoctetes* and Gide's *Philoctète*', *Studi italiani di filologia classica*, 11 (1), 5–41.
Alvares, J. (2006), 'Reading Longus' *Daphnis and Chloe* and Achilles Tatius' *Leucippe and Clitophon* in Counterpoint', in S. N. Byrne, E. P. Cueva, and J. Alvares (eds.), *Authors, Authority, and Interpreters in the Ancient Novel* (Ancient Narrative Supplementum 5; Groningen: Barkhuis), 1–33.
Anderson, G. (1979a), 'Themes and Composition in Lucian's *Podagra*', *Rheinisches Museum für Philologie*, 122, 149–54.
Anderson, G. (1979b), 'The Mystic Pomegranate and the Vine of Sodom: Achilles Tatius 3.6', *American Journal of Philology*, 100, 516–18.
Anderson, G. (1986), *Philostratus: Biography and Belles Lettres in the Third Century* A.D. (London: Croom Helm).
Anton, J. P. and Kustas, G. L. (eds.) (1971), *Essays in Ancient Greek Philosophy* (Albany: State University of New York Press).
Armstrong, N. (1987), *Desire and Domestic Fiction: A Political History of the Novel* (Oxford: Oxford University Press).
Aujoulat, N. (1990), 'La phantasia dans le *De Anima* d'Aristote', *Pallas*, 36, 19–51.
Ayache, L. (1997), 'L'animal, les hommes et l'ancienne médecine', in B. Cassin, J.-L. Labarrière, and G. Romeyer Dherbey (eds.), *L'animal dans l'antiquité* (Paris: J. Vrin), 55–74.
Aydede, M. (ed.) (2005), *Pain: New Essays on Its Nature and the Methodology of Its Study* (Cambridge, MA: MIT Press).
Babut, D. (1969), *Plutarque et le stoïcisme* (Paris: Presses Universitaires de France).

Ballengee, J. R. (2005), 'Below the Belt: Looking into the Matter of Adventure-Time', in R. Bracht Branham (ed.), *The Bakhtin Circle and Ancient Narrative* (Ancient Narrative Supplementum 3; Groningen: Barkhuis), 130–63.

Ballengee, J. R. (2009), *The Wound and the Witness: The Rhetoric of Torture* (Albany: State University of New York Press).

Barnes, J. (1991), 'Galen on Logic and Therapy', in F. Kudlien and R. Durling (eds.), *Galen's Method of Healing* (Leiden: Brill), 50–102.

Barnes, J., Brunschwig, J., Burnyeat, M. F., and Schofield, M. (eds.) (1982), *Science and Speculation. Studies in Hellenistic Theory and Practice* (Cambridge: Cambridge University Press).

Barnouw, J. (2002), *Propositional Perception: Phantasia, Predication, and Sign in Plato, Aristotle and the Stoics* (Lanham: University Press of America).

Barrow, R. (1967), *Plutarch and his Times* (London: Chatto and Windus).

Barton, C. A. (1992), *The Sorrows of the Ancient Romans: The Gladiator and the Monster* (Princeton, NJ: Princeton University Press).

Barton, T. (1994), *Power and Knowledge: Astrology, Physiognomics, and Medicine under the Roman Empire* (Body in Theory; Ann Arbor, MI: University of Michigan Press).

Bartsch, S. (1989), *Decoding the Ancient Novel: The Reader and the Role of Description in Heliodorus and Achilles Tatius* (Princeton, NJ: Princeton University Press).

Bartsch, S. (2006), *The Mirror of the Self: Sexuality, Self-Knowledge, and the Gaze in the Early Roman Empire* (Chicago: University of Chicago Press).

Bartsch, S. (2007), '"Wait a moment, Phantasia": Ekphrastic Interference in Seneca and Epictetus', in S. Bartsch and J. Elsner (eds.), *Ekphrasis* (Chicago: University of Chicago Press), 83–95. (= *Classical Philology,* 102 (1)).

Bates, D. (ed.) (1995), *Knowledge and the Scholarly Medical Traditions* (Cambridge: Cambridge University Press).

Baumann, M. (2011), *Bilder Schreiben: Virtuose Ekphrasis in Philostrats Eikones* (Berlin: De Gruyter).

Beall, S. M. (1993), 'Word-Painting in the *Imagines* of the Elder Philostratus', *Hermes,* 121 (3), 350–63.

Beare, J. (1906), *Greek Theories of Elementary Cognition* (Oxford: Clarendon Press).

Beaujour, M. (1981), 'Some Paradoxes of Description', *Yale French Studies,* 61, 27–59.

Beer, M. (2007), 'The Role of Dietary Restriction in the Construction of Identity in the Graeco-Roman World' (PhD thesis; University of Exeter).

Beer, M. (2008), 'The Question is not, *Can they Reason*? nor, *Can They Talk*? but, *Can they Suffer*?: The Ethics of Vegetarianism in the Writings of Plutarch', in R. Muers and D. Grumett (eds.), *Eating and Believing: Interdisciplinary Perspectives on Vegetarianism and Theology* (New York: T&T Clark), 96–109.

Beer, M. (2009), *Taste or Taboo: Dietary Choices in Antiquity* (Totnes: Prospect).
Behr, C. (1968), *Aelius Aristides and The Sacred Tales* (Amsterdam: Hakkert).
Behr, C. (trans.) (1981-6), *P. Aelius Aristides: The Complete Works*, 2 vols. (Leiden: Brill).
Behr, J. (1999), 'The Rational Animal: A Rereading of Gregory of Nyssa's *De hominis Opificio*', *Journal of Early Christian Studies*, 7 (2), 219-47.
Beil, U. J. (1993), 'Rhetorische Phantasia: Ein Beitrag zur Archäologie des Erhabenen', *Arcadia*, 28 (3), 225-55.
Bending, L. (2000), *The Representation of Bodily Pain in Late Nineteenth-Century English Culture* (Oxford: Oxford University Press).
Bendz, G. (1956), 'Ὀλιγοποσία (-ποτίη) καὶ Ὑδροποσία (-ποτίη)? (Zu Sor. *Gyn.* II,49,6 und Aret. VII,2,14)', *Eranos*, 54, 121-2.
Bernard-Donals, M. F. and Glejzer, R. R. (2003), *Witnessing the Disaster: Essays on Representation and the Holocaust* (Madison, WI: University of Wisconsin Press).
Berryman, S. A. (2002), 'Aristotle on *pneuma* and Animal Self-Motion', *Oxford Studies in Ancient Philosophy*, 23, 85-97.
Betts, E. (ed.) (2017), *Senses of the Empire: Multisensory Approaches to Roman Culture* (Abingdon: Routledge).
Billault, A. (1979), 'Approche du problème de l' Ἔκφρασις dans les romans grecs', *Bulletin de l'Association Guillaume Budé*, 2, 199-204.
Birchall, J. (1996), 'The Lament as a Rhetorical Feature in the Greek Novel', *Groningen Colloquia on the Novel*, VII, 1-17.
Blank, D. L. (2011), 'Reading between the Lies: Plutarch and Chrysippus on the Uses of Poetry', *Oxford Studies in Ancient Philosophy*, 40, 237-64.
Blowers, P. (2010), 'Pity, Empathy, and the Tragic Spectacle of Human Suffering: Exploring the Emotional Culture of Compassion in Late Ancient Christianity', *Journal of Early Christian Studies*, 18 (1), 1-27.
Bollack, J. (1997), 'L'homme entre son semblable et le monstre', in B. Cassin, J.-L. Labarrière, and G. Romeyer Dherbey (eds.), *L'animal dans l'antiquité* (Paris: J. Vrin), 377-94.
Bompaire, J. (1989), 'Le sacré dans les discours d'Aelius Aristide (XLVII-LII Keil)', *Revue des Études Grecques*, 102, 28-39.
Bompaire, J. (1993), 'Quatre styles d'autobiographie au IIe siècle après J.-C.: Aelius Aristide, Lucien, Marc-Aurèle, Galien', in M.-F. Baslez, P. Hoffmann, and L. Pernot (eds.), *L'invention d'autobiographie d'Hésiode à Saint Augustin* (Études de Littérature Ancienne 5; Paris: Presses de l'École Normale Supérieure), 199-209.
Bos, A. (2002), '"Fire above": The Relation of Soul to its Instrumental Body in Aristotle's *De Longitudine et brevitate vitae* 2—3', *Ancient Philosophy*, 22 (2), 303-17.

Boudon, V. (1993), 'Médecine et enseignement dans l'*Art médical* de Galien', *Revue des Études Grecques,* 106, 120–41.

Boudon, V. (1994), 'Loisir et création littéraire chez Galien', *Bulletin de l'Association Guillaume Budé,* 1, 154–68.

Boudon, V. (2000), 'Galien par lui-même: les traités bio-bibliographiques (*De Ordine Librorum Suorum* et *De Libris Propriis*)', in D. Manetti (ed.), *Studi su Galeno: Scienza, filosofia, retorica e filologia* (Firenze: Università di Firenze), 119–33.

Boudon, V. (2003a), 'Art, science et conjecture chez Galien', in J. Barnes and J. Jouanna (eds.), *Galien et la Philosophie* (Vandoeuvres-Genève: Fondation Hardt), 269–98.

Boudon, V. (2003b), 'Le rôle de la sensation dans la définition galénique de la maladie', in I. Boehm and P. Luccioni (eds.), *Les cinq sens dans la médecine de l'époque Impériale: Sources et développements* (Paris: de Boccard), 21–30.

Boudon-Millot, V. (2007), 'Une traité perdu de Galien miraculeusement retrouvé, le *Sur l'inutilité de se chagriner*: Texte grec et traduction française', in V. Boudon-Millot, A. Guardasole, and C. Magdelaine (eds.), *La science médicale antique: Nouveaux regards* (Paris: Beauchesne), 72–123.

Boudon-Millot, V. (2012a), *Galien de Pergame, un médecin grec à Rome* (Paris: Les Belles Lettres).

Boudon-Millot, V. (2012b), 'Vision and Vision Disorders: Galen's Physiology of Sight', in M. Horstmanshoff, H. King, and C. Zittel (eds.), *Blood, Sweat and Tears: The Changing Concepts of Physiology from Antiquity into Early Modern Europe* (Leiden: Brill), 551–67.

Boulanger, A. (1968), *Aelius Aristide et la sophistique dans la province d'Asie au IIe siècle de notre ère* (Paris: de Boccard). (Orig. publ.: 1923).

Bourke, J. (2014), *The Story of Pain: From Prayer to Painkillers* (Oxford: Oxford University Press).

Bowersock, G. W. (1969), *Greek Sophists in the Roman Empire* (Oxford: Clarendon Press).

Bowersock, G. W. (1994), *Fiction as History: Nero to Julian* (Sather Classical Lectures; Berkeley, CA: University of California Press).

Bowie, E. L. (1978), 'Apollonius of Tyana: Tradition and Reality', *ANRW,* II.16.2, 1652–99.

Bowie, E. L. (1994), 'Philostratus: Writer of Fiction', in J. Morgan and R. Stoneman (eds.), *Greek Fiction: The Greek Novel in Context* (London: Routledge), 181–99.

Bowie, E. L. (1999), 'The Greek Novel: The Genre', in S. Swain (ed.), *Oxford Readings in the Greek Novel* (Oxford: Oxford University Press), 39–59.

Bowie, E. L. (2009), 'Philostratus: The Life of a Sophist', in E. L. Bowie and J. Elsner (eds.), *Philostratus* (Cambridge: Cambridge University Press), 19–32.

Bowie, E. L. and Elsner, J. (eds.) (2009), *Philostratus* (Cambridge: Cambridge University Press).

Bracht Branham, R. (ed.) (2005), *The Bakhtin Circle and Ancient Narrative* (Ancient Narrative Supplementum 3; Groningen: Barkhuis).
Bradley, M. (ed.) (2015), *Smell and the Ancient Senses* (Abingdon: Routledge).
Braund, S. M. and Gill, C. (eds.) (1997), *The Passions in Roman Thought and Literature* (Cambridge: Cambridge University Press).
Breivik, H., Borchgrevink, P., Allen, S., Rosseland, L., Romundstad, L., Breivik Hals, E., Kvarstein, G., and Stubhaug, A. (2008), 'Assessment of Pain', *British Journal of Anaesthesia*, 101 (1), 17–24.
Brenk, F. (1977), *In Mists Apparelled: Religious Themes in Plutarch's* Moralia *and* Lives (Leiden: Brill).
Brethes, R. (2007), '*Poiein aischra kai legein aischra*, est ce vraiment la même chose? Ou la bouche souillée de Chariclée', in V. Rimell (ed.), *Seeing Tongues, Hearing Scripts: Orality and Representation in the Ancient Novel* (Ancient Narrative Supplementum 7; Groningen: Barkhuis), 223–56.
Brown, P. (1978), *The Making of Late Antiquity* (Cambridge, MA: Harvard University Press).
Brown, P. (1988), *The Body and Society: Men, Women, and Sexual Renunciation in Early Christianity* (New York: Columbia University Press).
Bryson, N. (1994), 'Philostratus and the Imaginary Museum', in S. Goldhill and R. Osborne (eds.), *Art and Text in Ancient Greek Culture* (Cambridge: Cambridge University Press), 255–83.
Budelmann, F. (2006), 'Körper und Geist in tragischen Schmerz-Szenen', in B. Seidensticker and M. Vöhler (eds.), *Gewalt und Ästhetik: Zur Gewalt und ihrer Darstellung in der griechischen Klassik* (Berlin: De Gruyter), 123–48.
Budelmann, F. (2007), 'The Reception of Sophocles' Representation of Physical Pain', *American Journal of Philology*, 128, 443–67.
Budelmann, F. (2014), 'Pain', in H. Roisman (ed.), *The Encyclopedia of Greek Tragedy* (vol. 2; Chichester: Wiley-Blackwell), 941–3.
Burnyeat, M. F. (1982), 'The Origins of Non-Deductive Inference', in J. Barnes, J. Brunschwig, M. F. Burnyeat, and M. Schofield (eds.), *Science and Speculation. Studies in Hellenistic Theory and Practice* (Cambridge: Cambridge University Press), 193–238.
Burrus, V. (2004), *The Sex Lives of Saints: An Erotics of Ancient Hagiography* (Philadelphia, PA: University of Pennsylvania Press).
Burrus, V. (2005), 'Mimicking Virgins: Colonial Ambivalence and the Ancient Romance', *Arethusa*, 38 (1), 49–88.
Burrus, V. (2008), *Saving Shame: Martyrs, Saints, and Other Abject Subjects* (Philadelphia, PA: University of Pennsylvania Press).
Butler, A. and Purves, A. (eds.) (2014), *Synaesthesia and the Ancient Senses* (Abingdon: Routledge).

Byl, S. (1992), 'Le traitement de la douleur dans le Corpus hippocratique', in J. Lopez-Ferez (ed.), *Tratados hipocráticos. Estudios acerca de su contenido, forma y influencia,* (Madrid: UNED), 203–13.

Byrne, S. N., Cueva, E. P., and Alvares, J. (eds.) (2006), *Authors, Authority, and Interpreters in the Ancient Novel* (Ancient Narrative Supplementum 5; Groningen: Barkhuis).

Cairns, D. (2013), 'A Short History of Shudders', in A. Chaniotis and P. Ducrey (eds.), *Unveiling Emotions II: Emotions in Greece and Rome: Texts, Images, and Material Culture* (Stuttgart: Franz Steiner), 85–107.

Cairns, F. (ed.) (2005), *Greek and Roman Poetry, Greek and Roman Historiography* (Papers of the Langford Latin Seminar, 12; Liverpool: Liverpool University Press).

Calder, L. (2011), *Cruelty and Sentimentality: Greek Attitudes to Animals, 600–300 BC* (Studies in Classical Archaeology, 5; Oxford: Archaeopress).

Calderón Dorda, E., Morales Ortiz, A., and Valverde Sánchez, M. (eds.) (2006), *Koinòs lógos: Homenaje al profesor José García López* (Murcia: Universidad de Murcia, Servicio de Publicaciones).

Cartledge, P., Millett, P., and von Reden, S. (eds.) (1998), *Kosmos: Essays in Order, Conflict and Community in Classical Athens* (Cambridge: Cambridge University Press).

Caruth, C. (ed.) (1995), *Trauma: Explorations in Memory* (Baltimore, MD: Johns Hopkins University Press).

Caruth, C. (1996), *Unclaimed Experience: Trauma, Narrative, and History* (Baltimore, MD: Johns Hopkins University Press).

Cassell, E. (1985), *Talking With Patients* (MIT Press Series on the Humanistic and Social Dimensions of Medicine, 1–2; Cambridge, MA: MIT Press).

Cassin, B., Labarrière, J.-L., and Romeyer Dherbey, G. (eds.) (1997), *L'animal dans l'antiquité* (Paris: J. Vrin).

Castelli, E. (2005), 'Persecution and Spectacle. Cultural Appropriation in the Christian Commemoration of Martyrdom', *Archiv für Religionsgeschichte*, 7, 102–36.

Chaniotis, A. (1995), 'Illness and Cures in the Greek Propitiatory Inscriptions and Dedications of Lydia and Phrygia', in P. van der Eijk, H. Horstmanshoff, and P. Schrijvers (eds.), *Ancient Medicine in Its Socio-Cultural Context 2* (Amsterdam: Rodopi), 323–44.

Chaniotis, A. (ed.) (2012), *Unveiling Emotions: Sources and Methods for the Study of Emotions in the Greek World* (Stuttgart: Franz Steiner).

Chaniotis, A. and Ducrey, P. (eds.) (2013), *Unveiling Emotions II: Emotions in Greece and Rome: Texts, Images, and Material Culture* (Stuttgart: Franz Steiner).

Cherniss, H. and Helmbold, W. (trans.) (1957), *Plutarch.* Moralia XII (Loeb Classical Library; Cambridge, MA.: Harvard University Press).

Chew, K. (2000), 'Achilles Tatius and Parody', *Classical Journal*, 96, 57–70.

Chew, K. (2003), 'The Representation of Violence in the Greek Novels and Martyr Accounts', in S. Panayotakis, M. Zimmerman, and W. Keulen (eds.), *The Ancient Novel and Beyond* (Mnemosyne Supplementum 241; Leiden: Brill), 129–41.
Chinn, C. (2007), 'Before Your Very Eyes: Pliny *Epistulae* 5.6 and the Ancient Theory of Ekphrasis', *Classical Philology*, 102 (3), 265–80.
Coakley, S. (2007), 'Introduction', in S. Coakley and K. Shelemay (eds.), *Pain and Its Transformations: The Interface of Biology and Culture* (Cambridge, MA: Harvard University Press), 1–16.
Coakley, S. and Shelemay, K. (eds.) (2007), *Pain and Its Transformations: The Interface of Biology and Culture* (Cambridge, MA: Harvard University Press).
Coleman, K. (1990), 'Fatal Charades: Roman Executions Staged as Mythological Enactments', *Journal of Roman Studies*, 80, 44–73.
Constantinidou, S. (2008), *Logos into Mythos: The Case of Gorgias' Encomium of Helen* (Athens: Kardamitsa).
Cooper, K. (1998), 'The Voice of the Victim: Gender, Representation and Early Christian Martyrdom', *Bulletin of the John Rylands Library*, 80 (3), 147–57.
Cosans, C. E. (1997), 'Galen's Critique of Rationalist and Empiricist Anatomy', *Journal of the History of Biology*, 30 (1), 35–54.
Cosans, C. E. (1998), 'The Experimental Foundations of Galen's Teleology', *Studies in History and Philosophy of Science*, 29 (1), 63–80.
Costantini, M., Graziani, F., and Rolet, S. (2006), *Le défi de l'art: Philostrate, Callistrate et l'image sophistique* (Rennes: Presses Universitaires de Rennes).
Couch, H. N. (1934), 'A Medical Commentary on the Classical References of Aretaeus of Cappadocia', *Transactions of the American Philological Association*, 65, 45–6.
Coulmas, F. (1986), 'Reported Speech: Some General Issues', in F. Coulmas (ed.), *Direct and Indirect Speech* (Trends in Linguistics, Studies and Monographs 31; Berlin: De Gruyter), 1–28.
Cribiore, R. (2007), *The School of Libanius in Late Antique Antioch* (Princeton, NJ: Princeton University Press).
Cronjé, J. (1993), 'The Principle of Concealment (*TO ΛΑΘΕΙΝ*) in Greek Literary Theory', *Acta Classica*, 36, 55–64.
Crowther, P. (1993), *Critical Aesthetics and Post-Modernism* (Oxford: Clarendon).
Cueva, E. (2001), 'Euripides, Human Sacrifice, Cannibalism, Humor and the Ancient Greek Novel', *The Classical Bulletin*, 77 (1), 103–14.
D'Alconzo, N. (2014a), 'Works of Art in the Ancient Greek Novels', (PhD thesis; Swansea University).
D'Alconzo, N. (2014b), 'A Diptych by Evanthes: Andromeda and Prometheus (Ach. Tat. 3, 6–8)', *Ancient Narrative*, 11, 75–91.

Das, V. (1997), 'Language and Body: Transactions in the Construction of Pain', in A. Kleinman, V. Das, and M. Lock (eds.), *Social Suffering* (Berkeley, CA: University of California Press), 67–92.

Dean-Jones, L. (1995), '*Autopsia, Historia* and What Women Know: The Authority of Women in Hippocratic Gynaecology', in D. Bates (ed.), *Knowledge and the Scholarly Medical Traditions* (Cambridge: Cambridge University Press), 41–59.

Debru, A. (1995), 'Les démonstrations médicales à Rome au temps de Galien', in P. van der Eijk, H. Horstmanshoff, and P. Schrijvers (eds.), *Ancient Medicine in Its Socio-Cultural Context 1* (Amsterdam: Rodopi), 69–81.

Debru, A. (2008), 'Physiology' in R. J. Hankinson (ed.), *The Cambridge Companion to Galen* (Cambridge: Cambridge University Press), 263–82.

Debru, A., Palmieri, N., and Jacquinod, B. (eds.) (2001), '*Docente natura*': *Mélanges de médecine ancienne et médiévale offerts à Guy Sabbah* (Saint-Étienne: Publications de l'Université de Saint-Étienne).

Deichgräber, K. (1971), *Aretaeus von Kappadozien als medizinischer Schriftsteller* (Berlin: Akademie-Verlag).

De Lacy, P. (1966), 'Galen and the Greek Poets', *Greek, Roman and Byzantine Studies*, 7, 259–66.

De Lacy, P. (1979), 'Galen's Concept of Continuity', *Greek, Roman and Byzantine Studies*, 20, 355–69.

DelVecchio Good, M.-J., Brodwin, P., Good, B., and Kleinman, A. (eds.) (1992), *Pain as Human Experience: An Anthropological Perspective* (Berkeley, CA: University of California Press).

De Temmerman, K. and Demoen, K. (2011), 'Less than Ideal Paradigms in the Greek Novel', in K. Doulamis (ed.), *Echoing Narratives: Studies of Intertextuality in Greek and Roman Prose Fiction* (Ancient Narrative Supplementum 13; Groningen: Barkhuis), 1–20.

Didsbury, G. (1936), 'Considérations sur la migraine d'après Arétée de Cappadoce', *Bulletin de la Société française d'histoire de la médecine*, 34, 260–7.

Dillon, J. and Long, A. A. (eds.) (1988), *The Question of Eclecticism: Studies in Later Greek Philosophy* (Berkeley, CA: University of California Press).

Dodds, E. R. (1951), *The Greeks and the Irrational* (Sather Classical Lectures; Berkeley, CA: University of California Press).

Dodds, E. R. (1965), *Pagan and Christian in an Age of Anxiety* (Cambridge: Cambridge University Press).

Doherty, L. (1995), *Siren Songs: Gender, Audiences, and Narrators in the Odyssey* (Ann Arbor, MI: University of Michigan Press).

Doulamis, K. (ed.), (2011), *Echoing Narratives: Studies of Intertextuality in Greek and Roman Prose Fiction* (Ancient Narrative Supplementum 13; Groningen: Barkhuis).

Downie, J. (2013), *At the Limits of Art: A Literary Study of Aelius Aristides' Hieroi Logoi* (Oxford: Oxford University Press).

Drabkin, I. E. (ed. and trans.) (1950), *Caelius Aurelianus*: On Acute Diseases *and* On Chronic Diseases (Chicago: University of Chicago Press).

Dressler, A. (2011), 'The Sophist and the Swarm: Feminism, Platonism and Ancient Philosophy in Achilles Tatius' *Leucippe and Clitophon*', *Ramus*, 40 (1), 33–72.

Drozdek, A. (2009), 'Metempsychosis and Animals in Plato', *Maia*, 61 (1), 77–82.

Dubel, S. (2009), 'Colour in Philostratus' *Imagines*', in E. L. Bowie and J. Elsner (eds.), *Philostratus* (Cambridge: Cambridge University Press), 309–21.

duBois, P. (1991), *Torture and Truth* (London: Routledge).

Dugré, F. (1990), 'Le rôle de l'imagination dans le mouvement animal et l'action humaine chez Aristote', *Dialogue*, 29 (1), 65–78.

Durham, D. (1938), 'Parody in Achilles Tatius', *Classical Philology*, 33 (1), 1–19.

Durling, R. (1991), "Endeixis' as a Scientific Term: B) Endeixis in Authors Other than Galen and Its Medieval Latin Equivalents', in F. Kudlien and R. Durling (eds.), *Galen's Method of Healing* (Leiden: Brill), 112–13.

Easterling, P. (1997), 'From Repertoire to Canon', in P. Easterling (ed.), *The Cambridge Companion to Greek Tragedy* (Cambridge: Cambridge University Press), 211–27.

Ebstein, E. (1931), 'Klassische Krankengeschichten: I: Die Diphtherie bei Aretaios', *Kinderärtzliche Praxis*, 2, 42–5.

Edelstein, L. (1967), 'Greek Medicine in Relation to Religion and Magic', in O. Temkin and C. Temkin (eds.), *Ancient Medicine: Selected Papers of Ludwig Edelstein* (Baltimore, MD: Johns Hopkins University Press), 205–46.

Edlow, R. (1977), *Galen on Language and Ambiguity: An English Translation of Galen's* De captionibus (On Fallacies), *with Introduction, Text, and Commentary* (Leiden: Brill).

Egger, B. (1994), 'Looking at Chariton's *Callirhoe*', in J. Morgan and R. Stoneman (eds.), *Greek Fiction: The Greek Novel in Context* (London: Routledge), 31–48.

Einarson, B. and De Lacy, P. (trans.) (1967), *Plutarch. Moralia XIV* (Loeb Classical Library; Cambridge, MA.: Harvard University Press).

Ellis, J. (1993), *Ancient Minds* (Memphis, TN: Tennessee State University Department of Philosophy).

Elsner, J. (1993), 'Seductions of Art: Encolpius and Eumolpus in a Neronian Picture Gallery', *Proceedings of the Cambridge Philological Society*, 39, 30–47.

Elsner, J. (1994), 'From the Pyramids to Pausanias and Piglet: Monuments, Travel and Writing', in S. Goldhill and R. Osborne (eds.), *Art and Text in Ancient Greek Culture* (Cambridge: Cambridge University Press), 224–54.

Elsner, J. (1995), *Art and the Roman Viewer: The Transformation of Art from the Pagan World to Christianity* (Cambridge: Cambridge University Press).

Elsner, J. (ed.) (1996a), *Art and Text in Roman Culture* (Cambridge: Cambridge University Press).
Elsner, J. (1996b), 'Naturalism and the Erotics of the Gaze: Intimations of Narcissus', in N. Kampen (ed.), *Sexuality in Ancient Art* (Cambridge: Cambridge University Press), 247–61.
Elsner, J. (2000), 'Between Mimesis and Divine Power: Visuality in the Greco-Roman World', in R. Nelson (ed.), *Visuality before and beyond the Renaissance* (Cambridge: Cambridge University Press), 45–69.
Elsner, J. (ed.) (2002a), *The Verbal and the Visual: Cultures of Ekphrasis in Antiquity* (Bentleigh, Victoria: Aureal Publications). (= *Ramus*, 31 (1–2)).
Elsner, J. (2002b), 'Introduction: The Genres of Ekphrasis', in J. Elsner (ed.), *The Verbal and the Visual: Cultures of Ekphrasis in Antiquity* (Bentleigh, Victoria: Aureal Publications), 1–18.
Elsner, J. (2004), 'Seeing and Saying: A Psychoanalytic Account of Ekphrasis', *Helios*, 31 (1), 157–85.
Elsner, J. (2007), 'Philostratus Visualizes the Tragic: Some Ecphrastic and Pictorial Representations of Greek Tragedy in the Roman Era', in C. Kraus, S. Goldhill, H. Foley, and J. Elsner (eds.), *Visualizing the Tragic: Drama, Myth, and Ritual in Greek Art and Literature* (Oxford: Oxford University Press), 309–37.
Elsner, J. (2009), 'A Protean corpus', in E. L. Bowie and J. Elsner (eds.), *Philostratus* (Cambridge: Cambridge University Press), 3–18.
Elsom, H. (1992), '*Callirhoe*: Displaying the Phallic Woman', in A. Richlin (ed.), *Pornography and Representation in Greece and Rome* (Oxford: Oxford University Press), 212–30.
Enge, M. (1991), 'Psychische Erkrankungen bei Hippokrates, Celsus und Aretaios' (Diss. Med. Dent; Frankfurt am Main).
Evans, M. (2007), 'Plato and the Meaning of Pain', *Apeiron*, 40 (1), 71–93.
Everson, S. (ed.) (1990), *Epistemology* (Companions to Ancient Thought 1; Cambridge: Cambridge University Press).
Everson, S. (ed.) (1994), *Language* (Companions to Ancient Thought 3; Cambridge: Cambridge University Press).
Fairbanks, A. (trans.) (1931), *Philostratus the Elder, Imagines. Philostratus the Younger, Imagines. Callistratus, Descriptions* (Loeb Classical Library; Cambridge, MA: Harvard University Press).
Faraone, C. A. and Naiden, F. S. (eds.) (2011), *Greek and Roman Animal Sacrifice: Ancient Victims, Modern Observers* (Cambridge: Cambridge University Press).
Ferber, I. (2010), 'Herder: On Pain and the Origin of Language', *The Germanic Review*, 85 (3), 205–23.
Festugière, A. (1986), *Aelius Aristide, Discours sacrés: Rêve, religion, médecine au IIe siècle après J.-C.* (Collection Propylées; Paris: Macula).

Fields, H. (2007), 'Setting the Stage for Pain: Allegorical Tales from Neuroscience', in S. Coakley and K. Shelemay (eds.), *Pain and Its Transformations: The Interface of Biology and Culture* (Cambridge, MA: Harvard University Press), 36–61.
Finkelberg, A. (1997), 'Xenophanes' Physics, Parmenides' Doxa and Empedocles' Theory of Cosmogonical Mixture', *Hermes,* 125 (1), 1–16.
Fitzgerald, W. (2000), *Slavery and the Roman Literary Imagination* (Cambridge: Cambridge University Press).
Flemming, R. (2008), 'Commentary', in R. J. Hankinson (ed.), *The Cambridge Companion to Galen* (Cambridge: Cambridge University Press), 323–54.
Flinterman, J.-J. (1995), *Power, Paideia and Pythagoreanism: Greek Identity, Conceptions of the Relationship between Philosophers and Monarchs and Political Ideas in Philostratus'* Life of Apollonius (Amsterdam: J. C. Gieben).
Flory, D. (1996), 'Stoic Psychology, Classical Rhetoric, and Theories of Imagination in Western Philosophy', *Philosophy and Rhetoric,* 29 (2), 147–67.
Fortenbaugh, W. W. (1971), 'Aristotle: Animals, Emotion, and Moral Virtue', *Arethusa,* 4 (2), 137–65.
Foucault, M. (1986), *The History of Sexuality III: The Care of the Self,* trans. R. Hurley (London: Penguin).
Foucault, M. (1991), *Discipline and Punish. The Birth of the Prison,* trans. A. Sheridan (London: Penguin).
Francis, J. (1998), 'Truthful Fictions: New Questions to Old Answers on Philostratus' *Life of Apollonius*', *American Journal of Philology,* 119 (3), 419–41.
Frank, A. (1995), *The Wounded Storyteller: Body, Illness, and Ethics* (Chicago: University of Chicago Press).
Frankfurter, D. (2009), 'Martyrology and the Prurient Gaze', *Journal of Early Christian Studies,* 17 (2), 215–45.
Frede, M. (1981), 'On Galen's Epistemology', in V. Nutton (ed.), *Galen: Problems and Prospects* (London: Wellcome Institute for the History of Medicine), 65–86. (= repr. as Frede (1987), 279–98).
Frede, M. (1982), 'The Method of the So-Called Methodical School of Medicine', in J. Barnes, J. Brunschwig, M. F. Burnyeat, and M. Schofield (eds.), *Science and Speculation. Studies in Hellenistic Theory and Practice* (Cambridge: Cambridge University Press), 1–23.
Frede, M. (1987), *Essays in Ancient Philosophy* (Oxford: Clarendon Press).
Frede, M. (1994), 'The Stoic Notion of a Lekton', in S. Everson (ed.), *Language* (Companions to Ancient Thought 3; Cambridge: Cambridge University Press), 109–28.
Frilingos, C. (2009), '"It Moves Me to Wonder": Narrating Violence and Religion under the Roman Empire', *Journal of the American Academy of Religion,* 77 (4), 825–52.

Frixione, E. (2013), 'Pneuma—Fire Interactions in Hippocratic Physiology', *Journal of the History of Medicine and Allied Sciences,* 68 (4), 505–28.
Fusillo, M. (1989), *Il romanzo greco: Polifonia ed eros* (Venice: Marsilio).
Fusillo, M. (1991), *Naissance du roman,* trans. M. Abrioux (Paris: Seuil).
Fusillo, M. (1997), 'How Novels End: Some Patterns of Closure in Hellenistic Narrative', in D. Roberts, F. Dunn, and D. Fowler (eds.), *Classical Closure: Reading the End in Greek and Latin Literature* (Princeton, NJ: Princeton University Press), 209–27.
Fusillo, M. (1999), 'The Conflict of Emotions: A *Topos* in the Greek Erotic Novel', in S. Swain (ed.), *Oxford Readings in the Greek Novel* (Oxford: Oxford University Press), 60–82.
García Ballester, L. (1981), 'Galen as a Medical Practitioner: Problems in Diagnosis', in V. Nutton (ed.), *Galen: Problems and Prospects* (London: Wellcome Institute for the History of Medicine), 13–46.
García Ballester, L. (1988), 'Soul and Body, Disease of the Soul and Disease of the Body in Galen's Medical Thought', in P. Manuli and M. Vegetti (eds.), *Le opere psicologiche di Galeno* (Naples: Bibliopolis), 117–52.
García Ballester, L. and Moreno Rodriguez, R. (1982), 'El dolor en la teoría y práctica médicas de Galeno', *Acta Hispanica ad Medicinae Scientiarumque Historiam llustrandam,* 2, 3–24.
Garrison, D. (2012), *A Cultural History of the Human Body in Antiquity* (Oxford: Bloomsbury).
Garson, R. (1978), 'Works of Art in Achilles Tatius' *Leucippe and Clitophon*', *Acta Classica,* 21, 83–6.
Gärtner, F. (2014), 'Galen *De locis affectis* I–II Kritische Edition—Übersetzung—Kommentar' (PhD diss.; Humboldt University).
Gasco, F. (1989), 'The Meeting between Aelius Aristides and Marcus Aurelius in Smyrna', *American Journal of Philology,* 110 (3), 471–8.
Gill, C. (2010), *Naturalistic Psychology in Galen and Stoicism* (Oxford: Oxford University Press).
Gill, C., Whitmarsh, T., and Wilkins, J. (eds.) (2009), *Galen and the World of Knowledge* (Cambridge: Cambridge University Press).
Gillespie, C. (1912), 'The Use of Εἶδος and Ἰδέα in Hippocrates', *Classical Quarterly,* 6 (3), 179–203.
Gleason, M. (1995), *Making Men: Sophists and Self-Presentation in Ancient Rome* (Princeton, NJ: Princeton University Press).
Gleason, M. (2001), 'Mutilated Messengers: Body Language in Josephus', in S. Goldhill (ed.), *Being Greek under Rome: Cultural Identity, the Second Sophistic and the Development of Empire* (Cambridge: Cambridge University Press), 50–85.
Gleason, M. (2009), 'Shock and Awe: The Performance Dimension of Galen's Anatomy Demonstrations', in C. Gill, T. Whitmarsh, and J. Wilkins (eds.), *Galen and the World of Knowledge* (Cambridge: Cambridge University Press), 85–114.

Glucklich, A. (2001), *Sacred Pain: Hurting the Body for the Sake of the Soul* (New York: Oxford University Press).
Goldhill, S. (1994), 'The Naive and Knowing Eye: Ecphrasis and the Culture of Viewing in the Hellenistic World', in S. Goldhill and R. Osborne (eds.), *Art and Text in Ancient Greek Culture* (Cambridge: Cambridge University Press), 197–223.
Goldhill, S. (1995), *Foucault's Virginity: Ancient Erotic Fiction and the History of Sexuality* (Cambridge: Cambridge University Press).
Goldhill, S. (ed.) (2001a), *Being Greek under Rome: Cultural Identity, the Second Sophistic and the Development of Empire* (Cambridge: Cambridge University Press).
Goldhill, S. (2001b), 'The Erotic Eye: Visual Stimulation and Cultural Conflict', in S. Goldhill (ed.), *Being Greek under Rome: Cultural Identity, the Second Sophistic and the Development of Empire* (Cambridge: Cambridge University Press), 154–94.
Goldhill, S. (2002), 'The Erotic Experience of Looking: Cultural Conflict and the Gaze in Empire Culture', in M. C. Nussbaum and J. Sihvola (eds.), *The Sleep of Reason: Erotic Experience and Sexual Ethics in Ancient Greece and Rome* (Chicago: University of Chicago Press), 374–99.
Goldhill, S. (2007), 'What Is Ekphrasis for?', in S. Bartsch and J. Elsner (eds.), *Ekphrasis* (Chicago: University of Chicago Press), 1–19 (= *Classical Philology*, 102 (1)).
Goldhill, S. (2012), 'Forms of Attention: Time and Narrative in Ecphrasis', *Cambridge Classical Journal*, 58, 88–114.
Goldhill, S. and Osborne, R. (eds.) (1994), *Art and Text in Ancient Greek Culture* (Cambridge: Cambridge University Press).
Gourevitch, D. (2001), 'Un éléphant peut en cacher un autre, ou comment sauter du coq à l'âne peut mettre la puce à l'oreille', in A. Debru, N. Palmieri, and B. Jacquinod (eds.), *'Docente natura': Mélanges de médecine ancienne et médiévale offerts à Guy Sabbah* (Saint-Étienne: Publications de l'Université de Saint-Étienne), 156–76.
Griffin, M. and Barnes, J. (eds.) (1989), *Philosophia Togata: Essays on Philosophy and Roman Society* (Oxford: Clarendon).
Gritzalis, K., Karamanou, M., and Androutsos, G. (2011), 'Gout in the Writings of Eminent Greek and Byzantine Physicians', *Acta Medico-Historica Adriatica*, 9 (1), 83–8.
Gumpert, M. (2001), *Grafting Helen: The Abduction of the Classical Past* (Madison, WI: University of Wisconsin Press).
Gunderson, E. (1996), 'The Ideology of the Arena', *Classical Antiquity*, 15, 113–51.
Gunderson, E. (2000), *Staging Masculinity: The Rhetoric of Performance in the Roman World* (Ann Arbor, MI: University of Michigan Press).

Gutzwiller, K. (2002), 'Art's Echo: The Tradition of Hellenistic Ecphrastic Epigram', in M. Harder, R. Regtuit, and G. Wakker (eds.), *Hellenistic Epigrams* (Leuven: Peeters), 85–112.

Hägg, T. (1971), *Narrative Technique in Ancient Greek Romances: Studies of Chariton, Xenophon Ephesius, and Achilles Tatius* (Lund: P. Astrom).

Halliwell, S. (2002), *The Aesthetics of Mimesis: Ancient Texts and Modern Problems* (Princeton, NJ: Princeton University Press).

Hankinson, R. J. (ed.) (1988), *Method, Medicine and Metaphysics: Studies in the Philosophy of Ancient Science* (Edmonton: Academic Printing and Publishing). (= *Apeiron*, 21(2)).

Hankinson, R. J. (1989), 'Galen and the Best of all Possible Worlds', *Classical Quarterly*, 39 (1), 206–27.

Hankinson, R. J. (1991), 'Galen's Anatomy of the Soul', *Phronesis*, 36 (3), 197–233.

Hankinson, R. J. (1994a), 'Usage and Abusage: Galen on Language', in S. Everson (ed.), *Language* (Companions to Ancient Thought 3; Cambridge: Cambridge University Press), 166–87.

Hankinson, R. J. (1994b), 'Galen's Anatomical Procedures: A Second-Century Debate in Medical Epistemology', *ANRW*, II.37.2, 1834–55.

Hankinson, R. J. (1994c), 'Galen's Concept of Scientific Progress', *ANRW*, II.37.2, 1775–89.

Hankinson, R. J. (1995), 'The Growth of Medical Empiricism', in D. Bates (ed.), *Knowledge and the Scholarly Medical Traditions* (Cambridge: Cambridge University Press), 60–83.

Hankinson, R. J. (1997), 'Le phénomène et l'obscur: Galien et les animaux', in B. Cassin, J.-L. Labarrière, and G. Romeyer Dherbey (eds.), *L'animal dans l'antiquité* (Paris: J. Vrin), 75–93.

Hankinson, R. J. (2005), 'Prédiction, prophétie, pronostic: La gnoséologie de l'avenir dans la divination et la médecine antique', in J. Kany-Turpin (ed.), *Signes et prédiction dans l'antiquité* (Saint-Étienne: Publications de l'Université de Saint-Étienne), 147–62.

Hankinson, R. J. (2006), 'Body and Soul in Galen', in R. King (ed.), *Common to Body and Soul: Philosophical Approaches to Explaining Living Behaviour in Greco-Roman Antiquity* (Berlin: De Gruyter), 231–58.

Hankinson, R. J. (ed.) (2008a), *The Cambridge Companion to Galen* (Cambridge: Cambridge University Press).

Hankinson, R. J. (2008b), 'The Man and His Work', in R. J. Hankinson (ed.), *The Cambridge Companion to Galen* (Cambridge: Cambridge University Press), 1–33.

Hankinson, R. J. (2008c), 'Epistemology', in R. J. Hankinson (ed.), *The Cambridge Companion to Galen* (Cambridge: Cambridge University Press), 157–83.

Hankinson, R. J. (2008d), 'Philosophy of Nature', in R. J. Hankinson (ed.), *The Cambridge Companion to Galen* (Cambridge: Cambridge University Press), 210–41.

Hardcastle, V. (1999), *The Myth of Pain* (Cambridge, MA: MIT Press).

Harlan, E. (1965), 'The Description of Paintings as a Literary Device and Its Application in Achilles Tatius' (PhD diss.; Columbia University).

Harloe, K. (2013), *Winckelmann and the Invention of Antiquity: History and Aesthetics in the Age of Altertumswissenschaft* (Oxford: Oxford University Press).

Harris, H. A. (1961), 'Philostratus, *Imagines* i, 24, 2', *Classical Review*, 11 (1), 3–5.

Harris, W. and Holmes, B. (eds.) (2008), *Aelius Aristides between Greece, Rome, and the Gods* (Leiden: Brill).

Harrison, S. (2000), 'Apuleius, Aelius Aristides and Religious Autobiography', *Ancient Narrative*, 1, 245–59.

Heath, J. (2005), *The Talking Greeks: Speech, Animals, and the Other in Homer, Aeschylus, and Plato* (Cambridge: Cambridge University Press).

Heinemann, K. (1941), 'Aus der Frühgeschichte der Lehre von den Drüsen im menschlichen Körper', *Janus*, 45, 137–65.

Heinrichs, A. (2003), '"Hieroi Logoi" and "Hierai Bibloi": The (Un)Written Margins of the Sacred in Ancient Greece', *Harvard Studies in Classical Philology*, 101, 207–66.

Herbst, W. (1911), *Galeni Pergameni de atticissantium studiis testimonia* (Leipzig: Teubner).

Herder, J. and Suphan, B. (ed.) (1967–8), *Sämtliche Werke* (Hildesheim: Georg Olms Verlagsbuchhandlung).

Hide, L., Bourke, J., and Mangion, C. (2012), 'Perspectives on Pain: Introduction', *19 Interdisciplinary Studies on the Long 19th Century*, 15, 1–8.

Hodkinson, O., Rosenmeyer, P., and Bracke, E. (eds.) (2013), *Epistolary Narratives in Ancient Greek Literature* (Leiden: Brill).

Holmes, B. (2007), 'The *Iliad*'s Economy of Pain', *Transactions of the American Philological Association*, 137 (1), 45–84.

Holmes, B. (2008), 'Aelius Aristides' Illegible Body', in W. Harris and B. Holmes (eds.), *Aelius Aristides between Greece, Rome, and the Gods* (Leiden: Brill), 81–113.

Holmes, B. (2010), *The Symptom and the Subject: The Emergence of the Physical Body in Ancient Greece* (Princeton, NJ: Princeton University Press).

Holmes, B. (2015), 'Medicine and Misfortune: *Symptōma* in Greek Medical Writing', in B. Holmes and K. Fischer (eds.), *The Frontiers of Ancient Science: Essays in Honor of Heinrich von Staden* (Berlin: De Gruyter), 191–209.

Horden, P. (2008), 'Pain in Hippocratic Medicine', in P. Horden (ed.), *Hospitals and Healing from Antiquity to the Later Middle Ages* (Aldershot: Ashgate Variorum), 295–315.

Horstmanshoff, M., King, H., and Zittel, C. (eds.) (2012), *Blood, Sweat and Tears: The Changing Concepts of Physiology from Antiquity into Early Modern Europe* (Leiden: Brill).

Huby, P. M. (1969), 'The Epicureans, Animals, and Freewill', *Apeiron*, 3 (1), 17–19.

Hude, C. (1958), *Aretaeus* (CMG II; Berlin: Akademie Verlag).

Hunter, K. (1991), *Doctors' Stories: The Narrative Structure of Medical Knowledge* (Princeton, NJ: Princeton University Press).

Hunter, R. L. (2004), 'Homer and Greek Literature', in D. Fowler (ed.), *The Cambridge Companion to Homer* (Cambridge: Cambridge University Press), 235–53.

Hunter, R. L. (2009), *Critical Moments in Classical Literature: Studies in the Ancient View of Literature and Its Uses* (Cambridge: Cambridge University Press).

Hurwit, J. (1995), 'The Doryphoros: Looking Backward', in W. Moon (ed.), *Polykleitos, the Doryphoros, and Tradition* (Madison, WI: University of Wisconsin Press), 3–18.

Ihm, S. (1996), 'Archigenes als Verfasser des Traktates περὶ τῶν ἰοβόλων θηρίων και δηλητηρίων φαρμάκων?', *Sudhoffs Archiv*, 80 (2), 220–8.

Ilberg, G. (1923), 'Das neurologisch-psychiatrische Wissen und Können des Aretäus von Kappadokien', *Zeitschrift fur die gesamte Neurologie und Psychiatrie*, 86, 227–46.

Israelowich, I. (2012), *Society, Medicine and Religion in the Sacred Tales of Aelius Aristides* (Mnemosyne Supplements 341; Leiden: Brill).

Israelowich, I. (2015), *Patients and Healers in the High Roman Empire* (Baltimore, MD: Johns Hopkins University Press).

Jay, M. (2003), *Refractions of Violence* (New York: Routledge).

Jennison, G. (1937), *Animals for Show and Pleasure in Ancient Rome* (Manchester: Manchester University Press).

Johnston, I. (trans.) (2006), *Galen: On Diseases and Symptoms* (Cambridge: Cambridge University Press).

Jones, C. (2008), 'Aristides' First Admirer', in W. Harris and B. Holmes (eds.), *Aelius Aristides between Greece, Rome, and the Gods* (Leiden: Brill), 253–62.

Jones, C. and Porter, R. (eds.) (1994), *Reassessing Foucault: Power, Medicine and the Body* (London: Routledge).

Jouanna, J. (2001), 'Histoire du mot αἱμάλωψ d'Hippocrate à Galien et à la médecine tardive: Contribution à l'étude des dérivés en -αλ- de la famille de αἷμα et des termes techniques en -ωψ', *Revue des Études Grecques*, 114 (1), 1–23.

Jouanna, J. (2002), 'Le vin chez Arétée de Cappadoce', in J. Jouanna, L. Villard, and D. Béguin (eds.), *Vin et santé en Grèce ancienne* (Athens: École Française d'Athènes), 113–26.

Jouanna, J. and Leclant, J. (eds.) (2004), *Colloque La médecine grecque antique* (Paris: de Boccard).

Jouanna, J. and Villard, L. (eds.) (2002), *Vin et santé en Grèce ancienne* (Athens: École Française d'Athènes).

Ju, A. E. (2007), 'Chrysippus on Nature and Soul in Animals', *Classical Quarterly*, 57 (1), 97–108.

Kampen, N. B. (ed.) (1996), *Sexuality in Ancient Art: Near East, Egypt, Greece, and Italy* (Cambridge: Cambridge University Press).

Karavas, O. (2005), *Lucien et la tragédie* (Berlin: De Gruyter).

Kim, L. (2010), *Homer between History and Fiction in Imperial Greek Literature* (Cambridge: Cambridge University Press).

Kindstrand, J. (1973), *Homer in der zweiten Sophistik. Studien zu der Homerlektüre und dem Homerbild bei Dion von Prusa, Maximos von Tyros und Ailios Aristeides* (Stockholm: Almqvist & Wiksell).

King, D. (2012), 'Taking It like a Man: Gender, Body and Identity in Achilles Tatius' *Leucippe and Clitophon*', in M. Futre Pinheiro, M. Skinner, and F. Zeitlin (eds.), *Narrating Desire: Eros, Sex, and Gender in the Ancient Novel* (Berlin: De Gruyter), 147–57.

King, D. (2015), 'Galen and Grief: The Construction of Grief in Galen's Clinical Work', in A. Chaniotis and P. Ducrey (eds.), *Unveiling Emotions II: Emotions in Greece and Rome: Texts, Images, and Material Culture* (Stuttgart: Franz Steiner), 251–72.

King, H. (1988), 'The Early Anodynes: Pain in the Ancient World', in R. Mann (ed.), *The Management of Pain: The Historical Perspective* (Carnforth: Parthenon), 51–62.

King, H. (2002), 'Chronic Pain and the Creation of Narrative', in J. Porter (ed.), *Constructions of the Classical Body* (Ann Arbor, MI: University of Michigan Press), 269–86.

Kirmayer, L. (2007), 'On the Cultural Mediation of Pain', in S. Coakley and K. Shelemay (eds.), *Pain and Its Transformations: The Interface of Biology and Culture* (Cambridge, MA: Harvard University Press), 363–401.

Kleinman, A. (1980), *Patients and Healers in the Context of Culture: An Exploration of the Borderland between Anthropology, Medicine, and Psychiatry* (Comparative Studies of Health Systems and Medical Care 3; Berkeley, CA: University of California Press).

Kleinman, A. (1988), *The Illness Narratives: Suffering, Healing, and the Human Condition* (New York: Basic Books).

Kleinman, A. (2007), 'Opening Remarks: Pain and Experience', in S. Coakley and K. Shelemay (eds.), *Pain and Its Transformations: The Interface of Biology and Culture* (Cambridge, MA: Harvard University Press), 17–20.

Kleinman, A. and Kleinman, J. (1994), 'How Bodies Remember: Social Memory and Bodily Experience of Criticism, Resistance, and Delegitimation Following China's Cultural Revolution', *New Literary History*, 25, 707–23.

Kleinman, A. and Kleinman, J. (1997), 'The Appeal of Experience, the Dismay of Images: Cultural Appropriations of Suffering in Our Times', in A. Kleinman, V. Das, and M. Lock (eds.), *Social Suffering* (Berkeley, CA: University of California Press), 1–23.

Kleinman, A., Das, V., and Lock, M. (eds.) (1997), *Social Suffering* (Berkeley, CA: University of California Press).

Kleywegt, A. (1984), 'Cleanthes and the "Vital Heat"', *Mnemosyne*, 37 (1/2), 94–102.

Knust, J. W. and Várhelyi, Z. (eds.) (2011), *Ancient Mediterranean Sacrifice* (Oxford: Oxford University Press).

Koehler, P. and van de Wiel, T. (2001), 'Aretaeus on Migraine and Headache', *Journal of the History of the Neurosciences: Basic and Clinical Perspectives*, 10 (3), 253–61.

Kollesch, J. (1997), 'Die anatomischen Untersuchungen des Aristoteles und ihr Stellenwert als Forschungsmethode in der aristotelischen Biologie', in W. Kullmann and S. Föllinger (eds.), *Aristotelische Biologie: Intentionen, Methoden, Ergebnisse* (Stuttgart: Franz Steiner), 367–74.

Kollesch, J. and Nickel, D. (1979), *Antike Heilkunst: Ausgewählte Texte aus dem medizinischen Schrifttum der Griechen und Römer* (Leipzig: Phillip Reclam).

Kollmann, B. (1993), 'Eine Mysterienweihe bei Aretaios von Kappadokien', *Philologus*, 137 (2), 252–7.

König, J. (2005), *Athletics and Literature in the Roman Empire* (Cambridge: Cambridge University Press).

König, J. (2008), 'Body and Text', in T. Whitmarsh (ed.), *The Cambridge Companion to the Greek and Roman Novel* (Cambridge: Cambridge University Press), 127–44.

Konstan, D. (1994), *Sexual Symmetry: Love in the Ancient Novel and Related Genres* (Princeton, NJ: Princeton University Press).

Konstan, D. (2001), *Pity Transformed* (Classical Inter/Faces; London: Duckworth).

Konstan, D. (2003a), 'Before Jealousy', in D. Konstan and K. Rutter (eds.), *Envy, Spite and Jealousy: The Rivalrous Emotions in Ancient Greece* (Edinburgh: Edinburgh University Press), 7–27.

Konstan, D. (2003b), 'Translating Ancient Emotions', *Acta Classica*, 46, 5–19.

Konstan, D. (2004), '"The Birth of the Reader": Plutarch as Literary Critic', *Scholia*, 13 (1), 3–27.

Konstan, D. (2005), 'The Pleasures of the Ancient Text or the Pleasure of Poetry from Plato to Plutarch', in F. Cairns (ed.), *Greek and Roman Poetry, Greek and Roman Historiography* (Papers of the Langford Latin Seminar, 12; Cambridge: Cambridge University Press), 1–17.

Konstan, D. (2006), *The Emotions of the Ancient Greeks: Studies in Aristotle and Greek Literature* (Toronto: University of Toronto Press).

Konstan, D. (2007), 'Rhetoric and Emotion', in I. Worthington (ed.), *A Companion to Greek Rhetoric* (Oxford: Blackwell), 411–25.

Konstan, D. and Rutter, K. (eds.) (2003), *Envy, Spite and Jealousy: The Rivalrous Emotions in Ancient Greece* (Edinburgh: Edinburgh University Press).

Konstantinova, R. H. (2000), 'Emotions and Their Functions in Achilles Tatius' *Leucippe*' (PhD diss.; University of California, Berkeley).

Kosak, J. B. C. (1994), 'The Pain of the Living: Suffering and Healing in Euripidean Tragedy' (PhD diss.; University of Michigan).

Kosak, J. B. C. (2005), 'A Crying Shame: Pitying the Sick in the Hippocratic Corpus and Greek Tragedy', in R. Sternberg (ed.), *Pity and Power in Ancient Athens* (Cambridge: Cambridge University Press), 253–76.

Koskenniemi, H. (1956), *Studien zur Idee und Phraseologie des griechischen Briefes bis 400 n. Chr.* (Helsinki: Akateeminen Kirjakauppa).

Kostopoulou, V. (2009), 'Philostratus' *Imagines* 2.18: Words and Images', *Greek, Roman and Byzantine Studies,* 49 (1), 81–100.

Kotsopoulos, S. (1986), 'Aretaeus the Cappadocian on Mental Illness', *Comprehensive Psychology,* 27 (2), 171–9.

Kottek, S. and Horstmanshoff, M. (eds.) (2000), *From Athens to Jerusalem: Medicine in Hellenized Jewish Lore and in Early Christian Literature* (Rotterdam: Erasmus).

Kraus, C., Goldhill, S., and Foley, H. P. (eds.) (2007), *Visualizing the Tragic: Drama, Myth, and Ritual in Greek Art and Literature* (Oxford: Oxford University Press).

Krauss, F. (1912), 'Die rhetorischen Schriften Plutarchs und ihre Stellung im plutarchischen Schriftenkorpus' (PhD diss.; Nurnberg).

Kudlien, F. (1956), 'Zu Aretaeus', *Philologus,* 100 (1–2), 316.

Kudlien, F. (1964), *Untersuchungen zu Aretaios von Kappadokien* (Wiesbaden: Steiner).

Kudlien, F. (1974), 'Die Pneuma-Bewegung: ein Beitrag zum Thema Medizin und Stoa', *Gesnerus,* 31, 86–98.

Kudlien, F. (1991), '"Endeixis" as a Scientific Term: A) Galen's Usage of the Word (in Medicine and Logic)', in F. Kudlien and R. Durling (eds.), *Galen's Method of Healing* (Leiden: Brill), 103–11.

Kudlien, F. and Durling, R. (eds.) (1991), *Galen's Method of Healing* (Leiden: Brill).

Kumar, P. and Tripathi, L. (2014), 'Challenges in Pain Assessment: Pain Intensity Scales', *Indian Journal of Pain,* 28 (2), 61–70.

Kupreeva, I. (2014), 'Galen's Theory of Elements', in P. Adamson, R. Hansberger, and J. Wilberding (eds.), *Philosophical Themes in Galen* (London: Institute of Classical Studies), 153–96.

Kyle, D. (1998), *Spectacles of Death in Ancient Rome* (London: Routledge).
Labarrière, J.-L. (1997), 'Logos endiathetos et logos prophorikos dans la polémique entre le Portique et la Nouvelle-Académie', in B. Cassin, J.-L. Labarrière, and G. Romeyer Dherbey (eds.), *L'animal dans l'antiquité* (Paris: J. Vrin), 259–79.
LaCapra, D. (1998), *History and Memory after Auschwitz* (Ithaca, NY: Cornell University Press).
LaCapra, D. (2001), *Writing History, Writing Trauma* (Baltimore, MD: Johns Hopkins University Press).
LaCapra, D. (2009), *History and Its Limits: Human, Animal, Violence* (Ithaca, NY: Cornell University Press).
LaCourse Munteanu, D. (2013), *Emotion, Genre and Gender in Classical Antiquity* (London: Bloomsbury).
Lain Entralgo, P. (1970), *The Therapy of the Word in Classical Antiquity*, trans. L. Rather and J. Sharp (London: Yale University Press).
Lami, A. (2003), 'Areteo e i delicati di stomaco (IV 6, 2)', *Filologia Antica e Moderna*, 13 (24), 5–10.
Langholf, V. (1990), *Medical Theories in Hippocrates: Early Texts and the 'Epidemics'* (Berlin: De Gruyter).
Laplace, M. M. J. (1983), 'Achilleus Tatios, *Leucippé et Clitophon*. P. Oxyrhynchos 1250', *Zeitschrift für Papyrologie und Epigraphik*, 53, 53–9.
Laplace, M. M. J. (1993), 'À propos du P. Robinson-Coloniensis d'Achille Tatius, *Leucippé et Clitophon*', *Zeitschrift für Papyrologie und Epigraphik*, 98, 43–56.
Laplace, M. M. J. (2006), 'Achille Tatios, *Leucippé et Clitophon*, VII, 6, 7: Sur la beauté de Syrinx', *Revue des Études Grecques*, 119 (1), 436–9.
Laskaris, J. (2002), '"Acute" and "Chronic" in *On the Sacred Disease*', in A. Thivel and A. Zucker (eds.), *Le normal et le pathologique dans la collection hippocratique* (Nice: Faculté des Lettres, Arts et Sciences Humaines de Nice-Sophia Antipolis), 539–50.
Leach, E. W. (2000), 'Narrative Space and the Viewer in Philostratus' *Eikones*', *Mitteilungen des Deutschen Archäologischen Instituts, Römische Abteilung*, 107, 237–51.
Le Blay, F. (2006), 'Penser la douleur dans l'antiquité: enjeu médical ou enjeu philosophique?', in F. Prost and J. Wilgaux (eds.), *Penser et représenter le corps dans l'antiquité: actes du colloque international de Rennes, 1–4 septembre 2004* (Rennes: Presses Universitaires de Rennes), 79–92.
Leftwich, G. (1995), 'Polykleitos and Hippokratic Medicine', in W. Moon (ed.), *Polykleitos, the Doryphoros, and Tradition* (Madison, WI: University of Wisconsin Press), 38–51.
Lehmann-Hartleben, K. (1941), 'The *Imagines* of the Elder Philostratus', *The Art Bulletin*, 23 (1), 16–44.

Leigh, M. (1995), 'Wounding and Popular Rhetoric at Rome', *Bulletin of the Institute of Classical Studies*, 40 (1), 195–215.
Leopold, E. J. (1930), 'Aretaeus the Cappadocian: His Contribution to Diabetes Mellitus', *Annals of Medical History*, 2, 424–35.
Lessing, G. (1984), *Laocoon: An Essay on the Limits of Painting and Poetry*, trans. E. McCormick (Baltimore, MD: Johns Hopkins University Press).
Lessing, G. and von Barner, W. (1987–2003), *Werke und Briefe, in zwölf Bänden*. (Frankfurt am Main: Deutscher Klassiker Verlag).
Létoublon, F. (1993), *Les Lieux communs du roman. Stéréotypes grecs d'aventure et d'amour* (Mnemosyne Supplements 23; Leiden: Brill).
Letts, M. (2014), 'Rufus of Ephesus and the Patient's Perspective in Medicine', *British Journal for the History of Philosophy*, 22 (5), 996–1020.
Letts, M. (2015), 'Questioning the Patient, Questioning Hippocrates: Rufus of Ephesus and the Pursuit of Knowledge', in G. Petridou and C. Thumiger (eds.), *Homo Patiens: Approaches to the Patient in the Ancient World* (Leiden: Brill), 81–103.
Lévy, C. and Pernot, L. (1997), *Dire l'évidence: philosophie et rhétorique antiques* (Paris: L'Harmattan).
Lewis, O. (2015), 'The Practical Application of Ancient Pulse-Lore and Its Influence on the Patient–Doctor Interaction', in G. Petridou and C. Thumiger (eds.), *Homo Patiens: Approaches to the Patient in the Ancient World* (Leiden: Brill), 345–64.
Liviabella Furiani, P. (1985), 'Achille Tazio 8.9.9 sgg. e Platone, *Leggi* 12.961 A–B: Un esempio di imitazione e deformazione', *Prometheus*, 11, 179–82.
Lloyd, G. E. R. (1997), 'Les animaux de l'antiquité étaient bons à penser: Quelques points de comparaison entre Aristote et le Huainanzi', in B. Cassin, J.-L. Labarrière, and G. Romeyer Dherbey (eds.), *L'animal dans l'antiquité* (Paris: J. Vrin), 545–62.
Lloyd, G. E. R. (2008), 'Galen and His Contemporaries', in R. J. Hankinson (ed.), *The Cambridge Companion to Galen* (Cambridge University Press), 34–48.
Lloyd, G. E. R. (2009), 'Galen's un-Hippocratic case-histories', in C. Gill, T. Whitmarsh, and J. Wilkins (eds.), *Galen and the World of Knowledge* (Cambridge: Cambridge University Press), 115–31.
Long, A. A. (1971), *Problems in Stoicism* (London: Athlone Press).
López Férez, J. A. (ed.) (1991), *Galeno: Obra, pensamiento e influencia* (Madrid: UNED).
López Férez J. A. (ed.) (1992), *Tratados hipocráticos. Estudios acerca de su contenido, forma y influencia* (Madrid: UNED).
Luján Martínez, E. R. (2006), 'Cuatro notas críticas', in E. Calderón Dorda, A. Morales Ortiz, and M. Valverde Sánchez (eds.), *Koinòs lógos: Homenaje*

al profesor José García López (Murcia: Universidad de Murcia, Servicio de Publicaciones), 543–9.

McGill, S. (2000), 'The Literary Lives of a *Scheintod*: *Clitophon and Leucippe* 5.7 and Greek Epigram', *Classical Quarterly*, 50 (1), 323–6.

McLeod, A. M. G. (1969), 'Physiology and Medicine in a Greek Novel. Achilles Tatius' *Leucippe and Clitophon*', *The Journal of Hellenic Studies*, 89, 97–105.

MacLeod, M. (trans.) (1967), *Lucian Soloecista. Lucius or The Ass. Amores. Halcyon. Demosthenes. Podagra. Ocypus. Cyniscus. Philopatris. Charidemus. Nero.* (Loeb Classical Library; Cambridge, MA.: Harvard University Press).

Manetti, D. (2009), 'Galen and Hippocratic Medicine: Language and Practice', in C. Gill, T. Whitmarsh, and J. Wilkins (eds.), *Galen and the World of Knowledge* (Cambridge: Cambridge University Press), 157–74.

Manuli, P. (1988), 'La passione nel *De placitis hippocratis et platonis*', in P. Manuli and M. Vegetti (eds.), *Le opere psicologiche di Galeno* (Naples: Bibliopolis), 185–214.

Marzullo, B. (1999), 'Il "dolore" in Ippocrate', *Quaderni Urbinati di Cultura Classica*, 63 (3), 123–8.

Mattern, S. (2008), *Galen and the Rhetoric of Healing* (Baltimore, MD: Johns Hopkins University Press).

Mattern, S. (2013), *Prince of Medicine* (Princeton, NJ: Princeton University Press).

Mattern, S. (2015), 'Galen's Anxious Patients: Lypē as Anxiety Disorder', in G. Petridou and C. Thumiger (eds.), *Homo Patiens: Approaches to the Patient in the Ancient World* (Leiden: Brill), 203–23.

Mattingly, C. and Garro, L. (eds.) (2000), *Narrative and the Cultural Construction of Illness and Healing* (Berkeley, CA: University of California Press).

Mavroudis, A. D. (1986), 'Arétée de Cappadoce bibliographie analytique 1552–1986', *Ellenica*, 37, 26–68.

Mavroudis, A. D. (2000), Ἀρχιγένης Φιλίππου Ἀπαμεύς: ὁ βίος και τὰ ἔργα ἑνὸς Ἕλληνα γιατροῦ στὴν αὐτοκρατορικὴ Ῥώμη (Athens: Akadimia Athinon).

Mechley, B. J. (1998), 'Reading (with) the Animals: Lucretius' Creatures and his Poetic Program' (PhD diss.; University of Washington).

Melzack, R. (1975), 'The McGill Pain Questionnaire: Major Properties and Scoring Methods', *Pain*, 1 (3), 277–99.

Meyer, B. (ed.) (2009), *Aesthetic Formations: Media, Religion, and the Senses* (London: Macmillan).

Michenaud, G. and Dierkens, J. (1972), *Les rêves dans les* Discours Sacrés *d'Aelius Aristide, IIe siècle ap. J.-C. Essai d'analyse psychologique* (Mons: Université de Mons).

Mignogna, E. (1997), 'Leucippe in Tauride (Ach. Tat. 3, 15–22): mimo e "pantomimo" tra tragedia e romanzo', *Materiali e Discussioni per l'Analisi dei Testi Classici,* 38, 225–36.
Miguélez Cavero, L. (2010), 'Rhetorical Displays of Knowledge in *Leucippe and Clitophon*: Animal Talk', *Prometheus,* 36 (3), 263–83.
Miller, H. W. (1962), 'The Aetiology of Disease in Plato's *Timaeus*', *Transactions of the American Philological Association,* 93, 175–87.
Misch, G. (1950), *A History of Autobiography in Antiquity,* trans. E. Dickes (Cambridge, MA: Harvard University Press).
Montiglio, S. (2005), *Wandering in Ancient Greek Culture* (Chicago: University of Chicago Press).
Morales, H. (1996), 'The Torturer's Apprentice: Parrhasius and the Limits of Art', in J. Elsner (ed.), *Art and Text in Roman Culture* (Cambridge: Cambridge University Press), 182–209.
Morales, H. (2000), 'Sense and Sententiousness in the Greek Novels', in A. Sharrock and H. Morales (eds.), *Intratextuality: Greek and Roman Textual Relations* (Oxford: Oxford University Press), 67–88.
Morales, H. (2004), *Vision and Narrative in Achilles Tatius'* Leucippe and Clitophon (Cambridge: Cambridge University Press).
Moraux, P. (1981), 'Galien comme philosophe; la philosophie de la nature', in V. Nutton (ed.), *Galen: Problems and Prospects* (London: Wellcome Institute for the History of Medicine), 87–116.
Morgan, J. R. (1993), 'Make-Believe and Make Believe: The Fictionality of the Greek Novels', in C. Gill and T. Wiseman (ed.), *Lies and Fiction in the Ancient World* (Exeter: Exeter University Press), 175–229.
Morgan, J. R. (1996), 'Erotika Mathemata: Greek Romance as Sentimental Education', in A. Sommerstein and C. Atherton (eds.), *Education in Greek Fiction* (Bari: Levante Editori), 163–89.
Morgan, J. R. and Jones, M. (2007), *Philosophical Presences in the Ancient Novel* (Ancient Narrative Supplementum 10; Groningen: Barkhuis).
Morris, D. (1991), *The Culture of Pain* (Berkeley, CA: University of California Press).
Morris, D. (1997), 'About Suffering: Voice, Genre, and Moral Community', in A. Kleinman, V. Das, and M. Lock (eds.), *Social Suffering* (Berkeley, CA: University of California Press), 25–45.
Morison, B. (2008), 'Language', in R. J. Hankinson (ed.), *The Cambridge Companion to Galen* (Cambridge: Cambridge University Press), 116–56.
Mossman, J. M. (2005), 'Plutarch on Animals: Rhetorical Strategies in *de sollertia animalium*', *Hermathena,* 179, 141–63.
Moxon, I. S., Smart, J. D., and Woodman, A. J. (eds.) (1986), *Past Perspectives: Studies in Greek and Roman Historical Writing* (Cambridge: Cambridge University Press).
Mulvey, L. (1975), 'Visual Pleasure and Narrative Cinema', *Screen,* 16 (3), 6–18.

Neumayr, J. (1963), 'Plutarch, Aristotle and the Nature of Poetry (1)', *Laval Théologique et Philosophique*, 19 (2), 305-34.
Newby, Z. (2009), 'Absorption and erudition in Philostratus' *Imagines*', in E. L. Bowie and J. Elsner (eds.), *Philostratus* (Cambridge: Cambridge University Press), 322-42.
Newmyer, S. (1992), 'Plutarch on Justice toward Animals: Ancient Insights on a Modern Debate', *Scholia*, 1 (1), 38-54.
Newmyer, S. (1995), 'Plutarch on the Moral Grounds for Vegetarianism', *The Classical Outlook*, 72 (2), 41-3.
Newmyer, S. (1999), 'Speaking of Beasts: The Stoics and Plutarch on Animal Reason and the Modern Case against Animals', *Quaderni Urbinati di Cultura Classica*, 63 (3), 99-110.
Newmyer, S. (2000), 'Philo on Animal Psychology: Sources and Moral Implications', in S. Kottek and M. Horstmanshoff (eds.), *From Athens to Jerusalem: Medicine in Hellenized Jewish Law and Early Christian Literature* (Rotterdam: Erasmus), 143-55.
Newmyer, S. (2003), 'Paws to Reflect: Ancients and Moderns on the Religious Sensibilities of Animals', *Quaderni Urbinati di Cultura Classica*, 75 (3), 111-29.
Newmyer, S. (2005), 'Tool Use in Animals: Ancient and Modern Insights and Moral Consequences', *Scholia*, 14 (1), 3-17.
Newmyer, S. (2006), *Animals, Rights and Reason in Plutarch and Modern Ethics* (London: Routledge).
Newmyer, S. (2007), '*Just Beasts?*: Plutarch and Modern Science on the Sense of Fair Play in Animals', *The Classical Outlook*, 74 (3), 85-8.
Newmyer, S. (2010), *Animals in Greek and Roman Thought: A Sourcebook* (London: Routledge).
Nijhuis, K. (1995), 'Greek Doctors and Roman Patients: A Medical Anthropological Approach', in P. van der Eijk, H. Horstmanshoff, and P. Schrijvers (eds.), *Ancient Medicine in Its Socio-Cultural Context 1* (Amsterdam: Rodopi), 49-68.
NíMheallaigh, K. (2007), 'Philosophical Framing: The Phaedran Setting of *Leucippe and Cleitophon*', in J. Morgan and M. Jones (eds.), *Philosophical Presences in the Ancient Novel* (Ancient Narrative Supplementum 10; Groningen: Barkhuis), 231-44.
Nimis, S. (1994), 'The Prosaics of Ancient Novel', *Arethusa*, 27, 387-411.
Nussbaum, M. C. (2001), *Upheavals of Thought: The Intelligence of Emotions* (Cambridge: Cambridge University Press).
Nussbaum, M. C. and Sihvola, J. (2002), *The Sleep of Reason: Erotic Experience and Sexual Ethics in Ancient Greece and Rome* (Chicago: University of Chicago Press).
Nutton, V. (1973), 'The Chronology of Galen's Early Career', *Classical Quarterly*, 23 (1), 158-71.

Nutton, V. (ed.) (1981), *Galen: Problems and Prospects* (London: Wellcome Institute for the History of Medicine).
Nutton, V. (1993), 'Galen at the Bedside: The Methods of a Medical Detective', in W. Bynum and R. Porter (eds.), *Medicine and the Five Senses* (Cambridge: Cambridge University Press), 7–16.
Nutton, V. (1995), 'The Medical Meeting Place', in P. van der Eijk, H. Horstmanshoff, and P. Schrijvers (eds.), *Ancient Medicine in Its Socio-Cultural Context 1* (Amsterdam: Rodopi), 3–26.
Nutton, V. (ed.) (2002), *The Unknown Galen* (Bulletin of the Institute of Classical Studies Supplement 77; London: Institute of Classical Studies).
Nutton, V. (2004), *Ancient Medicine* (London: Routledge).
Oberhelman, S. M. (1994), 'On the Chronology and Pneumatism of Aretaios of Cappadocia', *ANRW*, II.2.37, 941–66.
Palazzini, S. (1996), 'Il vocabolario della vista nelle *Imagines* di Filostrato', *Annali della Facoltà di Lettere e Filosofia della Università di Macerata*, 29, 113–28.
Panayotakis, S., Zimmerman, M., and Keulen, W. (eds.) (2003), *The Ancient Novel and Beyond* (Mnemosyne Supplementum 241; Leiden: Brill).
Papadi, D. (2007), 'Tragedy and Theatricality in Plutarch' (PhD. thesis; University of London).
Paschalis, M., Panayotakis, S., and Schmeling, G. (eds.) (2009), *Readers and Writers in the Ancient Novel* (Ancient Narrative Supplementum 12; Groningen: Barkhuis).
Pasquier, A. (2011), 'Une écriture du visuel au temps de la Seconde Sophistique: Clément d'Alexandrie (*Protreptique*) et Philostrate (*Images*)', in T. Schmidt and P. Fleury (eds.), *Perceptions of the Second Sophistic and its Times—Regards sur la Seconde Sophistique et son époque* (Toronto: University of Toronto Press), 87–102.
Paz de Hoz, M. (2014), 'Lucian's *Podagra*, Asclepius and Galen. The Popularisation of Medicine in the Second Century AD', in L. Arturo Guichard, J. García Alonso, and M. Paz de Hoz (eds.), *The Alexandrian Tradition: Interactions between Science, Religion, and Literature* (Bern: Peter Lang), 175–210.
Pearcy, L. T. (1983), 'Galen and Stoic Rhetoric', *Greek, Roman and Byzantine Studies*, 24, 259–72.
Pearcy, L. T. (1988), 'Theme, Dream, and Narrative: Reading the *Sacred Tales* of Aelius Aristides', *Transactions of the American Philological Association*, 118, 377–91.
Pearcy, L. T. (1992), 'Diagnosis as Narrative in Ancient Literature', *American Journal of Philology*, 113 (4), 595–616.
Pearcy, L. T. (2012), 'Does Dying Hurt?: Philodemus of Gadara, *De morte* and Asclepiades of Bithynia', *Classical Quarterly*, 62 (1), 211–22.
Peck, A. L. (1971), 'Aristotle on κίνησις', in J. P. Anton and G. L. Kustas (eds.), *Essays in Ancient Greek Philosophy* (Albany, NY: State University of New York Press), 478–90.

Pelling, C. B. R. (1988), 'Aspects of Plutarch's Characterisation', *Illinois Classical Studies,* 13 (2), 257-74.
Pelling, C. B. R. (1989), 'Plutarch: Roman Heroes and Greek Culture', in M. Griffin and J. Barnes (eds.), *Philosophia Togata: Essays on Philosophy and Roman Society* (Oxford: Clarendon Press), 199-232.
Pelling C. B. R. (1990), *Characterization and Individuality in Greek Literature* (Oxford: Clarendon).
Pelling, C. B. R. (ed.) (1997), *Greek Tragedy and the Historian* (Oxford: Clarendon).
Pelling, C. B. R. (2002), *Plutarch and History: Eighteen Studies* (Swansea: Classical Press of Wales).
Pelling, C. B. R. (2005), 'Pity in Plutarch', in R. Sternberg (ed.), *Pity and Power in Ancient Athens* (Cambridge: Cambridge University Press), 277-312.
Pelling C. B. R. (2016), 'Tragic Colouring in Plutarch', in J. Opsomer, G. Roskam, and F. Titchener (eds.), *A Versatile Gentleman: Consistency in Plutarch's Writings* (Leuven: Leuven University Press), 113-33.
Pérez Jiménez, A., García López, J., and Aguilar, M. (eds.) (1999), *Plutarco, Platón y Aristóteles: Actas del V Congreso Internacional de la I.P.S* (Madrid: Ed. Clásicas).
Pérez Molina, M. E. (1991), 'Algunas carácterísticas lingüísticas de la obra médica de Areteo de Capadocia', *Myrtia,* 6, 83-94.
Pérez Molina M. E. (1992), 'Paralelismos sintomatológicos entre el corpus hippocraticum y la obra médica de Areteo de Capadocia', in J. López Férez (ed.), *Tratados hipocráticos. Estudios acerca de su contenido, forma y influencia* (Madrid: UNED), 585-95.
Pérez Molina, M. E. (2005), 'El léxico homérico en Areteo de Capadocia', *Myrtia,* 20, 63-85.
Perkins, J. (1995), *The Suffering Self: Pain and Self-Representation in the Early Christian Era* (London: Routledge).
Pernot, L. (2002), 'Les *Discours sacrés* d'Aelius Aristide entre médecine, religion et rhétorique', *Atti della Accademia Pontaniana, Napoli,* 51, 369-83.
Peterson, D. (1977), 'Observations on the Chronology of the Galenic Corpus', *Bulletin of the History of Medicine,* 51 (3), 484-95.
Petridou, G. and Thumiger, C. (eds.) (2015), *Homo Patiens: Approaches to the Patient in the Ancient World* (Leiden: Brill).
Petsalis-Diomidis, A. (2005), 'The Body in Space: Visual Dynamics in Graeco-Roman Healing Pilgrimage', in J. Elsner and I. Rutherford (eds.), *Seeing the Gods: Patterns of Pilgrimage in Antiquity* (Oxford: Oxford University Press), 183-218.
Petsalis-Diomidis, A. (2006), 'Sacred Writing, Sacred Reading: The Function of Aelius Aristides' Self-Presentation as Author in the *Sacred Tales*', in

J. Mossman and B. McGing (eds.), *The Limits of Ancient Biography* (Swansea: University of Wales Press), 193–211.

Petsalis-Diomidis, A. (2008), 'The Body in the Landscape: Aristides' *Corpus* in the Light of the *Sacred Tales*', in W. Harris and B. Holmes (eds.), *Aristides between Greece, Rome, and the Gods* (Leiden: Brill), 131–50.

Petsalis-Diomidis, A. (2010), *Truly beyond Wonders: Aelius Aristides and the Cult of Asklepios* (Oxford: Oxford University Press).

Phillips, K. M. (1968), 'Perseus and Andromeda', *American Journal of Archaeology*, 72 (1), 1–23.

Picone, M. and Zimmermann, B. (eds.) (1997), *Der antike Roman und seine mittelalterliche Rezeption* (Basel: Birkhäuser).

Pigeaud, J. (1987), *Folies et cures de la folie chez les médecins de l'antiquité gréco-romaine: La manie* (Paris: Les Belles Lettres).

Pigeaud, J. (2004), 'La rhétorique d'Arétée', in J. Jouanna and J. Leclant (eds.), *Colloque La médecine grecque antique* (Paris: de Boccard), 177–97.

Pleket, H. (1995), 'The Social Status of Physicians in the Graeco-Roman World', in P. van der Eijk, H. Horstmanshoff, and P. Schrijvers (eds.), *Ancient Medicine in Its Socio-Cultural Context 1* (Amsterdam: Rodopi), 27–34.

Porter, A. (2014), 'Empathy and Compassion in the Medicine and Literature of the First and Second Centuries AD' (PhD diss.; University of Calgary).

Porter, J. (1986), 'The Material Sublime: Towards a Reconstruction of a Materialist Critical Discourse and Aesthetics in Antiquity' (PhD diss.; University of California, Berkeley).

Porter, J. (ed.) (2002), *Constructions of the Classical Body* (Body in Theory; Ann Arbor, MI: University of Michigan Press).

Porter, J. (2010), *The Origins of Aesthetic Thought in Ancient Greece: Matter, Sensation, and Experience* (Cambridge: Cambridge University Press).

Porter, J. (2012), 'Is the Sublime an Aesthetic Value?', in I. Sluiter and R. Rosen (eds.), *Aesthetic Value in Classical Antiquity* (Mnemosyne Supplements 350; Leiden: Brill), 47–70.

Porter, J. (2016), *The Sublime in Antiquity* (Cambridge: Cambridge University Press).

Porter, R. (1991), 'History of the Body', in P. Burke (ed.), *New Perspectives on Historical Writing* (Philadelphia, PA: Pennsylvania State University Press), 206–32.

Potter, D. (1993), 'Martyrdom as Spectacle', in R. Scodel (ed.), *Theater and Society in the Classical World* (Ann Arbor, MI: University of Michigan Press), 53–88.

Prioux, É. (2013), 'Emotions in Ecphrasis and Art Criticism', in D. LaCourse Munteanu (ed.), *Emotions, Genre, and Gender in Classical Antiquity* (London: Bloomsbury), 135–74.

Prost, F. and Wilgaux, J. (2006), *Penser et représenter le corps dans l'antiquité: actes du colloque international de Rennes, 1–4 septembre 2004* (Rennes: Presses Universitaires de Rennes).

Quet, M. (1993), 'Parler de soi pour louer son dieu: le cas d'Aelius Aristide', in M. Baslez, P. Hoffman, and L. Pernot (eds.), *L'invention d'autobiographie d'Hésiode à Saint Augustin* (Études de Littérature Ancienne 5; Paris: Presses de l'École Normale Supérieure), 211–51.

Reardon, B. (1991), *The Form of Greek Romance* (Princeton, NJ: Princeton University Press).

Reardon, B. (1993), 'L'autobiographie à l'epoque de la Seconde Sophistique: Quelques conclusions', in M. Baslez, P. Hoffman, and L. Pernot (eds.), *L'invention d'autobiographie d'Hésiode à Saint Ausgustin* (Études de Littérature Ancienne 5; Paris: Presses de l'École Normale Supérieure), 279–84.

Reardon, B. (1994), 'Achilles Tatius and the Ego-Narrative', in J. Morgan and R. Stoneman (eds.), *Greek Fiction: The Greek Novel in Context* (London: Routledge), 80–96.

Reeves, B. (2007), 'The Role of the *Ekphrasis* in Plot Development: The Painting of Europa and the Bull in Achilles Tatius' *Leucippe and Clitophon*', *Mnemosyne*, 60 (1), 87–101.

Reinhardt, T. (2011), 'Galen on Unsayable Properties', *Oxford Studies in Ancient Philosophy*, 40, 297–317.

Renehan, R. (1981), 'The Greek Anthropocentric View of Man', *Harvard Studies in Classical Philology*, 85, 239–59.

Repath, I. (2005), 'Achilles Tatius' *Leucippe and Cleitophon*: What Happened Next?', *Classical Quarterly*, 55 (1), 250–65.

Repath, I. (2007), 'Emotional Conflict and Platonic Psychology in the Greek Novel', in J. Morgan and M. Jones (eds.), *Philosophical Presences in the Ancient Novel* (Ancient Narrative Supplementum 10; Groningen: Barkhuis), 53–84.

Repath, I. (2013), 'Yours Truly?: Letters in Achilles Tatius', in O. Hodkinson, P. Rosenmeyer, and E. Bracke (eds.), *Epistolary Narratives in Ancient Greek Literature* (Leiden: Brill), 237–62.

Rey, R. (1992), 'Les significations de la douleur dans le monde grec antique', in B. Claverie, D. Le Bars, N. Zavialoff, and R. Dantzer (eds.), *Douleurs, sociétés, personne et expressions* (Paris: Eschel), 179–96.

Rey, R. (1995), *The History of Pain*, trans. L. Wallace, J. Cadden, and S. Cadden (Cambridge, MA: Harvard University Press).

Riches, D. (ed.) (1986), *The Anthropology of Violence* (Oxford: Blackwell).

Richlin, A. (ed.) (1992), *Pornography and Representation in Greece and Rome* (Oxford: Oxford University Press).

Richter, S. (1992), *Laocoon's Body and the Aesthetics of Pain: Winckelmann, Lessing, Herder, Moritz, Goethe* (Detroit, MI: Wayne State University Press).

Riese, W. (1968), 'The Structure of Galen's Diagnostic Reasoning', *Bulletin of the New York Academy of Medicine*, 44 (7), 778–91.

Rimell, V. (2002), *Petronius and the Anatomy of Fiction* (Cambridge: Cambridge University Press).

Robiano, P. (2007), 'La voix et la main: La lettre intime dans *Chéréas et Callirhoé*', in V. Rimell (ed.), *Seeing Tongues, Hearing Scripts: Orality and Representation in the Ancient Novel* (Ancient Narrative Supplementum 7; Groningen: Barkhuis), 201–22.

Roby, C. (2015), 'Galen on the Patient's Role in Pain Diagnosis: Sensation, Consensus, and Metaphor', in G. Petridou and C. Thumiger (eds.), *Homo Patiens: Approaches to the Patient in the Ancient World* (Leiden: Brill), 304–22.

Rocca, J. (2003), *Galen on the Brain: Anatomical Knowledge and Physiological Speculation in the Second Century* AD (Leiden: Brill).

Rocca, J. (2008), 'Anatomy', in R. J. Hankinson (ed.), *The Cambridge Companion to Galen* (Cambridge: Cambridge University Press), 242–62.

Rohde, E. (1876), *Der griechische Roman und seine vorläufer* (Leipzig: Breitkopf and Härtel).

Romeyer Dherbey, G. (1996), 'La construction de la théorie aristotélicienne du sentir', in C. Viano and G. Romeyer Dherbey (eds.), *Corps et âme, sur le De anima d'Aristote* (Paris: J. Vrin), 127–47.

Romeyer Dherbey, G. and Gourinat, J.-B. (2005), *Les Stoïciens* (Paris: J. Vrin).

Roselli, A. (2001), 'Le doti del medico nella cura delle malattie croniche: Aretaeus III, 1, 2 (p. 36, 11–13 Hude)', in A. Debru, N. Palmieri, and B. Jacquinod (eds.), *'Docente Natura': Mélanges de médecine ancienne et médiévale offerts à Guy Sabbah* (Saint-Étienne: Publications de l'Université de Saint-Étienne), 247–55.

Roselli, A. (2004a), 'Galen and the Ambiguity of Written Language: The 'De captionibus' and the Commentaries on Hippocrates', in R. Petrilli and D. Gambarara (eds.), *Actualité des anciens sur la théorie du langage* (Materialien zur Geschichte der Sprachwissenschaft und der Semiotik 14; Munster: Nodus), 51–63.

Roselli, A. (2004b), 'Les éditions d'Arétée de Cappadoce et le commentaire de Pierre Petit', in V. Boudon, G. Guy Cobolet, H. Ferreira-Lopes, and A. Guardasole (eds.), *Lire les médecins grecs à la Renaissance* (Paris: de Boccard), 99–112.

Roselli, A. (2004c), 'Les malades d'Arétée de Cappadoce', in J. Jouanna and J. Leclant (eds.), *Colloque La médecine grecque antique* (Paris: de Boccard), 163–76.

Roselli, A. (2005), 'I malati e il medico: il caso di Areteo di Cappadocia', *Temi di medicina antica*, 1, 27–34.

Rosenmeyer, P. (2001), *Ancient Epistolary Fictions: The Letter in Greek Literature* (Cambridge: Cambridge University Press).

Roskam, G. and Van der Stockt, L. (eds.) (2011), *Virtues for the People: Aspects of Plutarchan Ethics* (Leuven: Leuven University Press).
Russell, D. (1968), 'On Reading Plutarch's *Moralia*', *Greece and Rome*, 15 (2), 130–46.
Sacks, O. (1998), *The Man Who Mistook His Wife for a Hat and Other Clinical Tales* (New York: Touchstone).
Sandbach, F. H. (1971), 'Phantasia Katalēptikē', in A. A. Long (ed.), *Problems in Stoicism* (London: Athlone Press), 9–21.
Scarborough, J. (1981), 'The Galenic Question', *Sudhoffs Archiv*, 65, 1–30.
Scarry, E. (1985), *The Body in Pain: The Making and Unmaking of the World* (Oxford: Oxford University Press).
Schäffer, E. (1941), 'Aus Galens schrift: Über die verschiedenheiten des Pulses. Beurteilung der lehren des Archigenes, Athenaios, Magnus, Moschion und Apollonius. Übersetzung und Kommentar aus Claudius Galenus gleichnamigem Werk' (Diss. Med.; Munich).
Schlange-Schöningen, H. (2003), *Die römische Gesellschaft bei Galen: Biographie und sozialgeschichte* (Berlin: De Gruyter).
Schmidt, T. and Fleury, P. (eds.) (2011), *Perceptions of the Second Sophistic and its Times—Regards sur la Seconde Sophistique et son époque* (Toronto: University of Toronto Press).
Schmitz, T. (1997), *Bildung und Macht: zur sozialen und politischen Funktion der zweiten Sophistik in der griechischen Welt der Kaiserzeit* (Munich: C. H. Beck).
Schröder, H. (1987), 'Das Odysseusbild des Ailios Aristides', *Rheinisches Museum*, 130 (3/4), 350–6.
Schweitzer, B. (1934), 'Mimesis und Phantasia', *Philologus*, 89 (3), 286–300.
Sedley, D. N. (2005), 'La définition de la 'Phantasia Katalêptikê' par Zénon', in G. Romeyer Dherbey and J.-B. Gourinat (eds.), *Les Stoïciens* (Paris: J. Vrin), 75–92.
Semenzato, C. (2006), 'Muses, *enthousiasmos* et *phantasia* chez Plutarque', *Incontri triestini di filologia classica*, 4, 291–300.
Shapiro, M. (1988), *The Politics of Representation: Writing Practices in Autobiography, Photography, and Policy Analysis* (Madison, WI: Wisconsin University Press).
Shaw, B. (1996), 'Body/Power/Identity: Passions of the Martyrs', *Journal of Early Christian Studies*, 4 (3), 269–312.
Shelton, J.-A. (1996), 'Lucretius on the Use and Abuse of Animals', *Eranos*, 94 (1), 48–64.
Siegel, R. (1970), *Galen On Sense Perception: His Doctrines, Observations and Experiments on Vision, Hearing, Smell, Touch and Pain, and their Historical Sources* (Basel: S Karger).
Sihvola, J. (1996), 'Emotional Animals: Do Aristotelian Emotions Require Beliefs?', *Apeiron*, 29 (2), 105–44.

Singer, P. N. (1997), 'Levels of Explanation in Galen', *Classical Quarterly*, 47 (2), 525–42.
Slater, N. W. (1997), 'Vision, Perception and Phantasia in the Roman Novel', in M. Picone and B. Zimmermann (eds.), *Der antike Roman und seine mittelalterliche Rezeption* (Basle: Birkhäuser), 89–105.
Sluiter, I. (1995a), 'The Embarrassment of Imperfection: Galen's Assessment of Hippocrates' Linguistic Merits', in P. van der Eijk, H. Horstmanshoff, and P. Schrijvers (eds.) (1995), *Ancient Medicine in Its Socio-Cultural Context 2* (Amsterdam: Rodopi), 519–35.
Sluiter, I. (1995b), 'The Poetics of Medicine', in J. Abbenes, S. Slings, and I. Sluiter (eds.), *Greek Literary Theory after Aristotle: A Collection of Papers in Honour of D. M. Schenkeveld* (Amsterdam: Vanderbilt University Press), 193–213.
Sluiter, I. and Rosen, R. (eds.) (2012), *Aesthetic Value in Classical Antiquity* (Leiden: Brill).
Solmsen, F. (1957), 'The Vital Heat, the Inborn Pneuma and the Aether', *The Journal of Hellenic Studies*, 77 (1), 119–23.
Solmsen, F. (1961), 'Greek Philosophy and the Discovery of the Nerves', *Museum Helveticum*, 18 (3), 150–67.
Sontag, S. (2003), *Regarding the Pain of Others* (New York: St Martin's Press).
Sorabji, R. (1993a), 'Animal Minds', *The Southern Journal of Philosophy*, 31, 1–18.
Sorabji, R. (1993b), *Animal Minds and Human Morals: The Origins of the Western Debate* (Ithaca, NY: Cornell University Press).
Sorabji, R. (1997), 'Esprits d'animaux', in B. Cassin, J.-L. Labarrière, and G. Romeyer Dherbey (eds.), *L'animal dans l'antiquité* (Paris: J. Vrin), 355–73.
Sorabji, R. (2002), *Emotion and Peace of Mind: From Stoic Agitation to Christian Temptation* (Oxford: Oxford University Press).
Squire, M. (2009), *Image and Text in Graeco-Roman Antiquity* (New York: Cambridge University Press).
Squire, M. (2011a), 'Reading a View: Poem and Picture in the *Greek Anthology*', *Ramus*, 39 (2), 73–103.
Squire, M. (2011b), *The Art of the Body: Antiquity and its Legacy* (London: I. B. Tauris).
Squire, M. (2013), 'Apparitions Apparent: Ekphrasis and the Parameters of Vision in the Elder Philostratus's *Imagines*', *Helios*, 40 (1–2), 97–141.
Stannard, J. (1964), 'Materia Medica and Philosophic Theory in Aretaeus', *Sudhoffs Archiv für Geschichte der Medizin und Naturwissenschaften*, 48, 27–53.
Steiner, G. (2009), 'Plutarch on the Question of Justice for Animals', *Ploutarchos*, 7, 73–82.

Sternberg, R. H. (2005a), 'The Nature of Pity', in R. H. Sternberg (ed.), *Pity and Power in Ancient Athens* (Cambridge: Cambridge University Press), 15–47.
Sternberg, R. H. (ed.) (2005b), *Pity and Power in Ancient Athens* (Cambridge: Cambridge University Press).
Stevens, B. (2008), 'Symbolic Language and Indexical Cries: A Semiotic Reading of Lucretius 5.1028-90', *American Journal of Philology*, 129 (4), 529–57.
Studtmann, P. H. (2004), 'Living Capacities and Vital Heat in Aristotle', *Ancient Philosophy*, 24 (2), 365–79.
Swain, S. (1996), *Hellenism and Empire: Language, Classicism, and Power in the Greek World*, AD 50–250 (Oxford: Oxford University Press).
Swain, S. (ed.) (1999), *Oxford Readings in the Greek Novel* (Oxford: Oxford University Press).
Swain, S., Harrison, S. J., and Elsner, J. (eds.) (2007), *Severan Culture* (Cambridge: Cambridge University Press).
Tagliabue, A. (2016), 'Aelius Aristides' *Sacred Tales*: A Study of the Creation of the "Narrative about Asclepius"', *Classical Antiquity*, 35 (1), 126–46.
Taylor, A. (1928), *A Commentary on Plato's* Timaeus (Oxford: Clarendon Press).
Temkin, O. (1971), *The Falling Sickness: A History of Epilepsy from the Greeks to the Beginnings of Modern Neurology* (Baltimore, MD: Johns Hopkins University Press).
Teodorsson, S.-T. (1989–96), *A Commentary on Plutarch's* Table Talks *I–III* (Goteborg: Acta Universitatis Gothoburgensis).
Thivel, A. and Zucker, A. (eds.) (2002), *Le normal et le pathologique dans la Collection hippocratique* (Nice: Faculté des Lettres, Arts et Sciences Humaines de Nice-Sophia Antipolis).
Throop, C. (2010), *Suffering and Sentiment: Exploring the Vicissitudes of Experience and Pain in Yap* (Berkeley, CA: University of California Press).
Tieleman, T. (1996), *Galen and Chrysippus on the Soul: Argument and Refutation in the* De placitis, *Books II–III* (Leiden: Brill).
Tieleman, T. (2003), 'Galen's Psychology', in J. Barnes and J. Jouanna (eds.), *Galien et la philosophie* (Geneve: Vandoeuvres), 131–61.
Townsend, P. (2011), 'Bonds of Flesh and Blood: Porphyry, Animal Sacrifice, and Empire', in J. W. Knust and Z. Várhelyi (eds.), *Ancient Mediterranean Sacrifice* (Oxford: Oxford University Press), 214–31.
Toye, D. (2000), 'Plutarch on Poetry, Prose, and Politeia', *The Ancient World*, 31 (2), 173–81.
Tsoukanelis, A. (1988), 'Concerning Archigenes and Galen: Correcting an Historical Error', *Bulletin of the History of Dentistry*, 36 (2), 87–90.
Tsouna, V. (1998), *The Epistemology of the Cyrenaic School* (Cambridge: Cambridge University Press).
Tümpel, K. (1893), 'Alkinou Apologos', *Philologus*, 52, 522–33.

Ullmann, M. (1978), *Rufus von Ephesos: Krankenjournale* (Wiesbaden: Harrassowitz).
Urmson, J. (1990), *The Greek Philosophical Vocabulary* (London: Duckworth).
van der Eijk, P., Horstmanshoff, H., and Schrijvers, P. (eds.) (1995), *Ancient Medicine in its Socio-Cultural Context 1-2* (Amsterdam: Rodopi).
Van der Stockt, L. (1990), 'L'Expérience esthétique de la mimèsis selon Plutarque', *Quaderni Urbinati di Cultura Classica*, 36 (3), 23–31.
Van der Stockt, L. (1992), *Twinkling and Twilight: Plutarch's Reflections on Literature* (Brussels: Paleis der Academiën (AWLSK)).
Van der Stockt, L., Titchener, F. B., Ingenkamp, H. G., and Pérez Jiménez, A. (eds.) (2010), *Gods, Daimones, Rituals, Myths and History of Religions in Plutarch's Works: Studies Devoted to Professor Frederick E. Brenk by the International Plutarch Society* (Malaga: Universidad de Málaga).
van Nuffelen, P. (2014), 'Galen, Divination and the Status of Medicine', *Classical Quarterly*, 64 (1), 337–52.
Vegetti, M. (1981), 'Modelli di medicina in Galeno', in V. Nutton (ed.), *Galen: Problems and Prospects* (London: Wellcome Institute for the History of Medicine), 47–63.
Vilborg, E. (1955), *Achilles Tatius, Leucippe and Clitophon* (Stockholm: Almqvist & Wiksell).
Villard, L. (2006), 'Vocabulaire et représentation de la douleur dans la Collection hippocratique', in F. Prost and J. Wilgaux (eds.), *Penser et représenter le corps dans l'antiquité* (Rennes: Presses Universitaires de Rennes), 61–78.
Vogliano, A. (1938), 'Un papiro di Achille Tazio', *Studi Italiani di Filologia Classica*, 15, 121–30.
von Staden, H. (1975), 'Experiment and Experience in Hellenistic Medicine', *Bulletin of the Institute of Classical Studies*, 22, 178–99.
von Staden, H. (1989), *Herophilus: The Art of Medicine in Early Alexandria* (Cambridge: Cambridge University Press).
von Staden, H. (1995a), 'Science as Text, Science as History: Galen on Metaphor' in P. van der Eijk, H. Horstmanshoff, and P. Schrijvers (eds.), *Ancient Medicine in Its Socio-Cultural Context 2* (Amsterdam: Rodopi), 499–518.
von Staden, H. (1995b), 'Anatomy as Rhetoric: Galen on Dissection and Persuasion', *Journal of the History of Medicine and Allied Sciences*, 50 (1), 47–66.
von Staden, H. (1997a), 'Galen and the "Second Sophistic"', in R. Sorabji (ed.), *Aristotle and After* (Bulletin of the Institute of Classical Studies Supplement 68; London: Institute of Classical Studies), 33–54.
von Staden, H. (1997b), 'Teleology and Mechanism: Aristotelian Biology and Early Hellenistic Medicine', in W. Kullmann and S. Föllinger (eds.), *Aristotelische Biologie: Intentionen, Methoden, Ergebnisse* (Stuttgart: Franz Steiner), 183–208.

von Staden, H. (2000), 'Body, Soul, and Nerves: Epicurus, Herophilus, Erasistratus, the Stoics, and Galen', in J. Wright and P. Potter (eds.), *Psyche and Soma: Physicians and Metaphysicians on the Mind-Body Problem from Antiquity to Enlightenment* (Oxford: Oxford University Press), 79–116.

Warren, J. (2013), 'Epicureans and Cyrenaics on Pleasure as a Pathos', in S. Marchand and F. Verde (eds.), *Épicurisme et scepticisme* (Rome: Sapienza Università Editrice), 127–44.

Watson, G. (1988a), 'Discovering the Imagination: Platonists and Stoics on Phantasia', in J. Dillon and A. A. Long (eds.), *The Question of Eclecticism: Studies in Later Greek Philosophy* (Berkely, CA: University of California Press), 208–33.

Watson, G. (1988b), *Phantasia in Classical Thought* (Galway: Galway University Press).

Waugh, P. (1984), *Metafiction: The Theory and Practice of Self-Conscious Fiction* (London: Routledge).

Webb, R. (1997a), 'Mémoire et imagination: Les limites de l'*enargeia* dans la théorie rhétorique grecque', in C. Lévy and L. Pernot (eds.), *Dire l'évidence: philosophie et rhétorique antiques* (Paris: L'Harmattan), 229–48.

Webb, R. (1997b), 'Imagination and the Arousal of the Emotions in Greco-Roman Rhetoric', in S. M. Braund and C. Gill (eds.), *The Passions in Roman Thought and Literature* (Cambridge: Cambridge University Press), 112–27.

Webb, R. (2006), 'The *Imagines* as a Fictional Text: Ekphrasis, *Apatê* and Illusion', in M. Costantini, F. Graziani, and S. Rolet (eds.), *Le défi de l'art: Philostrate, Callistrate, et l'image sophistique* (Rennes: Presses Universitaires de Rennes), 113–33.

Webb, R. (2009), *Ekphrasis, Imagination and Persuasion in Ancient Rhetorical Theory and Practice* (Farnham: Ashgate).

Weber, G. (1996), *Areteo di Cappadocia: interpretazioni e aspetti della formazione anatomo-patologica del Morgagni* (Florence: Olschki).

Weissberg, L. (1989), 'Language's Wound: Philoctetes and the Origin of Language', *MLN,* 104 (3), 548–79.

Wellbery, D. (1984), *Lessing's Laocoon: Semiotics and Aesthetics in the Age of Reason* (Cambridge: Cambridge University Press).

Wellmann, M. (1895a), 'Aretaios', *Paulys Realencyclopädie der classischen Altertumswissenschaft,* 2 (1), 669–70.

Wellmann, M. (1895b), 'Die Pneumatische Schule bis auf Archigenes', *Philologische Untersuchungen* (14; Berlin: Weidmann).

Whitmarsh, T. (2001), *Greek Literature and the Roman Empire: The Politics of Imitation* (Oxford: Oxford University Press).

Whitmarsh, T. (2002), 'Written on the Body: Ekphrasis, Perception, and Deception in Heliodorus' *Aethiopika*', in J. Elsner (ed.), *The Verbal and the*

Visual: Cultures of Ekphrasis in Antiquity (Bendigo, Victoria: Aureal Publications), 111–25.
Whitmarsh, T. (2003), 'Reading for Pleasure: Narrative, Irony and Erotics in Achilles Tatius', in S. Panayotakis, M. Zimmerman, and W. Keulen (eds.), *The Ancient Novel and Beyond* (Mnemosyne Supplementum 241; Leiden: Brill), 191–205.
Whitmarsh, T. (2004), 'Aelius Aristides', in I. de Jong, R. Nünlist, and A. Bowie (eds.), *Narrators, Narratives, and Narratees in Ancient Greece* (Leiden: Brill), 441–7.
Whitmarsh, T. (ed.) (2008), *The Cambridge Companion to the Greek and Roman Novel* (Cambridge: Cambridge University Press).
Whitmarsh, T. (2011), *Narrative and Identity in the Ancient Greek Novel: Returning Romance* (Cambridge: Cambridge University Press).
Whitmarsh, T. (2013), *Beyond the Second Sophistic: Adventures in Greek Postclassicism* (Berkeley, CA: University of California Press).
Wilkins, J. (2008), 'Animals in the Romano-Greek Culture of the Second Century A.D.', in A. Alexandridis (ed.), *Mensch und Tier in der Antike: Grenzziehung und Grenzüberschreitung* (Wiesbaden: Reichert), 315–28.
Willis, W. H. (1984), 'Identifying and Editing a Papyrus of Achilles Tatius by Computer', in M. Gigante (ed.), *Atti del xvii Congresso Internazionale di Papirologia 1* (Naples: Centro Internazionale per lo Studio dei Papiri Ercolanesi), 163–6.
Willis, W. H. (1990), 'The Robinson-Cologne Papyrus of Achilles Tatius', *Greek, Roman and Byzantine Studies,* 31, 73–102.
Wilson, L. G. (1959), 'Erasistratus, Galen, and the Pneuma', *Bulletin of the History of Medicine,* 33, 293–314.
Winkler, J. (1980), 'Lollianos and the Desperadoes', *Journal of Hellenic Studies,* 100, 155–81.
Winkler, J. (1985), *Auctor and Actor: A Narratological Reading of Apuleius's The Golden Ass* (Berkeley, CA: University of California Press).
Wöhrle, G. (1990), 'Die medizinische Theorie in Lukians Abdicatus (lib. 54)', *Medizin-Historisches Journal,* 25, 104–14.
Woolf, C. (2007), 'Deconstructing Pain: A Deterministic Dissection of the Molecular Basis of Pain', in S. Coakley and K. Shelemay (eds.), *Pain and Its Transformations: The Interface of Biology and Culture* (Cambridge, MA: Harvard University Press), 27–35.
Worthington, I. (ed.) (2007), *A Companion to Greek Rhetoric* (Oxford: Blackwell).
Wright, J. P. and Potter, P. (eds.) (2000), *Psyche and Soma: Physicians and Metaphysicians on the Mind-Body Problem from Antiquity to Enlightenment* (Oxford: Oxford University Press).
Wyke, M. (ed.) (1998), *Gender and the Body in Mediterranean Antiquity* (Oxford: Blackwell).

Wyke, M. (ed.) (1998), *Parchments of Gender: Deciphering the Bodies of Antiquity* (Oxford: Clarendon).
Zanker, G. (1981), 'Enargeia in the Ancient Criticism of Poetry', *Rheinisches Museum für Philologie,* 124, 297–311.
Zanker, G. (2004), *Modes of Viewing in Hellenistic Poetry and Art* (Madison, WI: University of Wisconsin Press).
Zeitlin, F. (1996), *Playing the Other: Gender and Society in Classical Greek Literature* (Chicago: University of Chicago Press).
Zeitlin, F. (2001), 'Visions and Revisions of Homer', in S. Goldhill (ed.), *Being Greek under Rome: Cultural Identity, the Second Sophistic and the Development of Empire* (Cambridge: Cambridge University Press), 195–266.
Zeitlin, F. (2012), 'Gendered Ambiguities, Hybrid Formations, and the Imaginary Body in Achilles Tatius', in M. Pinheiro, M. Skinner, and F. Zeitlin (eds.), *Narrating Desire: Eros, Sex, and Gender in the Ancient Novel* (Berlin: De Gruyter), 105–26.

General Index

Aisthēsis (/*aisthēteria*) 12, 39, 45, 47, 50, 52, 53n25, 57, 59, 68, 68n3, 71nn7, 9, 79, 79n27, 85, 86n40, 93, 190, 223, 238, 241
ἄλγημα (*algēma*; 'pain') 16n45, 55, 55n28, 56n29, 78n24, 79n28, 81, 83, 132n11
ἄλγος (*algos*; 'pain') 47, 51n22, 74, 177, 177n6, 178n7, 188, 199, 200–1, 202, 230
Amazement (/shock/*explēxis*): *see* Emotions
Anatomico-aesthetic model of the body 12, 16, 17, 237
Anatomy 15, 16, 34–5, 35nn5–7, 36, 51–3, 56–8, 107, 109, 130, 131, 136, 219, 238–40
 (Classical) 13, 13nn30–2
 (dissections, performances, and demonstration) 14, 15nn36–7, 39, 70n6, 144–8, 167
 (Hellenistic) 14, 14nn33–4, 78
 (and pain symptoms) 35n6, 36, 52, 53, 56, 57–8, 66, 77, 79, 103, 201
 (as system of knowledge) 13, 13nn30–2, 14, 14nn33–4, 22, 34–5, 51–2, 56, 68–9, 69n4, 77, 78, 96, 99, 100, 101–2
 (and viewing) 15, 15nn37–9, 144–8, 164, 164n7, 165, 165n8, 168, 172, 200–1, 201n25, 209–10
Animals (and pain) 13, 15, 15n39, 48, 62–3, 124, 217–31
ἀνώδυνος (*anōdunos*; 'without pain') 54
Antilokhos 178n7, 179, 182–4
ἀπονίη (*aponiē*; 'without pain') 52, 53, 61, 64, 65
ἄπονος (*aponos*; 'without pain') 47, 53n24, 85, 86
Aretaios (of Kappodokia)
 (connection with Arkhigenes) 44, 44n3, 57
 (life) 43–4
 (and nosological tradition) 44
 (pneumatism) 43n2

Aristeides, Ailios
 (importance) 129, 129nn2–4
 (life) 129
 (rejected by modern scholars) 129, 129n5
Aristippos 47, 48n12
Aristotle 12–13, 25, 25n61, 26, 35, 35n5, 48n16, 49, 72n12, 94, 161, 161n3, 173
Arkhigenes (of Apamea) 42, 43n2, 44, 44n3, 57, 77, 77n21, 79, 79nn25, 27–8, 80n28, 81, 81n31, 83–4, 84n36, 85, 85n37, 86, 86n38, 87, 134, 144
Arthritis 46–9, 116, 164
Asklepieia 33
 (at Pergamon) 132, 146n44
Asklepios 108, 113, 130, 132, 139, 146, 147–50

Beauty 16, 16n44, 120–1, 173, 174, 179, 180–2, 184–5, 187, 189n19, 190–1, 194, 194n7, 195, 199, 199n23, 207, 207n33, 235, 236
Bravery 60–3

Case-history 38, 41n22, 69nn5–6, 89n46, 90, 90n50, 91, 91nn50, 53, 92, 93, 95, 98n63, 99, 138, 138n23, 139, 142–4
Christian culture 3, 5, 9, 26–30, 166–7, 193n1, 194n8, 195, 195n9, 236, 242

Demokritos 13, 48, 48n14, 73
Desensitization 221–4
Desire *See* Emotions
Despair *See* Emotions
Diagnosis 44, 103–4, 140, 141, 145, 237, 238
 (and narrative) 37–42, 68–9, 79, 80–8, 90–101
 (and pain types) 50–1, 53–5, 79, 83–7, 96–7
 (as rational categorisation) 7–8, 39, 44, 68, 76–8

General Index

Divine healing 34, 41, 108, 113, 136, 138n23, 139–41, 146, 151, 153
Divine punishment 5, 123–4, 172, 172n29, 198, 203, 205

Ekphrasis 162, 163, 165, 170, 170n20, 175, 175n2, 177n7, 178, 179, 181, 183, 187, 195, 195n11, 196n14, 198–203, 205–7, 214, 228–32
Emotions
  (desire) 24, 89, 111–12, 124, 163, 171, 171n24, 173–4, 179–83, 192, 202, 215, 231, 234, 235, 239
  (despair) 23, 62, 151, 153, 154, 155
  (distress) (See also λύπη) 19, 24, 24n58, 25n61, 26, 58, 64–5, 66, 75, 89, 111, 161, 164, 165, 169, 172, 177n6, 178, 179, 181–3, 184, 189, 191, 196, 200, 202, 204, 208, 209, 210, 213, 215, 218, 219n6, 221, 222, 230, 231, 236, 241
  (emotional *aporia*) 170, 196, 206–7, 208, 208n37, 209, 210, 215
  (fear) 23, 62, 89, 152, 169, 171n24, 172, 172n29, 173, 173n31, 181, 181n12, 199, 199n23, 202
  (hope) 23, 62, 123, 151–3, 202–3, 234
  (as part of pain experience) 10, 21–6, 58–64, 89–90, 92, 97, 151–4, 169–74, 177–8, 178n7, 182, 184, 189–90, 202, 214
  (philanthropy) 22
  (pity) 22, 24, 24n59, 25, 25nn61–2, 62, 64, 65, 90, 116–19, 164, 171, 171n24, 173, 173n32, 179, 187, 192, 196, 200, 202, 203, 210–12, 214, 215, 230, 236, 240, 241
  (pleasure) 24–6, 26n64, 27, 28, 60, 65, 71, 71n9, 127, 152, 162–4, 172, 174, 177, 177n6, 179–85, 189–92, 204, 208, 214–15, 218, 219, 220–4, 230, 231, 235–6, 241
  (shock/amazement/*ekplēxis*) 24, 63, 69n6, 90, 90n48, 171, 171n24, 172, 173n31, 197, 206, 207, 207nn32–3, 218, 221, 224, 225, 230, 231
ἐπιπόνος (*epiponos*; 'painful') 51n22
Erasistratos 14, 35, 51, 57, 78, 78n23, 95, 95n61

Fear: *See* Emotions
Foucault, Michel

  (and *Care of the Self*) 26–7, 27nn65–6, 68, 28, 30
  (and *Discipline and Punish*) 166, 166n10, 194, 194nn5–6

Galen
  (anatomical writings) 68–9
  (connection with Arkhigenes) 77–87
  (importance at Rome) 69n5
  (life) 67n1
  (and method of diagnosis) 8, 38–9, 68–9, 98–101
Gout (/*Podagra*)
  (condition) 17n45, 115, 115n1, 116, 116nn2–3, 5, 117, 121–7, 157–8
  (Lucianic work) 121–7
  (Personified deity) 122, 127

Heroes/Heroism 2, 2n4, 60, 60n34, 61, 63, 107, 110, 111, 115, 118–21, 124, 125, 130–1, 148, 150, 151–5, 177, 179, 180, 182, 183, 187
Herophilos 14, 35, 35n7, 51, 99
Hippokrates 7n19, 8n20, 12, 12n27, 24n59, 34, 34n4, 35, 35n5, 40, 41n22, 44n6, 47–8, 48n16, 49, 50–1, 51n21, 55n27, 59, 61, 69n6, 71, 71n8, 73, 73n14, 80n29, 88, 88n43, 89n46, 90n50, 91n50, 94, 123, 132–3, 133n15
Hope *See* Emotions

Images of pain (historical) 161n3, 198, 200n24

Khrysippos 48n12, 49, 49n17
Kleinman, Arthur 18–19, 37, 38, 38nn9–11, 39–41, 162n4, 169n17
Kleitophon 196–8, 214, 215, 234
  (and emotional *aporia*) 206–8, 209, 212–14
  (and viewing Leukippe) 204n29, 205–14
  (and viewing Prometheus) 199–203

Lacan, Jacques 235
Laokoon (all spellings) 1, 1n1, 2, 2nn2–5, 3–5
Lessing, Gotthold 1, 1n1, 2–5
Leukippe 29, 29n75, 193, 193n3, 194, 194nn4, 7–8, 195, 198, 199, 203–14
Leukippe and Kleitophon 193–5

General Index

λύπη ('distress'/'grief')
  See also Emotions (distress) 25n61,
  89, 122, 161n3, 200, 208, 209

Marsyas 5, 205
Martyrdom 5, 166, 167, 242
Menoikeus 179–82, 184, 185
Mulvey, Laura 235
Mystery cult 125–6, 151, 152n60

Narrative medicine 37–44

ὀδύνη (*odunē*; 'pain') 16n45, 34n4, 45n8,
  51n22, 55–6, 59, 60, 64–5, 71n8, 75,
  96–7, 132, 132n11, 133, 221
Odysseus 110–12, 136, 148, 148n51, 149

Pain
  (and *duskrasia*) 47–9, 74, 74n16
  (and external causes) 10, 46–8, 74–6
  (modern approaches to) 5–7
  (as movement or change) 47–8, 71–3
  (as perception of movement or
    change) 48n12, 71–4
  (and Western intellectual
    tradition) 1–5
Pain Experience
  (definition of) 10–11
Pain as ineffable 81, 82, 82n34, 83n35,
  84–6, 86n38, 143–4, 144n35
Pain and Language 17–21
  (and diagnosis) 37–42, 50–2, 76–88,
    96–9, 103–4
  (and patient language/narrative) 36,
    37–42, 52, 58, 76–88, 101, 103–4,
    120–1, 126–7, 137–51, 211–15, 225–8
  (scientific terms for) 50–2, 55–6,
    83–8, 132–6
  (screams) 2, 2n4, 4, 18, 20, 111, 112,
    112n10, 126, 126n32, 127, 143,
    154–5, 168, 181, 183, 188, 188n18,
    189, 206, 221, 222, 233
  See also Tragedy (and lamentation)
Pantheia 179, 184–92
Philoktetes 1, 2, 2n4, 4, 108n2, 110, 111,
  112, 112n10, 119–21, 125, 161,
  161n1
Philostratos
  (the *Imagines*) 175–6, 176–92
  (importance for Imperial
    culture) 175, 175n1
  (works) 175

Pity See Emotions
Plato 12, 12n27, 48, 71, 72n12, 92n54,
  120, 149, 180, 181
Pleasure
  (as emotion): See Emotions
  (as perception) 46, 71n9, 116–19, 219,
    219n6
Plutarch (of Khaironea)
  On Flesh-Eating 217, 217nn1–2,
    218–31
  (views on animals) 217n2
πόνος (*ponos*; 'pain') 46, 46n9, 47,
  50n19, 51n22, 53, 53n25, 54, 54n27,
  55, 55nn27, 28, 59, 61, 64, 71, 83,
  84n36, 117, 124, 200, 202
Prometheus 198–203, 204, 205, 206,
  208, 210, 211

Religion/religious experience 8n20,
  28n71, 33, 34n3, 107, 110, 113,
  113n12, 114, 120, 121–2, 125–6,
  127, 138–9, 142, 145, 145n40,
  152, 152n60 167
Rufus (of Ephesos) 14n34, 35, 40, 42,
  42n23, 91n50, 98n63, 115, 115n1, 123

Scarry, Elaine 2n5, 4, 4n10, 17, 17n47,
  18, 18nn49–51, 21, 112n10, 239,
  239n1
Sensory Perception
  (and affective response) 21–6
  (and language) 17–21
  (modern approaches to) 6, 6n14, 7
  (perception, process of) 10–13,
    13n28, 34–7, 45–9, 53–4, 56–7, 58,
    60, 66, 70–6, 77, 79, 79n27, 82–5,
    86n40, 89, 103, 109, 110–11,
    131–6, 153, 157–8, 164–5, 167,
    168n16, 190, 201, 219, 219n6,
    234, 237, 238, 241
Shock (/amazement/*explēxis*): See
  Emotions
Sontag, Susan 2n5, 4–5, 5n11–13
Soranos 50n20, 55
Suffering 1–5, 7, 9, 17, 18, 19, 25, 28,
  29, 30, 38, 54, 62, 85, 87, 108, 110,
  111, 118, 121, 123, 124, 136, 141,
  151, 166, 167, 206, 212, 212nn45–6,
  213, 214, 218, 220, 226, 228, 231,
  234, 236
  (Christian concern with) 9, 28–30
  (as metaphor) 9

συμμετρία ('symmetry'/'proportion') 16, 16nn41–3, 165, 180, 183, 187, 189, 189n19

Tatios, Akhilleus 193, 193n1
Theophrastos 48
Torture 5, 19, 29, 29n75, 30, 30n78, 166, 166nn10, 12, 167, 179, 193–4, 198, 202, 203–13, 218, 223, 225, 225n13, 226, 228, 238
Tragedy 1, 7n19, 17, 57, 63n37, 77, 167
  (and lamentation) 121, 126, 155, 183, 188, 197, 197n17, 209, 209n39, 210, 212n45
  (and language) 17, 121, 121n16, 125–6, 126n32, 153–4, 187, 188, 188n18, 197, 197n17, 210, 210n42
  (reception of) 65, 107, 108, 108nn1–2, 109–13, 115, 118, 119, 121–7, 154, 157–8, 174, 196–7, 204, 207–10, 234
  (Trauma) 10, 46, 131, 134, 136, 140, 140n28, 143, 161–6, 169–70, 171, 171n24, 174–7, 177n6, 179, 182, 183, 184, 186–9, 191–2, 194, 194n8, 195–8, 201, 202, 203–4, 206, 208, 210–11, 213, 215, 217, 218–20, 225, 227, 230, 231, 233–5, 238, 240

Viewing 14–17, 24, 24n58, 63–5, 152, 161–2, 163, 164–9, 233–6, 241
  (the anatomized body) 14–16, 144–8, 199–202, 204–7, 209, 228–9
  (the sick body) 63–5, 98, 151, 161–2, 164–5
  (*sophos theatēs*) 170–1
  (viewing artistic representations of the sick) 24–6, 161–2
  See also anatomico-aesthetic model; anatomy; ekphrasis, desire, distress, pleasure

Winckelmann, Johann 1–2, 2nn2–5, 3–5
Wound 14, 47, 96, 119, 162, 163, 166, 167–8, 168n16, 169, 174, 179, 181, 182, 183, 184, 186, 188, 189, 190, 192, 200–2, 202n26, 203, 206, 215, 223, 225, 227, 229, 231, 233–5

Index Locorum

AILIAN
On the Nature of Animals (NA.)
vii.38   63n37

AILIOS ARISTEIDES
17.18K	120
28.130	120n13
47.1K	148, 153n61
47.2K	139, 142n32
47.2–3	41n21
47.3K	136, 138
47.4K	139, 145, 164n7
47.55K	146, 147
47.62	132n11
47.68K	211n44
47.75	146n44
48.1K	143
48.2K	145, 145n39
48.6K	137n22, 144n36
48.9K	129n4
48.10K	145n40
48.23K	144n35, 152n58
48.31K	146
48.36K	146
48.38K	152n58
48.38–9K	153–4
48.39K	135
48.42K	149
48.49K	144, 151
48.56K	138n25
48.57K	132, 133
48.59K	141
48.60K	149
48.62K	133, 144n36
48.63K	133, 137, 137n21, 153
48.64–5K	149n54
48.68K	137
48.69K	141
48.70K	136n19
48.73K	152n58
48.75K	144n36
49.1K	137n21
49.13K	152n58
49.16	132n11, 137n21
49.17K	143, 144, 144n38
49.40K	150
49.44K	136n19
49.46K	144n36
49.48K	146n44
50.2K	152n58
50.7K	151–2
50.8K	151
50.14K	143n34
50.17K	143n34
50.20K	138n25
50.21K	146n44

AISKHYLOS
Agamemnon (Ag.)
209	63n37
1057	63n37
1092	63n37
1096	63n37
1278	63n37
1389	63n37
1433	63n37
1599	63n37

Libation Bearers (Ch.)
548	227n18
926	209n39

AKHILLEUS TATIOS
i.2.2	208n36
i.4	194n7
i.4.4	167n15, 207n33
i.4.5	207n33
i.9–10	194n4
i.10.4	207n33
ii.35–8	194n4
iii.2.5.1	136n20
iii.7.2–3	199n23
iii.8.1–5	199–200
iii.8.7	202
iii.10	209n39
iii.11.1	208n37, 209n39
iii.14–15	194n4
iii.15.4–5	205
iii.15.5–6	206

Index Locorum

AKHILLEUS TATIOS (*cont.*)
iii.15.6	207n33
iii.16	204
iii.16.1	208
iii.17	208
iii.17.2	208
iii.16.3	209
iv.14.5	207n33
v.7	194n4
v.17.3	211
v.17.6–7	211
v.18.2	212
v.18.3	212
v.18.4	212
v.18.5	212
v.18.6	212n46
v.19.6	213
v.23.5	207n33
vi.20–2	29n75
vi.21–2	194n4
vii.8.1	207n33
viii.1.2	195n9
viii.5.14	211n44
viii.6	194n4
viii.6.14–15	195n9
viii.11	194n4
viii.12.5–7	195n9
viii.13.2	195n9

ANTHOLOGIA PALATINA
ix.203	29n76
xi.414	116n4
xvi.111	120n12, 161n1
xvi.112	120n12

ARETAIOS
Causes and Signs of Acute Diseases (SA.)
i.	44n7
i.5.4.3	63n38
i.6.1.1	51n22
i.6.7.5	51n22
i.6.8.5–6	64n39
i.6.8.6	164n6
i.6.8.6–9.7	64, 109, 109n4
i.7.2.9	51n22
i.7.4.5–6	51n22
i.7.5.8	50n19
i.9.1.8	54
i.9.5.1–2	54
i.10.2.1	55
i.10.2.4–6	55
i.10.5.2	55
ii.1.2.5–6	52
ii.1.2.6–9	53n24
ii.2.9.6	50n19
ii.2.15.3–4	53n25
ii.2.16.1–2	53
ii.2.17	124n22
ii.2.17.6–7	62, 64n40
ii.2.17.7–8	62
ii.2.17.7–11	110n6
ii.2.17.9–11	63
ii.2.18.1–7	61–2, 109n4, 153n62
ii.3.5.1	50n19
ii.5.1.2–3	51n22
ii.4.8.3	57n31
ii.6.5.3	57n31
ii.7.3.4–5	50n19
ii.7.3.7	51n22
ii.7.3.9	51n22
ii.11.1.7	66n42
ii.12	116n2
ii.12.1.10	66n42
ii.12.4.3	51n22
ii.12.4.4	64n39

Causes and Signs of Chronic Diseases (SD.)
iii.1	44, 44n7, 62n36, 97n62
iii.1.1.1–2	59
iii.1.1.2-2.7	59–60, 152n59
iii.1.1.5	51n22
iii.2.1.1–5	52n23
iii.2.1.1–3	133n15
iii.2.1.2	46n8
iii.2.1.4–5	50n19
iii.2.2.9–10	51n22
iii.2.3.6	66n42
iii.2.3.6–7	64n40, 124n22
iii.4.1.4	52n23
iii.4.2.3	51n22
iii.4.3.3	64n39
iii.6.11.2–3	66n42
iii.13.6.3	51n22
iii.15.11.8	66n42
iv.1.9.6	64n40, 124n22
iv.2.1.7	51n22
iv.4.5.6	51n22
iv.4.8.2–3	52n23
iv.10	123n21
iv.12	17n45, 169n16

Index Locorum

iv.12.1.1–2	46n9, 117n7
iv.12.1.2–3	46n9
iv.12.1.6–7	46n9
iv.12.1.7–2.1	46n10
iv.12.2.2	46
iv.12.2.2–3	46
iv.12.3.1–2	46n11
iv.12.3.3	47
iv.12.3.4–5	47
iv.12.3.5–6	47
iv.12.3.6–7	47
iv.12.3.7–4.4	47
iv.13.8.2–3	50n19
iv.13.19.7	66n42
iv.13.20	44n5

On the Therapy of Acute Diseases (CA.)
v. praef.4	50n19
v.2.6.3	66n42
v.2.14.6	51n22
v.10.2.1–6	49n18
vi.5.1.10–11	64n40, 124n22
vi.8.6.2	51n22
vi.9.1.4	51n22
vi.11	49n18

On the Therapy of Chronic Diseases (CD.)
vii.4.1.2.	51n22

ARISTIPPOS
Frag. 197A	48n12

ARISTOTLE
On the Generation of Animals (GA.)
766a16–b13	48n16

On the Heavens (Mu.)
394b	94n59

On the Parts of Animals (PA.)
650a–b	48n16

On the Soul (de An.)
416b34–424b	13n28
416b28–9	48n16

On Youth and Old Age (Juv.)
469b1–20	48n16

Physics (Ph.)
226a–b	72n12

Poetics (Po.)
1448b10–12	26n63
1448b11–7	161n3

Rhetoric (Rh.)
1385b13–6	25n61

AULUS GELLIUS
2.26.1	116n3

CAELIUS ARELIANUS
On Chronic and Acute Diseases (CA.)
v.ii.43	17n45
v.ii.50–1	17n45

CELSUS
On Medicine (de Med.)
praef. 23–6	35n6
praef. 53–7	33n2

CHARITON
i.1.7	167n15
i.4.12	204n29, 210n41
viii.1.4	110n5

CICERO
On Ends (de Fin.)
ii.29	119

DEMOSTHENES
2.6	145n39
2.21	188n17
18.139	145n39
21.58	228n19

DIO (OF PRUSA)
1.25	173n31
16.2	169n17

DIOKLES
Frag. 165	13n32

DIONYSIOS (OF HALIKARNASSOS)
Roman Antiquities (Antiq. Rom.)
1.78.3	145n39

DIOSKOURIDES
ii.119.2	43n2

EMPEDOKLES
Frag. 154a	221n11

EPIKTETOS
Discourses
4.7.17	210n42

Encheiridon (Ench.)
1.1	172n26

ERASISTRATOS
  Frag. 293   95n61

EURIPIDES
Elektra (*El.*)
  824   225n13
Hekuba (*Hec.*)
  783   118n9
Hippolytos (*Hipp.*)
  1213   136n20
Phoinissai (*Ph.*)
  1449   208n38

FRONTO
Letters to Friends (*Amic.*)
  20   116n3
  34   116n3
  50   116n3

GALEN
The Best Doctor is also a Philosopher (*Opt. Med.*)
  i.53–63K   68n2
Introduction to the Sects (*Sect. Int.*)
  i.64–6K   68n2
Composition of the Art of Medicine (*CAM.*)
  i.274K   55–6
On the Art of Medicine (*Ars. Med.*)
  i.343.2K   16
On the Elements According to Hippocrates (*Hipp. Elem.*)
  i.418–9:   13n29, 74
  i.420K   74
On Temperaments (*Temp.*)
  i.565–6K: 16n41, 165n9
Natural Faculties (*Nat. Fac.*)
  ii.3K   72n12
  ii.89K   48–9
  ii.88–92K   48n15, 49n17
On Anatomical Procedures (*AA.*)
  ii.219K   15n39
  ii.220K   15n39
  ii.221–2K   15n39
  ii.223–4K   15n39
  ii.225K   15n39
  ii.282K   13n32
  ii.499K   145n42
  ii.603K   147n48
  ii.642–3K   15n37
  ii.652K   147n46
  ii.669K   15n38, 172n30
  ii.693K   172n30
  9.9   35n7
On the Anatomy of the Uterus (*Ut. Diss.*)
  ii.895–6K   35n7
Usefulness of Parts (*UP.*)
  iii.286–7K   69n5
  iii.631K   15n38
  iv.286K   210n42
On the Passions of the Soul (*Aff. Dig.*)
  v.19K   70n6
On the Opinions of Plato and Hippocrates (*PHP.*)
  v.543–4K   35n7
  v.636K   71, 71n9
  v.636–7K   12n27, 13n29, 48n12
On Hygiene (*San. Tu.*)
  vi.2K   16n42
  vi.7K   16n42
  vi.13K   16n42
  vi.278K   173n31
Properties of Food Stuffs (*Alim. Fac.*)
  vi.598–601K   91n52
On the Differences of Diseases (*Morb. Diff.*)
  vi.837–8K   72n10
On the Causes of Symptoms (*Caus. Symp.*)
  vii.115K   71, 71nn7–8
  vii.115–17K   12n27
  vii.116K   74n16
  vii.116–17K   74n15
  vii.117K   74n17
  vii.118K   75
  vii.119K   75
  vii.119–20K   75
  vii.175–7K   74n16
On the Differences of Symptoms (*Symp. Diff.*)
  vii.43K   72, 72n10
  vii.56–7K   74n15
On Affected Parts (*Loc. Aff.*)
  viii.1K   78n23
  viii.8K   98, 98n64
  viii.14K   69n4, 78n23

Index Locorum

viii.32K	72, 72nn11, 13	viii.629K	85n37
viii.56–7K	99, 99n65	viii.680K	83n35
viii.57K	99–101	viii.692K	83n35
viii.69K	78, 78n23		

On Crises (*Cris.*)

ix.554K	56n29
ix.682–3K	70n6
ix.756K	133n15

viii.69–70K	69n4, 79n26
viii.70K	78, 78n24, 80n28
viii.71–2K	134n17
viii.72K	79n27
viii.79K	35n5
viii.79–80K	79n26
viii.83K	79n26
viii.85K	79n26
viii.86K	55
viii.87K	76n19
viii.88–9K	80–1, 85, 86n38, 92, 110n7, 135n18, 142n31

Method of Healing (*MM.*)

x.71–5K	72n10
x.78–80K	72n10
x.232K	168n16, 202n26
x.382K	70n6
x.431K	132n12
x.636	49n17
x.676K	70n6
x.604K	82n33
x.731K	82n33
x.810K	82n33
x.814K	132n12
x.841K	132n12
x.854K	132n12

viii.89K	81n31
viii.89–90K	81n32
viii.100–1K	79n26
viii.101K	79n27
viii.103–4K	79n27
viii.108	55n29
viii.110K	83–4, 84n36
viii.111K	85, 145n43
viii.113K	41n20, 85
viii.114K	85
viii.116K	86, 86n39–40
viii.117K	81nn31–2, 86
viii.118K	87
viii.120K	79n27
viii.194K	92–3
viii.212K	14n34, 35n7
viii.212–3K	98
viii.213–14K	98–9
viii.231K	145n43
viii.293–6K	91n52
viii.301–2K	89n46, 92n55
viii.311K	145n43
viii.313K	145n43
viii.314K	145n43
viii.363–5K	70n6
viii.381K	145n43
viii.403K	132n12
viii.410K	145n43

On Simple Medicines (*SMT.*)

xii.312K	44n5

Composition of Drugs According to Kind (*Comp. Med. Gen.*)

xiii.599–601	14n35, 165n8

On Linguistic Sophisms (*Soph.*).

xiv.582K	80n29

On Prognosis (*Praen.*)

xiv.605–19K	69n5, 70n6
xiv.606K	139n27
xiv.606–7K	91n52
xiv.606-16K	67n1
xiv.609K	93n57
xiv.612–13K	67n1
xiv.621–4K	91n52
xiv.625–6K	15n37, 69n5
xiv.631–3K	70n6
xiv.631–4K	89n46
xiv.656–7K	70n6
xiv.657–61K	70n6
xiv.659K	93n57

On the Differences of Pulses (*Diff. Puls.*)

viii.508K	83n35
viii.525K	83n35
viii.572K	139n27

How to Detect Malingerers (*Sim. Morb.*)

xix.4K	95
xix.5K	79n25, 96
xix.6K	96–7

288 Index Locorum

GALEN (cont.)
Outline of Empiricism (*Subf. Emp.*)
  10   44n5
Commentary on Hippocrates Epidemics VI (*Hipp. Epid. VI.*)
  485.5–487.17   89n46
On Recognising the Best Physicians (*Opt. Med. Cogn.*)
  9.4–8   14n35
  9.6–7   15n37

HELIODOROS
  ii.3.5   204n29, 210n41
  viii.7.7   204n29, 210n41

HERMOGENES
On Styles (*Id.*)
  1.6.45–9   196n14
On the Pursuit of Intensity (*Meth.*)
  11.1–4   226n16

HERODOTOS
  2.57   226n14
  3.66   188n18
  3.132   228n19
  4.97   145n39

HIPPOKRATES
Affections (*Aff.*)
  2.3–4   34n4
Airs, Waters, and Places (*Aër.*)
  6.7   94n59
Aphorisms (*Aph.*)
  i.1   59n33
  i.14   48n16
Art of Medicine (*de Arte*)
  3   34n4
Breaths (*Flat.*)
  12   94n60
  14   94n60, 95n61
Diseases (*Morb.*)
  i.22   57n31
Epidemics (*Epid.*)
  i.2.9.29   51n21
  i.2.9.72   51n21
  i.3.13(9).1   132n12
  i.3.13(11).4   88n43
  ii.1.4.5   51n21
  ii.2.10.1   132n12
  iii.3.12.1   51n21
  iii.3.17(2).14   132n12
  iii.3.17(7).4   88n43
  v.1.64.5   88n43
Fleshes (*Carn.*)
  2–3   48n16
  6   48n16
Nature of Man (*Nat. Hom.*)
  12   48n16
  14.16   55n27
On Genitals (*Genit.*)
  15.30   54n27
  44.14   54n27
  48.13   54n27
  55.13   54n27
On Joints (*Fist.*)
  7   34n4
Places in Man (*Loc. Hom.*)
  14.13   132n12
Prognosis (*Prog.*)
  22.1   133n14
Prorrhetic (*Prorrh.*)
  ii.1.11   51n21
  ii.2.11   51n21
  ii.11.9   51n21
  ii.11.14   51n21
  ii.24.2   51n21

HOMER
Iliad (*Il.*)
  2.422   225n13
  4.141–2   183
  4.141–7   186n14
  4.190   34n4
  5.529   60n34
  6.437   60n34
  13.227   60n34
  17.53   187n15
  23.101   181, 181n11
Odyssey (*Od.*)
  4.235–64   148
  4.239   148
  4.245   148n51
  4.266   149
  9.19–20   112n11
  9.385   86
  10.19   225n13
  19.391   211n44
  19.393   211n44
  24.9   181n11

Index Locorum

ISOKRATES
  47.6   145n39

KHRYSIPPOS
  Frag. 411   48n12

LONGUS
Daphnis and Khloe (*D&C.*)
  Praef.   170n23, 195n11,
                      203n27
  i.7   194n7

LUCIAN
Encomium of Demonax (*Dem. Enc.*)
  33   136n20
On the Hall (*Dom.*)
  1–2   170n23

Podagra (*Pod.*)
  9   124n23
  13   124n23
  15   122
  16–21   122–3
  25   123
  26   123
  27–9   123
  42–4   126
  112   124n24,
                      125n27
  119–24   124
  125   125
  128   125n28
  175   126n32
  180–2   126
  289   126n32
  332   127
  332–5   121n15
  333   127
  334   127

True Histories (*VH.*)
  3   112n11

MENANDER RHETOR
  ii.390.2–3   175n2

PHILOSTRATOS
Imagines (*Im.*)
  294.9–10K   177n5
  294.18–19K   177
  294.19–20K   177
  295.10–12K   176
  295.15–16K   176
  296.22K   177n7
  299.16–300.22K 179

  299.24–5K   180
  300.7K   180
  300.9–10K   180
  300.14–22K   180–1
  305.10K   177n6
  349.29–30K   183
  349.30K   177n6
  350.1–2K   183
  350.7K   183
  350.14–15K   183
  350.15K   177n6
  350.19K   183
  350.22K   183
  350.31–2K   183
  351.2–8K   184
  351.6–8K   177n7
  353.1–2K   185
  353.17–18K   185
  353.29–354.6K 185–6
  354.13–19K   187–8
  354.18–24K   189
  354.28–30   189n20
  354.29–30K   190
  354.30–31K   191
  354.31–2K   191
  371.26K   188n17
  376.13–14K   188n17
  378.29K   188n17
  379.29–30K   177n6
  384.11K   188n17

Life of Apollonios of Tyana (*VA.*)
  3.45 (61–2K)   150n56
  4.30 (77K)   121n15
Lives of Sophists (*VS.*)
  487–8 (205–6K) 121n15
  577 (250K)   226n15
  581–2 (252–3K) 129n3

PLATO
Gorgias (*Grg.*)
  491b4   92n54
Parmenides (*Prm.*)
  138b–c   72n12
Philebos (*Phlb.*)
  32a–b   12n27
  64e   16n44
Republic (*R.*)
  387a–e   181n12
  474d–e   180
  614b   149

PLATO (cont.)
Symposium (*Smp.*)
217e   120n13

Timaios (*Ti.*)
64d: 12n27, 48n13, 71n8

Theatetos (*Tht.*)
182d-e   72n12

PLINY
Natural History (*HN.*)
35.79-80   16n43
35.129   16n43
35.138   161n1

PLUTARCH
Consolation to Apollonios (*Consol. ad Apoll.*)
108b7-8   173n31
118f   188n17

How One Might Tell a Flatterer from a Friend (*Adulat. Amic.*)
71a   15n37

How Young Men Should Listen to Poetry (*Quomodo Adulesc.*)
14d-f   221n10
15b   221n10
16b-d   207n35
16e   172n29
17a   172
17b   172n29
18c   120n12, 161
18c-d   26n64, 161n1
18d   161n2
22e   88n43
25b   172n27
25d   172n28, 207n33

On Flesh-Eating (*de Esu Carn.*)
993a-b   222n12
993b   225
993c   227, 229n20, 230
994e   224, 228, 230n23
996a   225n13
996d   221
996e   221, 222
996f   230
996f-997a   229, 230
997b   222, 223
997c   223
997e   230
998b   224
999a: 220n8
999b   220

On Whether Land or Sea Animals are Cleverer (*de Sollert. Anim.*)
959d-961a   219n6

Sympotic Questions (*Quaest. Conviv.*)
674a   24, 24n58
674b   24n58, 26n64
699b   117n6

That it is not Possible to Live According to Epikouros (*Non Posse.*)
1087-8   13n29
1087e   116
1087f   119
1088a   117

POLYBIOS
34.4.3   172n27

PS.-LONGINOS
On the Sublime (*Subl.*)
1.4   171, 207n32
9.14   196n14
12.3   207n32
15.2   171
15.3   226n16
15.11   207n32

QUINTILIAN
Principles of Oratory (*Inst.*)
9.3.30-4   226n17

RUFUS (OF EPHESOS)
Anatomy (*Anat.*)
71-5   14n34, 35n8

Medical Questions (*Quaest. Med.*)
1   40n18, 98n63
2-3   40n19
42-3   40n19

Names (*Onom.*)
149-50   14n34, 35n8

On Gout (*de Podagra*)
Praef.   123n21

SOPHOKLES
Ajax (*Aj.*)
632   209n39

Philoktetes (*Ph.*)
189-90   188n18
369   118n8
930   118n8

Index Locorum

Women of Trakhis (Tr.)
1083   57n31

SORANOS
Diseases of Women (Gyn.)
i.3.22   16n45
i.5.29   16n45
i.5.35   16n45
i.7.34   16n45
i.14.46   16n45
i.17.24   16n45
i.17.27   16n45
i.22.8   16n45
ii.3.5–6   16n45
ii.5.26   16n45
iii.2.50   16n45
iii.2.92   16n45
iii.2.106   16n45
iii.2.157   16n45
iii.4.21   16n45
iii.4.41   16n45
iii.4.79   16n45
iii.4.91   16n45
iii.5.26   16n45
iii.7.19   16n45
iii.11.19   16n45
iii.13.18   16n45
iii.37.15   55n28
iv.4.28   16n45
iv.6.30   16n45

Fractures (Fract.)
xvii.1.3   55n28
xviii.1.3   55n28
xv.1.4   55n28

STRABO
1.2.17   172n27

THEOKRITOS
i.56   227n18

THEOPHRASTOS
On the Causes of Plants (CP.)
iv.5.5   72n12

On Senses (Sens.)
63–4   48n14
65.2   48n14
66.11   48n14
67.9   48n14
73.3   48n14

XENOPHON (OF ATHENS)
Anabasis (An.)
1.2.8   225n13

Economics (Oec.)
i.19.4   92n54

Education of Kyros (Cyr.)
6.4.2   187n16

XENOPHON (OF EPHESOS)
i.7   208n37
iii.5.3   212n45
iii.5.11   204n29, 210n41
iii.7   210n41
v.3.2   194n7